Volume 19

DIRECTORY OF WORLD CINEMA
AUSTRALIA & NEW ZEALAND 2

Edited by Ben Goldsmith, Mark David Ryan
and Geoff Lealand

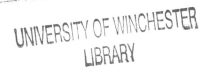

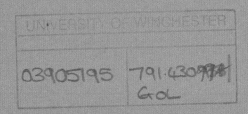
First published in the UK in 2015 by
Intellect Books, The Mill, Parnall Road, Fishponds, Bristol, BS16 3JG, UK

First published in the USA in 2015 by Intellect Books, The University of Chicago Press,
1427 E. 60th Street, Chicago, IL 60637, USA

Publisher: May Yao
Publishing Managers: Jelena Stanovik and Heather Gibson

Cover photograph: *Samson and Delilah*, 2009, Scarlett Pictures/The Kobal Collection
Cover designer: Holly Rose
Copy-editor: Emma Rhys
Typesetter: John Teehan

Directory of World Cinema ISSN 2040-7971
Directory of World Cinema eISSN 2040-798X

Directory of World Cinema: Australia & New Zealand 2 ISBN 978-1-84150-634-0
Directory of World Cinema: Australia & New Zealand 2 eISBN 978-1-78320-481-6

Printed and bound by Short Run Press, UK.

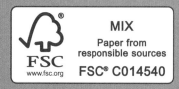

MIX
Paper from
responsible sources
FSC® C014540

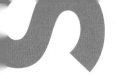

DIRECTORY OF WORLD CINEMA
AUSTRALIA & NEW ZEALAND 2

ACKNOWLEDGEMENTS

First and foremost, the editors would like to thank the contributors for all their hard work, their enthusiasm for Australian and New Zealand cinema, and their patience while waiting for the book's publication.

The editors would like to thank the Film, Screen and Animation Discipline in the School of Media, Entertainment, Creative Arts, Creative Industries Faculty, Queensland University of Technology, for its financial contribution to the book to purchase licensed images and to print this volume in colour. We are extremely grateful for this generous support. The colour version is striking and makes a huge difference to the text's visuals.

Thanks must also go to Heather Gibson, Jelena Stanovnik and Melanie Marshall for all their editorial work behind the scenes to prepare the directory for print.

Finally, Mark Ryan would like to thank Hal and Jim McElroy and Catherine Gillam from the AFI Research Collection for their permission to use the *Razorback* images.

INTRODUCTION:
BY BEN GOLDSMITH and MARK DAVID RYAN

The question of what exactly constitutes an 'Australian film' has long preoccupied those involved or interested in the films made either in this country, or those films made with Australian involvement elsewhere in the world. When Warwick Thornton's first film *Samson and Delilah* (2009) won the Camera d'Or at Cannes, there was no doubt that it clearly qualified as an Australian film. This story about two young Indigenous Australians living in an isolated community in the middle of the country, was written, directed and shot by Thornton, himself a Kaytetye man from the Northern Territory. But when another film by an Australian director won the Camera d'Or the following year, there was division among commentators and critics over whether this could be claimed as Australian. The Melbourne *Herald Sun* and the *Northern Territory News*, among others, were in no doubt that Melbournian Michael Rowe's *Año Bisiesta/Leap Year* (2010) – made in Spanish, in Mexico – is Australian, with the latter publication memorably headlining its story of Rowe's win 'Oz S&M Flick Cannes Pick' (Johnson 2010; Anon 2010a). Even one of the national public broadcasters described the film as an 'Oz-Mex sex thriller' in its news coverage (Vincent 2010). Rowe himself was careful to emphasize the 'Mexican resonance' of the film in interviews following his win (Wilson 2010), but he would also tell Australian film magazine *Encore* that 'I'm a son of Australia, of course [...] My artistic sensibility and narrative is incorruptibly Australian; that comes from the cradle and you can't get rid of it even if you wanted to' (Anon 2010b: 21). This is reminiscent of the view expressed by George (*Mad Max*) Miller in the early 1980s that:

> we are Australians, we are Australian film-makers. I think, without even trying, the Australianness comes through in the film, so you can't suddenly export yourself, as it were, and make film without that Australian point of view. Even though our culture reproduces to some degree the American, British, European and, in a little way, Asian culture, I think that makes us even in a very subtle way peculiarly Australian and you can never get around that. (Quoted in White 1984: 96)

The idea of a nation's cinema as a bounded, discrete and identifiable space neatly separated from the cinema of other nations has never been a reality. National cinemas are porous and leaky, inevitably multivalent, multiply connected to, influenced by, and impacting on narratives and styles, practices of film production and patterns of consumption beyond the national territory. Tom O'Regan locates the specificity of Australian cinema 'not in any particular set of attributes, so much as in its relational character' (O'Regan 1996: 7). Over the last few decades, Australian cinema's international relations in production and policy have expanded and become more complex. Deb Verhoeven's useful expansion of Susan Dermody and Elizabeth

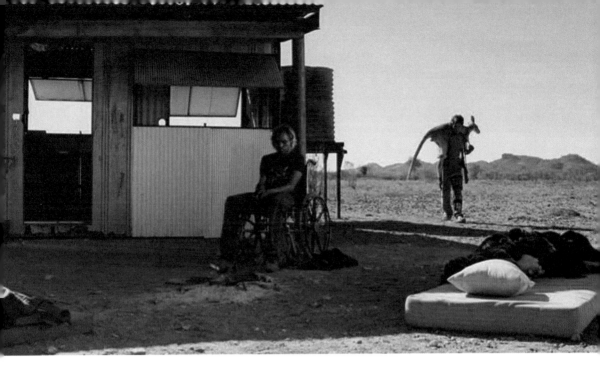

Samson and Delilah
(Warwick Thornton, 2009)

Jacka's influential 'Industry 1–Industry 2' model of Australian cinema elaborates these changes (Verhoeven 2010; Dermody and Jacka 1987). Verhoeven suggests a new model, 'Industry 3', which is characterized by the mixing of national and international elements, films and film-makers. Alongside the inward-looking Industry 1, which Dermody and Jacka classified as principally being concerned with Australian identity (albeit influenced by European-style art cinema and obsessed by local, social purpose), and the more outward-looking Industry 2, preoccupied with entertainment, internationalism, genre production and learning from Hollywood, Verhoeven argues that a third industry became evident by the end of the 1990s:

> [Industry 3] comprises films and film-makers happily embedded in *both* the local and global [and] typically [...] films initiated by Australians wanting to work with large budgets, international resources, high-profile actors and local content or personnel, and shooting either in Australia or offshore, or combining the two. (Verhoeven 2010: 141)

If the qualification 'initiated by Australians' were removed, this category could also include many of the international productions made in Australia. Moreover, as Ryan (2012) has argued, since the inception of the Producer Offset in 2007, policy priorities have shifted away from telling Australian stories without commercial imperatives towards fostering commercial productions that engage with audiences. A by-product of this policy shift, from largely cultural to industry policy, has been the renaissance of high-budget local blockbusters and genre movies (both dominant production strategies in the 1980s) which are for the most part embedded in the local and the global and draw upon codes, conventions and expectations that are not (only) set locally.

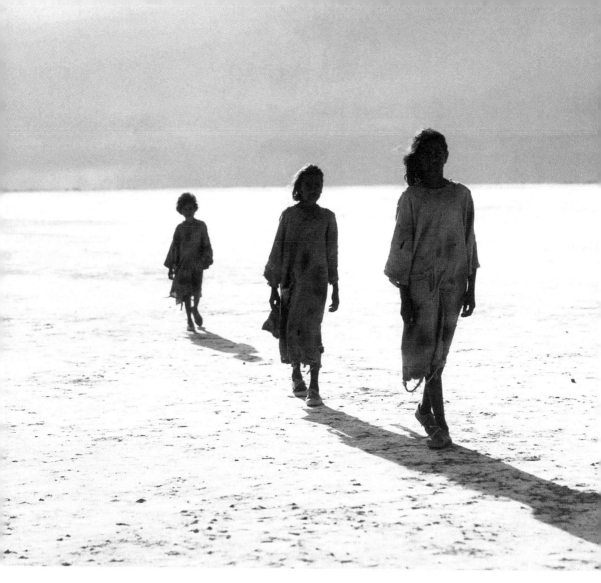

Rabbit-Proof Fence (Phillip Noyce, 2002). © Kobal Collection

The essays and reviews in this Australian section of the second volume of Intellect's *Directory of World Cinema: Australia and New Zealand* illuminate something of the particularity of Australian cinema, and also its connectedness through people, films, genres, to the cinema of the world. This volume complements and extends the first volume, published in 2010. There are several new sections (Film of the Year, Festival Focus, Locations, Marketing Mix, Star Study), articles on four Australian directors, original essays on eleven genres, and over sixty reviews of Australian films. We take a deliberately broad view of Australian cinema, and many of the essays take up and flesh out its relational character.

Kriv Stenders's *Red Dog* (2011) was an easy choice as 'Film of the Year'. The film is an amalgam of shaggy dog stories, adapted from English author Louis de Bernières's 2001 novel *Red Dog*, which itself was based on a series of tales about a famous canine inhabitant of the north-west of Western Australia in the 1970s. Immediately on its release the film struck a chord with Australian audiences and critics. As Anna Blagrove describes in her essay, the film was an enormous commercial success domestically, earning over AU$21 million at the Australian box office (making it the eighth highest grossing Australian film of all time), and millions more in DVD sales. *Red Dog* also won seven Inside Film (IF) Awards from nine nominations, and two Australian Academy of Cinema and Television Arts (AACTA) Awards (formerly the AFI Awards) including Best Film in 2011.

In 'Festival Focus', Tess Van Hemert recounts the history of the Brisbane International Film Festival (BIFF), which was held for the twenty-first time in 2012. BIFF has always had a strong focus on Asian cinema, and since 2010 it has coincided with the annual Asia Pacific Screen Awards, held on the Gold Coast. The festival has also long been an important venue for Australian films, many of which struggle to obtain wide release in local cinemas. It has also championed Australian documentaries; in 2012 the festival hosted the world premiere of *Show Me the Magic*, Cathy Henkel's film about the life and career of internationally renowned Australian cinematographer Don McAlpine. Several of the feature films shot by McAlpine over his long career are reviewed elsewhere in this volume.

The north of Western Australia, a vast, barren and sparsely populated region, has largely been out of bounds for Australian and international film-makers due to the area's remoteness and the attendant costs of production there. While several films have been set in the region, they have usually been shot in more accessible places. And yet as Jane Stadler illustrates in her essay on Australian film locations, a growing number of films have been shot in the Kimberley and Pilbara regions, including *Red Dog* and parts of *Australia* (Baz Luhrmann, 2008).

In her 'Marketing Mix' essay, Karina Aveyard examines the UK release of the road movie comedy *Charlie & Boots* (Dean Murphy, 2009) and discusses some of the difficulties Australian films face internationally. Despite the presence in leading roles of an iconic Australian comedian and actor well-known in the United Kingdom from his film and television work over several decades (Paul Hogan), and an actor who had earned recent renown for his role as the eponymous *Kenny* (Shane Jacobson, directed by his brother Clayton Jacobson, 2006) the film failed to receive a theatrical release in Britain. *Charlie & Boots* was, however, a hit at the annual London Australian Film Festival in 2010, with much of the audience coming from London's large expatriate Australian population.

An expatriate Australian and international star of a different order, Errol Flynn, is the subject of Adrian Danks's essay in the 'Star Study' section of this volume. Born in Tasmania, Flynn was one of the biggest stars in Hollywood in the 1930s and 1940s, perhaps best known for his performance in the title role in *The Adventures of Robin Hood* (Michael Curtiz and William Keighley, 1938). And yet as Danks describes, Flynn's career and achievements have not been widely celebrated in Australia, with 'only a nondescript seashore park and an isolated star outside the Theatre Royal [in Hobart] noticeably trading on his name'. Flynn only starred in one Australian film, Charles Chauvel's *In the Wake of the Bounty* (1933) before his departure for the United Kingdom and later Hollywood where, like many of his contemporaries, he was provided with a new identity and background by his studio employer, Warner Bros. Flynn was by no means the first Australian actor to seek fortune in Hollywood. The now defunct Australian journal *Picture Show* named over twenty Australian actors and actresses working in Hollywood at the time who attended a screening of Raymond Longford's *The Sentimental Bloke* (1919) in Los Angeles in 1922. But Flynn was undoubtedly by far the most well known of the so-called 'gum-leaf mafia' (Delamoir 2004) until the recent successes of Russell Crowe, Hugh Jackman, Cate Blanchett, Naomi Watts, Jacki Weaver and Toni Collette, among others. For the new generation of young Australian actors who are now coming to prominence in American cinema, many schooled in the long-running Australian soap operas *Neighbours* (Grundy Television, Seven Network 1985-86; Network Ten 1986-) and *Home and Away*, (Seven Network, 1988-), in the words of Danks, Flynn 'remains a salient and formative example of the fate that still awaits many Antipodean actors in the murky waters of international cinema'.

Antipodean directors have also earned great acclaim and success both for their work in local and international films, in Australia and New Zealand or overseas. The Directors section of this volume is bookended by two examples from different ends of the film-making spectrum, Jane Campion and Brian Trenchard-Smith. Sandwiched between them are three other film-makers whose work and careers were very much concentrated in Australia albeit with multiple external connections: Arthur and Corinne Cantrill, and Ken G Hall. The first essay in this section profiles perhaps the highest profile Antipodean art-film director who, among her many awards and plaudits, remains the only female director to win the Palme d'Or at Cannes. The film for which she won this award, *The Piano* (1993), is reviewed in the Gothic section of this volume. Deb Verhoeven describes the importance of the international film festival circuit in Campion's career, and the voluminous scholarly literature that has grown up around the auteur and her work. Arthur and Corinne Cantrill are without question the most important Australian experimental film-makers, as Adrian Danks elaborates in the second essay in this section. The Cantrills are enormously significant not only because of their many groundbreaking films made from 1960 onwards, but also for their contributions to Australian and international screen culture principally through the publication *Cantrills Filmnotes* (1971–2000). Another hugely important figure in Australian cinema – albeit one who is perhaps less well-remembered today than some more recent directors – is the subject of the third essay in this section. Ken G Hall was the producer and principal director of Australia's most prolific film studio, Cinesound Productions, from the 1930s to the 1950s. In part because his extraordinary career did not extend into the period of the revival of the Australian cinema from the 1970s onwards, and in part because his endorsement of Hollywood-style commercial film-making did not fit well with the cultural nationalism of the latter period, Hall is perhaps not as well known as he deserves to be. In her essay on Hall, Lesley Speed makes the point that despite his unabashed commercial emphasis and embrace of Hollywood, Hall made many important contributions to Australian film culture, not least through his work as producer of the newsreel *Cinesound Review* from 1932 to 1956. Hall both produced and edited the first Australian film to win an Academy Award, the Cinesound documentary *Kokoda Front Line!*, shot by Damien Parer in 1942. The final director profiled in this volume has long been well-known to cult film enthusiasts, but has enjoyed renewed fame in recent years after his work featured prominently, and was championed by Quentin Tarantino, in the documentary *Not Quite Hollywood: The Wild, Untold Story of Ozploitation!* (Mark Hartley, 2008). Brian Trenchard-Smith first came to prominence through his work directing action and stunt films in the 1970s and 1980s. He is also famous in the film industry for his work on film trailers – very much a hidden art – and for the many movies he has directed for American television.

The first of the genre sections of this volume, Action and Adventure, contains reviews of three of Brian Trenchard-Smith's films, *BMX Bandits* (1983), *Deathcheaters* (1976) and *Turkey Shoot* (1982). In his essay, Ben Goldsmith discusses the history of Action and Adventure films in Australian cinema, with particular attention paid to films featuring female protagonists, children's films, and large-scale international productions made in Australia in recent years. These various aspects are represented in the reviews in this section by the children's film *BMX Bandits* (notable as Nicole Kidman's debut film), the invasion story *Tomorrow, When the War Began* (Stuart Beattie, 2010) in which Ellie (Caitlin Stasey) leads a band of teenage resistance fighters, and the unofficial Australia-France coproduction *Walk into Paradise* (Lee Robinson, 1957). The latter film was made in Papua New Guinea, and stars one of the most recognizable Australian actors of the period, Chips Rafferty.

In his essay on Australian Animated Feature Films, Chris Carter describes the genre's long history here, and its close ties with American television animation. These ties were first forged by the pioneer animator Eric Porter whose film *Marco Polo Jnr Versus the*

Red Dragon (1972) was the first feature-length Australian animation. Eric Porter Studios worked on a range of animated children's television series for Hanna-Barbera Productions in the 1960s and 1970s, including *The Flintstones* (Hanna-Barbera Productions, ABC (USA), 1960-66) and *The Yogi Bear Show* (Screen Gems, ABC (USA), 1961-88). As Carter notes, the work generated by the presence of Hanna-Barbera and later Walt Disney Television in Australia helped to establish a local workforce with the capacity to produce animated feature films. Carter argues that the visual style of these cartoons limited the potential for a distinctive Australian style to emerge, at least until the production of *Dot and the Kangaroo* (Yoram Gross, 1977). Polish-born Gross formed Yoram Gross Film Studios in the 1970s, and produced fifteen feature-length animated films from 1977 to 1994, nine of which feature Dot, in Gross's signature style of cel animation matted onto live backgrounds. The reviews in this section highlight the diversity and variety of animation in Australia, from the live action/animatronics of *Babe* (Chris Noonan, 1995), and the traditional 2D hand-drawn animation of *FernGully: The Last Rainforest* (Bill Kroyer, 1992), to the CGI animation of *Legends of the Guardians: The Owls of Ga'Hoole* (Zack Snyder, 2010) and the claymation *Mary and Max* (Adam Elliot, 2009).

Razorback (Russell Mulcahy, 1984). Sourced from the AFI Research Collection with permission from Hal McElroy (McElroy All Media) and Jim McElroy (McElroy and McElroy)

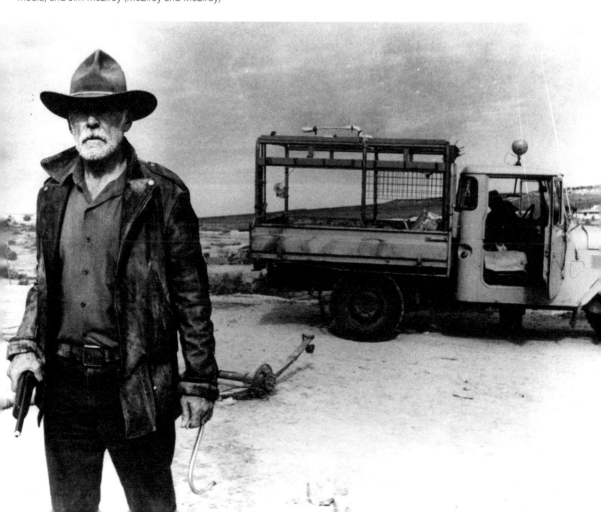

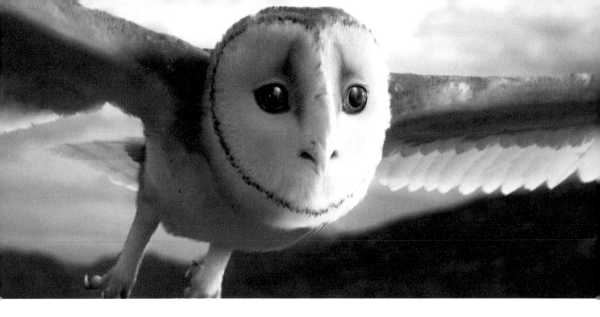

Legends of the Guardians: The Owls of Ga'Hoole
(Zack Snyder, 2010). © Kobal Collection

Building on her framing essay on Comedy in the first volume of the *Directory of World Cinema: Australia and New Zealand*, Lesley Speed delves in to the subgenre of Comedian Comedy in her essay for this volume. Tracing a genealogy from Pat Hanna's Diggers films (1931-33) and the several features starring George Wallace in the 1930s through to the present day, Speed describes the subgenre as existing in parallel with, but separate from, the American tradition of films featuring comedic performers famous from other entertainment media. The subgenre includes *Crocodile Dundee* (Peter Faiman, 1986), which is (still) the most successful Australian film of all time. Ensemble comedian comedies have appeared regularly in recent years, many starring or produced by the loose collective of comedians based in Melbourne that grew out of, or spun off from the ABC/Seven Network television series and breakfast radio show, *The D-Generation* (ABC (Australia), 1986–1989). As Speed notes,

> The ensemble form in Australian comedian comedy reflects both the abundance of local talent and the small size of the local production industry, in which casting more than one prominent comedian in a film is considered to maximize its audience appeal.

Three of the films reviewed for this section are ensemble comedian comedies – Tony Martin's *Bad Eggs* (2003), Ted Emery's *The Craic* (1999) and Wayne Blair's *The Sapphires* (2012).

Like comedy, Australian Crime movies have their own distinct style or accent while drawing upon universal codes and conventions. In his introductory essay, Greg Dolgopolov notes that Australian crime films feature 'criminals, gangsters and vengeful victims', and even on the rare occasions that films focus on the police, the force is invariably depicted as corrupt and criminal. Dolgopolov discusses the fascination in recent Australian film and television with 'true crime' stories, including the stand-out recent examples *Animal Kingdom* (David Michôd, 2011) and *Snowtown* (Justin Kurzel, 2011), both of which are reviewed in this volume. Dolgopolov's essay also highlights ethnic crime narratives in recent Australian cinema. Two films about crime and the Lebanese Australian community in western Sydney feature prominently, and both *The Combination* (David Field, 2009) and *Cedar Boys* (Serhat Caradee, 2009) are reviewed here.

More of a stylistic mode that distils elements from multiple genres, the Australian Gothic is, in Jonathan Rayner's words 'the most persistent, fertile, articulate and therefore significant trend within Australian cinema over the past forty or more years'. Rayner describes the variety of Australian Gothic, noting that while it distinguishes 'the brand of Australian horror overseas' neither is it confined to horror, nor do all horror films fit the Gothic bill. Elements of the Gothic can be identified in such seminal early revival films as *Walkabout* (Nicolas Roeg, 1971) and *Wake in Fright* (Ted Kotcheff, 1971), as well as in Peter Weir's *The Cars That Ate Paris* (1974). And, as Rayner describes, the Gothic 'permeates, complicates and articulates' the work of Australian directors in Hollywood, in such films as *The Truman Show* (Peter Weir, 1998) and *Hearts in Atlantis* (Scott Hicks, 2001). The films reviewed for this section provide a flavour of the diversity of the Australian Gothic, from Steve Jodrell's modern western *Shame* (1988) to Ann Turner's *Celia* (1988), which is set during the period in which anti-Communist hysteria was at its height in Australia, to Ray Lawrence's fantastical adaptation of Peter Carey's novel *Bliss* (1985).

The 'monstrous landscape', also a feature of the Australian Gothic, is the focus of Mark David Ryan's essay on Horror. Ryan describes the appearance of the landscape as a usually malevolent character in many horror films, before discussing the parallel theme of the revenge of nature. Reviews of Kimble Rendall's gory 'sharks in the supermarket' film *Bait* (2012), Colin Eggleston's *Long Weekend* (1978) about a couple's nightmare beach holiday, and Russel Mulcahy's cult classic *Razorback* (1984) flesh out the latter theme. The monstrous outback of *Primal* (Josh Reed, 2010) and the complementary terrors of subterranean Sydney in *The Tunnel* (Carlo Ledesma, 2011) are also reviewed, along with the torture horror *The Loved Ones* (Sean Byrne, 2009) and Philip Brophy's splatter comedy *Body Melt* (1994).

In her essay on Road Movies, Deborah J Thomas makes a case for the cultural specificity of the Australian genre in comparison with the American progenitor. Referencing in particular the work of Brian Trenchard-Smith and George Miller, Quentin Tarantino has claimed that 'nobody shoots a car the way Aussies do' (in *Not Quite Hollywood*). But it is not only the stunts, chases and crashes typical of Trenchard-Smith's and Miller's films that mark Australian road movies from those made elsewhere. Local road movies are often gentle, cerebral affairs, in which the confined space of the motor vehicle becomes the stage on which personal dramas are worked through and relationships worked out along the way. *Charlie & Boots* provides the example here, though there are many others, from *Travelling North* (Carl Schultz, 1986), to *Last Ride* (Glendyn Ivin, 2009). The latter film to some extent belies Thomas's claim that Australian road movies rarely feature the 'nihilistic rebel outlaw' so common in American genre films. There is also a greater tendency in Australian films to explore 'off road'; indeed Fiona Probyn (2005) has identified a specific local subgenre, the 'no road' film, exemplified here in the reviews of *Rabbit-Proof Fence* (Phillip Noyce, 2002) and *Walkabout* (Nicolas Roeg, 1971). Then there are films like *The Adventures of Priscilla: Queen of the Desert* (Stephan Elliott, 1994) which are aesthetic categories all of their own.

Science Fiction is a genre which has produced only a relatively small number of films and is less prominent than road movies in Australian cinema despite producing a handful of popular titles including *Mad Max Beyond Thunderdome* (George Miller, 1985) and *Dark City* (Alex Proyas, 1998). Unlike genres such as horror which have attracted considerable academic interest in recent years, discussion around local science fiction movies is still in its infancy. In recent years, authors who have explored the genre have tended to focus on both international 'runaway' productions that film in Australia and draw upon local crews, acting talent and heads of departments such as *The Matrix* (Andy and Lana Wachowski, 1999) and locally sourced productions which include independent titles, co-productions and higher-end titles produced within a globalized industry structure (see for example Moran and Vieth 2006; McMullen 2010). As such what constitutes a local tradition has been poorly defined. In their essay, while acknowledging the international dynamics of the genre, Peter Schembri and Mark David Ryan narrow their discussion to local movies sourced by Australian key creatives and 'officially recognized as "local productions" by government screen agencies'. For the authors, the move to '[shift] discussion away from international science fiction movies filmed in Australia (and the question of local input) to focus upon local science fiction production, provides a less impressive but more accurate picture of local production'. In doing so they find that 'Australia does not have sustained periods of production where the "science" in science fiction is taken seriously'. Rather local films with science fiction content are often hybrid genre movies combined with other genres (such as horror or action), or pertain more to the tendencies of 'soft' rather than 'hard' science fiction.

Although not always labelled as such at the time of release, Thrillers or films with recognizable thriller elements, are identifiable throughout the history of Australian narrative cinema, dating back to Charles Tait's groundbreaking *The Story of the Kelly Gang* (1906). Ben Goldsmith provides a brief genealogy in his essay on the genre, before discussing the eight-part thriller typology first proposed by Charles Derry, and elaborated by Albert Moran and Errol Vieth (2006). Goldsmith's chief interest is in the political thriller; despite noting the relative dearth of political thrillers in Australian cinema, Goldsmith discusses the variety of the subgenre, from nuclear thrillers (exemplified in reviews of *Ground Zero* [Michael Pattinson and Bruce Myles, 1987] and *The Chain Reaction* [Ian Barry, 1980]), to international scandals (*Balibo* [Robert Connolly, 2009]), and cover-ups closer to home (*The Killing of Angel Street* [Donald Crombie, 1981]).

Extending his discussion of First World War films in the first volume of the *Directory of World Cinema: Australia and New Zealand*, Daniel Reynaud examines recent and revisionist treatments of the Anzac legend in his essay on War cinema. Reynaud notes that the Second

The Castle
(Rob Sitch, 1997)

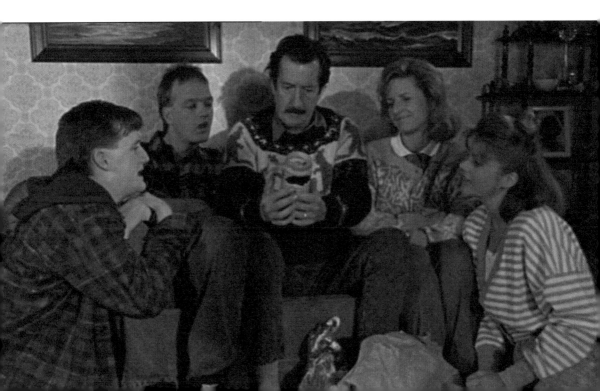

World War has always played second fiddle to the Great War in Anzac mythology, and this is reflected in the output of Australian film-makers. Reynaud identifies five films that have been made since 1982 that make some reference to the Second World War, but of these only two – *Attack Force Z* (Tim Burstall, 1982) and *Kokoda* (Alister Grierson, 2006) focus on the Anzac myth. The others – *Blood Oath* (aka *Prisoners of the Sun*; Stephen Wallace, 1990), *Paradise Road* (Bruce Beresford, 1997) and *Australia* – while set during or immediately after the war, use the conflict to interrogate a range of other issues. Importantly all of these films offer perspectives and insights into Australian military history and the mythology of Anzac while at the same time elaborating different international aspects of Australian screen culture.

The last section of this volume discusses another local variant of a familiar international genre, the western. Daniel Eisenberg argues that the Australian Western has played a key role in Australian cinema history, from its prototype in the bushranger films of the early 1900s, to more recent explorations of colonial relations and survival in the outback. Drawing on Peter Limbrick's work, Eisenberg maintains that unlike westerns made in other countries, the Australian western is not a local cinematic response to the 'myth of America', but rather is 'engaged in a dialogue with Australia's own myths and history'. This point is evident in different ways and to different degrees in each of the films reviewed in this section: Kriv Stenders's *Lucky Country* (2009), George Miller's *The Man from Snowy River* (1982), Harry Watt's *The Overlanders* (1946), John Hillcoat's *The Proposition* (2005) and Patrick Hughes's *Red Hill* (2010).

References

Anon (2010a) 'Oz S&M Flick Cannes Pick', *Northern Territory News*, 25 May, p. 16.

Anon (2010b) 'Rise of the Prodigal Son', *Encore*, July, p. 21.

Delamoir, Jeanette (2004) 'The First "Gum-Leaf Mafia": Australians in Hollywood, 1915–25', *Screening the Past*, 16, http://tlweb.latrobe.edu.au/humanities/screeningthepast/firstrelease/fr_16/jdfr16.html. Accessed 10 May 2013.

Dermody, Susan and Elizabeth Jacka (1987) *The Screening of Australia: Anatomy of a Film Industry*, Paddington: Currency Press.

Johnson, Neala (2010) 'Graphic is Good in Cannes', *Herald Sun* [Melbourne], 25 May, p. 2.

McMullen, Sean (2010) 'Science fiction and Fantasy', in Ben Goldsmith and Geoff Lealand (eds), *Directory of World Cinema: Australian and New Zealand*, Bristol: Intellect, pp. 224–35.

Moran, Albert and Vieth, Errol (2006) *Film in Australia: An introduction*, Cambridge, UK: Cambridge University Press.

O'Regan, Tom (1996) *Australian National Cinema*, London and New York: Routledge.

Probyn, Fiona (2005) 'An Ethics of Following and the No Road Film: Trackers, Followers and Fanatics', *Australian Humanities Review*, http://www.australianhumanitiesreview.org/archive/Issue-December-2005/Probyn.html. Accessed 28 September 2013.

Ryan, Mark David (2012) 'A silver bullet for Australian cinema? Genre movies and the audience debate', *Studies in Australasian Cinema*, 6: 2, pp. 141–57.

Verhoeven, Deb (2010) 'It was an experience that totally blew up in my face: Steve Railsback and Turkey Shoot', *Studies in Australasian Cinema*, 4: 1, pp. 73–79.

Vincent, Michael (2010) 'From Ballarat to Cannes: Oz-Mex Sex Thriller is a Winner', *ABC News*, 26 May. http://www.abc.net.au/news/2010-05-26/from-ballarat-to-cannes-oz-mex-sex-thriller-is-a/841306 Accessed 28 September 2013.

White, David (1984) *Australian Movies to the World: The International Success of Australian Films Since 1970*, Sydney and Melbourne: Fontana Australia and Cinema Papers.

Wilson, Jake (2010) 'Filmmaker Takes Leap and Reaps the Reward', *The Age*, 6 August, p. 19.

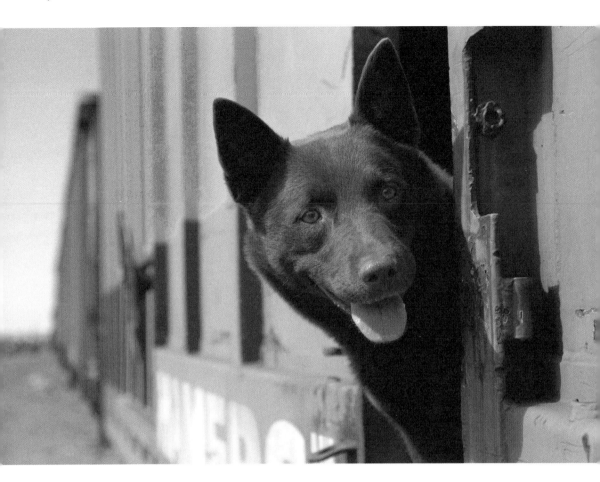

Red Dog (Kriv Stenders, 2011).
© Kobal Collection

FILM OF THE YEAR
RED DOG

Red Dog

Country of Origin:

Australia

Studio/Distributor:

Endymion Films
The Woss Group

Director:

Kriv Stenders

Producers:

Julie Ryan
Nelson Woss

Screenwriter:

Daniel Taplitz, based on the
2001 novel *Red Dog* by Louis
de Bernières

Director of Photography:

Geoffrey Hall

Production Designer:

Ian Gracie

Composer:

Cezary Skubiszewski

Editor:

Jill Bilcock

Duration:

92 minutes

Genres:

Comedy
Drama

Cast:

Koko
Rachael Taylor
Josh Lucas
Noah Taylor
Luke Ford
Rohan Nichol
John Batchelor
Arthur Angel
Radek Jonak
Costa Ronin

Format:

35mm

Year:

2011

Synopsis

Truck driver Thomas enters a roadhouse in Western Australia as the locals and workers from a nearby mine debate how to euthanize a dog. Seizing on the diversion, publican Jack Collins tells Thomas the story of Red Dog, who has brought the disparate people of the mining town of Dampier together as a community. In flashback, Red Dog befriends many locals, including the mining company's immigrant employees, but stays with no single master – he is a 'dog for everyone'. This changes when American traveller, John Grant, takes a job as the mine's bus driver. Red Dog develops a strong bond with Grant, who becomes his 'true master'. Grant develops a romance with sassy secretary Nancy Grey, but after proposing to Nancy, Grant is killed in a road accident. Red Dog is left to pine and wander all over the Pilbara desert and beyond in search of his absent master. Some time later, he returns to the town where he fights his arch enemy, Red Cat. After eating poisoned meat left by Red Cat's owners, Red Dog is taken to the roadhouse, where he lies when Thomas arrives. One of the miners proposes that they erect a statue of Red Dog. As they celebrate the idea, Red Dog leaves unnoticed. He is later found lying dead on John Grant's grave. A year later, Thomas returns with a puppy, as the statue of the original Red Dog is unveiled.

Critique

Red Dog is based on the many stories of a real life red kelpie dog that lived in northern Western Australia in the 1970s. Red Dog was renowned for his loyalty to his master and his habit of roaming the desert. In 2001, British author Louis de Bernières visited Dampier, heard the story and published a novella based on the legend, also called *Red Dog*. It was from this book that Daniel Taplitz adapted his screenplay. The film's producer, Nelson Woss, bought a red kelpie named Koko from a dog breeder two years before filming began and trained him to star as Red Dog. Australian rising star, Rachael Taylor (*Transformers* [Michael Bay, 2007]) plays Nancy and American, Josh Lucas (*Sweet Home Alabama* [Andy Tennant, 2002]) is John Grant. Director, Kriv Stenders, previously directed little-known, hard-hitting, urban drama *Boxing Day* (2007) and heritage thriller *Lucky Country* (2009) among other titles. Other collaborators were cinematographer, Geoffrey Hall (*Chopper* [Andrew Dominik, 2000] and *Dirty Deeds* [David Caesar, 2002]) and Baz Luhrmann's long-time editor Jill Bilcock (*Strictly Ballroom* [1992], *Moulin Rouge!* [2001]). Prolific screen composer Cezary Skubiszewski (*Two Hands* [Gregor Jordan, 1999], *Bran Nue Dae* [Rachel Perkins, 2009] and *The Sapphires* [Wayne Blair, 2012]), provided the score after the original choice, Martin Armiger, left the project. The film won seven Inside Film (IF) Awards from nine nominations, and two Australian Academy of Cinema and Television Arts (AACTA) Awards (formerly the AFI Awards) including Best Film, from eight nominations in 2011.

Red Dog had an estimated AU$8.5 million production budget and on release in 2011 made AU$21.3 million at the Australian box office (Screen Australia 2012), rendering the film a massive commercial success. It was the highest grossing domestic film of that year, and currently sits eighth on the list of top Australian films at the Australian box office (Screen Australia 2012). *Red Dog* is also the first Australian film not backed by a Hollywood studio to pass AU$20 million gross since *Strictly Ballroom* in 1992. It has since sold millions of copies on DVD, and is the third biggest selling DVD of all time in Australia behind only *Avatar* (James Cameron, 2009) and *Finding Nemo* (Andrew Stanton, 2003) (Bodey 2012).

What is it that struck a chord with Australian audiences? The backdrop for the story is the vast, red Pilbara desert with its immense iron-ore mines, and the beaches and turquoise ocean off the attractive Western Australian coast. The film showcases the natural beauty of the region which serves as a scenic background for the representation of close friendship in rural, working communities. The familiar theme of mateship, loyalty and respect between man and dog – a staple element of Australian working life – is highlighted, as is the central romance between John and Nancy and its bittersweet conclusion. Another emotional subplot involves one of the miners, Jocko, who experiences depression brought on by bereavement. Jocko attempts suicide by swimming with 'Lord Nelson', the resident shark off Dampier beach, and is saved by a heroic Red Dog. There is plenty of light relief in the form of broad, physical comedy provided by both Red Dog and the eclectic locals, and canine flatulence jokes. There is a distinct element of nostalgia for the 1970s exemplified by the 'Oz Rock' music on the soundtrack, the type of 'utes' the characters drive and the beer they drink in the pub. The theme of belonging is also explored via the only real villains in the film, a cantankerous, dog-hating couple, the Cribbages, who deny the existence of any kind of community in Dampier. In Mr Cribbage's words, 'there's just a bunch of dirty miners working, drinking and whoring.' This provides an opportunity for the townsfolk to rally in solidarity against the couple in support of Red Dog.

Red Dog has an inter-generational appeal, with animal action for young people (including the cartoon-like scraps between Red Cat and Red Dog), and nostalgic elements for older audiences that lived through the 1970s. Comedy generally has wide and broad appeal; the number one run-away Australian film-success of all time, *Crocodile Dundee* (Peter Faiman, 1986), was also a comedy about 'Australianness' set partly in stunning outback locations. The similar irreverent humour of the 'ocker' working-men is certainly one of *Red Dog*'s attractions, along with the romance and pathos.

Red Dog can be viewed as a much lighter version of *Wake in Fright* (Ted Kotcheff, 1971), a cult, outback-set film that both *Red Dog*'s producer, Nelson Woss, and director, Kriv Stenders, have referenced as an influence (Barkham 2012). This homage is most recognizable in a gambling scene in the pub. At first glance it evokes the game of 'two-up', that features so ominously in *Wake in Fright*, but is comically revealed to be the men of Dampier betting on how quickly Red can eat a bowl of dog food.

The supporting cast are mostly mining company employees ranging from good old 'ocker Aussie', Peeto (John Batchelor), and depressive Jocko (Rohan Nichol) to Italian immigrant Vanno (Arthur Angel) and Chuposki and Dzambaski (the Eastern European 'ski patrol', played by Radek Jonak and Costa Ronin). It is these characters that provide representations of nationalities that some audiences may see as affectionately comic, but others may view as shallow stereotypes. Peeto, the burly, bearded bloke from Melbourne, is exposed as having a penchant for relaxing with some knitting in his *donga* (a portable housing unit, typically for rural workers), while listening to jaunty jazz records – a comedic subversion of the tough, masculine working-class Australian stereotype. The supporting cast also features prolific character-actor Noah Taylor as the town publican, and a memorable cameo from Australian national treasure Bill Hunter as a Quint-from-*Jaws* type, in the last role he filmed before his death in 2011. New Zealand's Keisha Castle-Hughes (*Whale Rider* [Niki Caro, 2002]) also makes an appearance in a small role as a veterinary assistant and love-interest for the Italian romantic, Vanno.

Red Dog was released the same year as Steven Spielberg's *War Horse*, a similar tale that centred on an animal's heroic loyalty to its master, but manages to avoid that film's overt sentimentality and earnest tone. *Red Dog* received mostly positive reviews, exemplified by the declaration by a critic from *The Age* that it was an 'instant Aussie classic' (Schembri 2011). Other critics denounced its lack of Indigenous characters and its sentimentalizing of the mining industry (Burnside 2011). Defending the film, director Stenders argues that *Red Dog* is not a documentary and is instead intended as a feel-good 'celebration' of the birth of the modern mining boom, upon which Australia's latter-day economic success is based (Barkham 2012).

Red Dog can be viewed as a popular new outback legend that Australia has welcomed to its canon, alongside Waltzing Matilda, Ned Kelly and Crocodile Dundee. It features the universal narrative theme of a dog's loyalty for its master, in the style of Scotland's Greyfriars Bobby or Japan's Hachikō. It also has a postcolonial theme of 'damn the British' as exemplified in the key motivational speech that Jocko delivers to the community in the pub at the film's conclusion. He denounces the town's namesake, seventeenth-century English explorer William Dampier, whose written account of their part of the country amounts to 'too many flies'. A statue of William Dampier is about to be erected in the town and Jocko exclaims, 'Well I say, to hell with all that! Why should we have a statue honouring a poncey, pommie, fly-hating aristocrat? Or for that matter a fat general or, god help us, a stinking politician?' The Australian distrust of authority is also made clear here. Jocko instead suggests that they erect a statue to 'somebody who lives and breathes this vastness and desolation. Somebody that has red dust stuck up their nose, and in their eyes and in their ears and *up their arses!*' He goes on to highlight the Australian notion of mateship, delineating it from a British militaristic camaraderie; 'mates who are loyal by nature not design'. Jocko concludes by suggesting to unanimous approval that they should be honouring 'somebody that represents the Pilbara in all of us and I say that somebody, dammit, IS A DOG!'

The legacy of the film's success is already in evidence, as demonstrated by reports that a stage musical of *Red Dog* is in development – aligning *Red Dog* with *The Adventures of Priscilla: Queen of the Desert* (Stephan Elliot, 1994), another Australian film-comedy success that was adapted into a stage musical to great acclaim.

Anna Blagrove

References

Barkham, Patrick (2012) 'Red Dog: An Audience with Australia's Best Friend', *The Guardian*, 9 February, http://www.guardian.co.uk/film/2012/feb/09/red-dog-australia-best-friend. Accessed 28 September 2013.

Bodey, Michael (2012) 'Local hit reigns again as top selling DVD', *The Australian*, 8 February, http://www.theaustralian.com.au/business/opinion/local-hit-reigns-again-as-top-selling-dvd/story-e6frg9sx-1226265114081. Accessed 12 November 2012.

Burnside, Sarah (2011) 'Red Dog Whitewashes The Pilbara', *New Matilda*, 16 August, http://newmatilda.com. Accessed 12 November 2012.

Schembri, Jim (2011) 'Red Dog is an Instant Classic', *The Age*, 5 August, http://www.theage.com.au/entertainment/movies/red-dog-20110804-1id0c.html. Accessed 9 May 2013.

Screen Australia (2012) 'Number of Australian and overseas films released in Australian cinemas 1984–2011', http://www.screenaustralia.gov.au/research/statistics/wcfilmxcountry.asp. Accessed 13 October 2012.

FESTIVAL FOCUS
BRISBANE INTERNATIONAL FILM FESTIVAL

In 2012, the Brisbane International Film Festival (BIFF) officially came of age, celebrating its twenty-first birthday. The festival has emerged from a tumultuous adolescence and redefined its position on the Australian festival circuit as an advocate of locally made films and documentary film-making. BIFF was first held in 1992 and has since been attended by more than 400,000 filmgoers. The festival is held annually and showcases a diverse range of feature films, documentaries, short films, animation and experimental work, children's films and retrospectives.

Since the proliferation of film festivals in the 1980s and 1990s, local city-based festivals have emerged as a growing and integral component of the international film festival circuit (Stringer 2001). Local film-makers are increasingly taking advantage of these festivals to make industry connections, garner critical appraisal and showcase their films to audiences. Although local film festivals like BIFF are typically located on the periphery of the global festival circuit – with the 'centre' comprising larger and more prestigious festivals such as Cannes or Toronto (Stringer 2001: 138) – they play a significant role in showcasing international films to local audiences, especially those which are not usually accessible through commercial film outlets. Moreover, festivals such as the BIFF are arguably designed to appeal to a specific city's film culture and community. BIFF is the largest international film festival within the state of Queensland in terms of the audience numbers it attracts and the amount and variety of films screened. Other film festivals currently held in Queensland include the West End Film Festival, the Gold Coast Film Festival, the Brisbane Queer Film Festival, and a range of travelling film festivals including the Spanish Film Festival, the Lavazza Italian Film Festival and the Alliance Française French Film Festival.

During 2009/10, BIFF underwent a period of major change. In 2010, the festival changed dates to coincide with the Asia Pacific Screen Awards (APSA), held annually on the Gold Coast in November. According to the BIFF Festival Director and Screen Queensland's Head of Screen Culture, Richard Moore, the change in dates was an attempt to strengthen the links between the community importance of BIFF and the prestige of the awards (personal communication, 2012). The shift in festival dates from July to November, the introduction of a new Festival Director and the loss of the Regent Cinema – the festival's home since inception – have been the most significant changes BIFF has experienced throughout its history as a film festival. Understandably, these changes had a profound impact on BIFF's structure, agenda and festival image. Richard Moore moved to Brisbane in 2010 after four successful years at the helm of the Melbourne International Film Festival (MIFF). Moore was the Executive Director of MIFF from 2007 to 2010 and in that time was responsible for fostering the implementation of the MIFF Premiere Fund, the festival's film investment fund, and 37° South Market, MIFF's co-financing market. During this period, he also upheld MIFF's reputation as a festival for exciting programming and negotiated MIFF's dual image as both a community festival and industry event.

BIFF has been quite clearly positioned by Moore and Screen Queensland as a showcase for both international and local film-making. Each year the festival draws direct inspiration for its programming choices from national film festivals (Sydney and Melbourne) and international film festivals (such as Berlin, Venice and Cannes). It is also clearly defined as a city-based festival, with strong links to specific venues within the centre of the city, including Tribal Theatre, Palace Barracks and Palace Centro. In 2012, the festival also featured Fulldome screenings (movie projection within a dome-shaped environment) at the Brisbane Planetarium, in partnership with the Brisbane Open-air Cinema. BIFF's links to other key film events on Brisbane's industry calendar, such as the Asia Pacific Screen Awards and the Queensland New Filmmakers Awards, were also strengthened in 2012, with the prestigious APSA ceremony held in Brisbane for the first time at the end of the festival.

The festival's programme must appeal to the city's diverse demographics, and must bring the 'best' of world cinema to Brisbane. However, the personal preferences and politics of any festival's programmers are, (arguably) always, embedded in the design and choice of films. Previous festival director Anne Demy-Geroe carved out a distinct identity for BIFF, with a focus on Asian and Pacific cinema and retrospectives paying tribute to internationally acclaimed auteurs such as Dennis Hopper, Roman Polanski, Stanley Kubrick and Luis Buñuel. BIFF was also responsible for launching films such as *The Usual Suspects* (Bryan Singer, 1995), *Gettin' Square* (Jonathan Teplitzky, 2003), *A Prairie Home Companion* (Robert Altman, 2006) and *An Education* (Lone Scherfig, 2009) onto the national and international festival circuit. The current director, Richard Moore, had a specific vision to make the festival attractive to a younger audience and refocus the festivities within the cultural hub of the city. Moore also implemented significant changes in the agenda and structure of the festival's programme. He felt that it was particularly important to put a focus back on local film-making in his first year of programming, stating that, 'I think it's important that you really connect with the film-makers in the local community […] Whether it's a doco, or whether its shorts or whether they're features […] BIFF should be a platform for launching Queensland films' (personal communication, 2012).

In his first year in Brisbane, Moore identified documentary film-making as a strength of Queensland's film-makers and a favourite of the festival's audience. In 2010, seven of the top-ten audience favourites were documentary films. Moore further solidified the festival's new focus with the introduction of the BIFFDOCS prize in 2011. The prize of AU$25,000 is Australia's most lucrative award for documentary film-makers and recognizes excellence in documentary production. Moore's new focus on documentary is certainly a shift away from the festival's former agenda, but may work well in the long term to forge a place for BIFF that is distinct from other key film festivals in Australia.

In 2012, the festival programmed 136 feature films in total, with three world premiere screenings: Ai Weiwei's *Ping'an Yueqing* (2012) from China, and two Australian documentaries, *Waziz* (Julie Romaniuk, 2012) and *Show Me the Magic* (Cathy Henkel, 2012). BIFF also secured the Australian premieres of 46 feature films, representing a cross section of current international cinema. The festival showcased new releases from the United Kingdom, opening with *The Sweeney* (Nick Love, 2012), a remake of the 1970s television cop show and closing with Joe Wright's adaptation of the Leo Tolstoy novel, *Anna Karenina* (2012). The always popular gala events, Bubbles at BIFF, featured screenings of Michael Haneke's latest masterpiece, *Amour* (2012), a co-production between France, Germany and Austria; Jacques Audiard's *Rust and Bone* (2012), a co-production between Belgium and France; a contemporary adaptation of *Great Expectations* (Mike Newell, 2012) from the United Kingdom and the United States; and an unlikely Australian comedy about mateship and cricket, *Save your Legs* (Boyd Hicklin, 2012). The world premiere of the local Queensland documentary *Show Me the Magic*, featuring the life and career of internationally renowned Australian cinematographer Don McAlpine, was another highlight of the festival, with a memorable post-screening question-and-answer session revealing some of McAlpine's unique experiences working on the sets of iconic Australian films.

The festival's continued support of Australian content had been particularly evident in 2011, with the 'Local Heroes' section featuring seven Australian films and a further three local documentaries in competition for the BIFFDOCS prize. The festival stream, 'Let's Go Surfing', was a celebration of Australian beach culture and a tribute to the surf movie. This programme featured classics such as Bob Evans's *High on a Cool Wave* (1967) and Bruce Beresford's *Puberty Blues* (1981), as well as more recent films including a look at the world of women's wave-riding in *First Love* (Claire Gorman, 2011) and the controversial introduction of the shortboard in the feature-length documentary *Going Vertical: The Shortboard Revolution* (David Bradbury, 2010). BIFF also showcased local and national short films in three curated selections of Australian and Queensland shorts. The much loved film *Red Dog* (Kriv Stenders, 2011) was a highlight of the festival with a bring-your-own-dog-to-the-drive-in screening a great success with festival audiences. In 2012, however, there was a surprising lack of Australian content at the festival, with no specific section dedicated to local or national film-makers. Australian short films were well represented with two collections of shorts screened, and a collection dedicated to contemporary Indigenous cinema (through a partnership with Blackfella Films). Yet Australian feature films were under-represented, with only six full-length Australian features and two Australian/international co-productions included in the program. These included the bizarre Z-grade science fiction *The 25th Reich* (Stephen Amis, 2012) and the psychological thriller *Errors of the Human Body* (Eron Sheean, 2012). Shortly after the conclusion of the festival in 2012, Screen Queensland announced that Richard Moore would not be returning to BIFF, signalling further change for the festival in 2013.

BIFF prides itself on a diverse and internationally celebrated selection of films in its programme each year and the festival attracts film-makers, critics and industry professionals from around Australia and beyond these shores. As the festival continues to define its new position on the Australian festival circuit, particularly through its support of documentary film-making and growing alignment with the Asia Pacific Screen Awards, its audience numbers have also increased, with the festival attracting 25,000 people in 2012 (up from 22,600 people in 2011). In its 21 years to date, BIFF has established itself as a valuable institution in Queensland's film and festival culture.

Tess Van Hemert

Reference

Stringer, Julian (2001) 'Global Cities and International Film Festival Economy', in Mark Shiel and Tony Fitzmaurice (eds), *Cinema and the City: Film and Urban Societies in a Global Context*, Oxford: Blackwell, pp. 134–44.

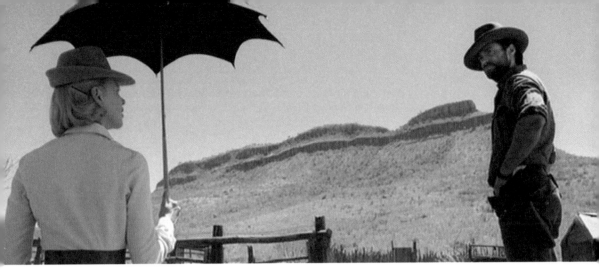

Australia (Baz Luhrmann, 2008)

AUSTRALIAN FILM LOCATIONS

Australia is well known for its distinctive film locations. Bushranger films dating from *The Story of the Kelly Gang* (Charles Tait, 1906) and early rural melodramas such as *The Squatter's Daughter* (Bert Bailey, 1910; remade by Ken G Hall in 1933) quickly established the historical and cultural importance of landscape to Australian cinema. In the first half of the twentieth century when most Hollywood films were shot in the controlled environment of studios, backlots or on nearby properties owned by the studio, the emphasis on location and landscape in Australian films was, and continues to be, noteworthy.

Location shooting became increasingly important as the Australian film industry matured, both in terms of exporting images of Australia to the world and framing narratives that reflected on Australian national identity. This is particularly evident in Charles Chauvel's films such as *Sons of Matthew* (1948), the story of pioneering Irish immigrants in Queensland, and *Jedda* (1955), which traverses the Northern Territory. In *Featuring Australia*, Stuart Cunningham uses the term 'locationism' to describe Chauvel's commitment to location shooting, stating 'the concept of locationism engages with Chauvel's nationalist desire to make Australia a film star' (1991: 126). Instead of the usual process of first securing actors to help promote and finance *Jedda*, Chauvel developed a story to 'match the magnificent backgrounds' of locations such as Nitmiluk National Park (Katherine Gorge) and Standley Chasm, then he sought non-professional actors to play roles consonant with their own backgrounds or professions (Cunningham 1991: 157).

The tradition of location shooting continued in a suite of nostalgic landscape films that rose to prominence during the Australian film revival in the 1970s and 1980s, including *Walkabout* (Nicholas Roeg, 1971), *Picnic at Hanging Rock* (Peter Weir, 1975) and *We of the Never Never* (Igor Auzins, 1982). The latter two period films were funded by the Australian Film Commission and shot on location in the bush and the outback with an aesthetic marked by the influence of the Heidelberg School of Australian landscape painting. However, location shooting also figures prominently in a wide range of contemporary and historical films and genres, to the extent that it has become something of a cliché for Australian directors to claim landscape is a character in the narrative – usually a harsh antagonist, beautiful virgin or nurturing motherland.

Of the ten highest grossing Australian films of all time, *Moulin Rouge!* (Baz Luhrmann, 2001) and *Happy Feet* (George Miller, 2006) are not set in Australia and *Strictly Ballroom* (Luhrmann,

1992) is a studio-based urban film. However, the overwhelming majority showcase locations from the Top End (the northernmost part of the Northern Territory) in *Crocodile Dundee* (Peter Faiman, 1986), *Crocodile Dundee II* (John Cornell, 1988) and *Australia* (Baz Luhrmann, 2008), through the Pilbara in *Red Dog* (Kriv Stenders, 2011), rural New South Wales in *The Dish* (Rob Stitch, 2000) and *Babe* (Chris Noonan, 1995), to the Victorian High Country in *The Man from Snowy River* (George Miller, 1982).

As Tom O'Regan and Rama Venkataswamy note, from the 1990s Australian film production aimed to appeal to a global audience by 'internationalising story properties', partly by filming in locations that did not look distinctively Australian and partly by using digital effects and studio sets to create possible worlds and storybook lands with a universal dimension (O'Regan and Venkataswamy 1999: 187–89). In films like *Babe: Pig in the City* (George Miller, 1998) and *Where the Wild Things Are* (Spike Jonze, 2009), 'Australian locations were valued for their capacity to double for somewhere else or be geographically unspecific' (O'Regan and Venkataswamy 1999: 192). Today iconic landmarks are significant for their recognizability and the potential to attract tourism, but there is still a need for locations to stand in for other places, as when Brisbane furnishes a futuristic American cityscape in the vampire film *Daybreakers* (Michael and Peter Spierig, 2009).

As the examples above suggest, locations are deployed in varied ways in contemporary cinema. Settings can play themselves (Tasmania's Central Plateau is both a narrative setting and a shooting location in Daniel Nettheim's *The Hunter* [2011]), or they can represent a generalized space (*Babe* was shot in Robertson, New South Wales, but its rural setting could be almost anywhere). A shooting location can also double for a named place: *Rabbit-Proof Fence* (Philip Noyce, 2002) is a stolen generation story set in the Moore River Native Settlement just north of Perth and in arid country on the way north to Jigalong, but it was mainly shot in McLaren Vale and the Flinders Ranges, South Australia. Similarly, a location might stand in for a genre's setting: the lunar landscape in the science fiction film *Pitch Black* (David Twohy, 2000) was shot at Moon Plains near Coober Pedy, South Australia. In addition, shooting locations can represent imaginary spaces such as the Never Never (an extremely remote location somewhere in the Outback), or fictional places like the town of Bundanyabba in *Wake in Fright* (Ted Kotcheff, 1971), filmed in Broken Hill, New South Wales.

Different uses of film locations in Australian cinema encompass actual locations and familiar landforms, set construction, as well as the modification and displacement of settings. However, demarcations between authentic and constructed settings are eroding, given the increasing prevalence of composite locations, virtual sets and computer-generated imagery. As Goldsmith, Ward and O'Regan put it, 'digitisation is blurring the never hard and fast distinction between purpose-built and existing natural and built environments' (2010: 188). For example, in *Australia* natural rock formations in the Bungle Bungles (Purnululu National Park, Western Australia) were augmented with computer-generated images of a ravine to stage a cattle stampede, and footage of Bowen, Queensland, was made to resemble Darwin in the 1940s with the addition of a digital escarpment rising up from the foreshore where historic buildings and purpose-built sets were filmed.

While it is difficult to single out one Australian site that is indicative of current trends in location shooting, the northern reaches of Western Australia have attracted a spate of productions in recent years, after previously being deemed too isolated and costly for feature film production. Unlike the Flinders Ranges near Adelaide Studios or production hubs near Sydney's Fox Studios, Melbourne's Docklands Studios, or Village Roadshow Studios in Queensland, Western Australia's dramatic, monsoonal, resource-rich and remote regions lack an established infrastructure to facilitate location shooting. Until recently, films that were set in Western Australia such as *Wolf Creek* (Greg McLean, 2005) and *Rabbit-Proof Fence* were filmed predominantly in South Australia. It is financially advantageous to have studio production facilities, postproduction facilities and location opportunities in the same area, supported by a trained screen production workforce: 'The most successful of the places competing for international production rely on a combination of built and natural environments, film services infrastructure including studios and a strong 'location interest', underwritten by a supportive policy and regulatory framework' (Goldsmith and O'Regan 2005: 41). Western Australia is the nation's largest state so it is expensive and time consuming to travel between far-flung locations and the limited production facilities in Perth. Yet the sparsely populated Kimberley and Pilbara regions in the far north with their fly-in-fly-out mine workers, small Aboriginal communities and isolated sheep and cattle stations are increasingly popular shooting locations for films set in the west.

A number of films that take place in Western Australia play on the Hollywood conventions of road movies and westerns, but reverse the established pattern of movement westward across the American frontier and south towards the Mexican border. Instead, Australian geography dictates that films follow their protagonists' journeys east in films like *The Overlanders* (Harry Watt, 1946), *Australia* and the Indigenous road comedy *Stone Bros* (Richard Frankland, 2009). Still more feature a northbound trajectory travelling over 2,000 km up the coast from Perth: consider, for instance, Sue Brooks's *Japanese Story* (2003), Rachel Perkins's Indigenous musical road movie *Bran Nue Dae* (2009), Brendan Fletcher's Indigenous drama, *Mad Bastards* (2010), and Katriona McKenzie's Aboriginal coming-of-age story, *Satellite Boy* (2012). Furthermore, two of the nation's highest grossing films, *Australia* and *Red Dog*, were shot in the northwest. Given that the south is far more populous, disproportionate representations of the northwest indicate that the region occupies an important place in the cultural imaginary.

In addition to the political-economy approach taken above, where location is understood as a narrative backdrop chosen or constructed for genre and budgetary reasons, researchers have analysed Australian cinema locations primarily in terms of narrative dichotomies like bush versus city, symbolic interpretations of screen aesthetics, or postcolonial critiques of settler culture and Indigenous land rights. Notably, chapters on the desert, the rural country town and the city in *Australian Cinema After Mabo* (Collins and Davis 2004) interpret the significance of film locations in light of a reconsideration of Australian colonial history and Indigenous heritage that finds expression on-screen in narratives exploring repressed traumatic memory, national self-recognition and dramas of origin. This is pertinent in relation to Western Australian cinema since so many of the films set there feature Aboriginal actors, film-makers and themes. This suggests a return to geographic specificity, an emerging focus on the connections between country and Indigenous culture and, perhaps, new ways of seeing and representing Australian film locations.

Jane Stadler

References

Cunningham, Stuart (1991) *Featuring Australia: The Cinema of Charles Chauvel*, Sydney: Allen & Unwin.

Goldsmith, Ben and O'Regan, Tom (2005) *The Film Studio: Film Production in the Global Economy*, Lanham: Rowman and Littlefield.

Goldsmith, Ben, Ward, Susan and O'Regan, Tom (2010) *Local Hollywood: Global Film Production and the Gold Coast*, Brisbane: University of Queensland Press.

O'Regan, Tom and Venkataswamy, Rama (1999) 'A Tale of Two Cities: *Dark City* and *Babe: Pig in the City*', in Deb Verhoeven (ed.), *Twin Peeks: Australian and New Zealand Feature Films*, Melbourne: Damned Publishing, pp. 187–203.

MARKETING MIX
FINDING INTERNATIONAL AUDIENCES: THE UK ROAD TRIP OF *CHARLIE & BOOTS*

The fate of *Charlie & Boots* (Dean Murphy, 2009) overseas provides an interesting case study of the complexities facing Australian films in international markets. It is not a film that fits readily into the specialist film market that numerous local films tap into. It is in many ways a very mainstream story but without the star power or budget to attract a wide audience outside Australia. Nevertheless the film has been screened in cinemas in both the United States and the United Kingdom. In America it was toured by Emerging Pictures as part of the 2010 USA-Australia Film Showcase, a subsidized initiative supported by Screen Australia (Screen Australia 2010b). In the United Kingdom the film was distributed independently and its fortunes there are the focus of this essay. The film's journey highlights the significance of broader industry structures in shaping the possibilities for Australian films. It also illustrates how it can be possible to circumvent some of these limitations, even if only on a relatively small scale.

Charlie & Boots was part of a slate of local films released in 2009 that helped deliver a strong domestic box office result for Australian-made titles after nearly a decade of poor returns. It had one of the best opening weekends for any Australian film that year and contributed a respectable AU$3.9 million to a total of AU$55 million in earnings for domestic releases (Swift 2009; Screen Australia 2010a). The film tells the story of a father ('Charlie' played by Paul Hogan) and son ('Boots' played by Shane Jacobson) who embark on a road trip from Victoria to Cape York in an attempt to deal with their grief following the death of Charlie's wife (Boots's mother). The film's trailer and other marketing materials positioned it squarely as comedy, highlighting a series of light-hearted adventures played out against rural and bush backdrops during their journey north in an iconic Holden Kingswood. However, the strained relationship between Charlie and Boots also provides some dramatic tension and a few poignant, albeit stiff, moments. Some news outlets celebrated the film as a story of the 'true Blue Aussie bloke' (Roach 2009). Indeed it drew heavily on the characterization of the Australian male portrayed by its lead actors in others films – such as *Crocodile Dundee* (Peter Faiman, 1986), *Kenny* (Clayton Jacobson, 2006) and *Strange Bedfellows* (Dean Murphy, 2004) – the slightly irreverent but endearing larrikin with an aversion to articulating emotions but who likes his beer and stands by his mates. Box office results indicate that the story resonated with some local audiences, although the overall total was perhaps slightly disappointing given the film's very promising start. But what of the film's potential in markets beyond Australia?

Language and cultural considerations mean that Australian films transfer most readily into English-speaking territories. Success in the premium markets of the United Kingdom and the United States is highly sought after, but not often achieved. Competition for locally made films is tough enough at home against the steady stream of Hollywood imports. Relatively low budgets and correspondingly minimalist production values make it difficult for Australian films to compete on an equal footing. It is often very difficult to secure screens with large mainstream cinema circuits, and instead local films are pushed through arthouse or specialist exhibitors and second-tier independents (see Aveyard 2011).

These problems are often compounded for films attempting to make inroads overseas. The international slate of 300 or so titles released in Australia each year (Screen Australia 2012), pales in comparison to the 600 + movies screened in cinemas each year in the United States and Canada (MPAA 2012), while in the United Kingdom the figure hovers above 500 annually (BFI 2012). In these markets Australian films again face competition from high-budget productions. They also cease to be distinguished culturally by their home-grown credentials, although this can hinder as well as boost a film's commercial chances. In foreign markets, Australian films may become exotic or 'othered' and this can sometimes enhance their prospects. More often, however, local titles circulate as one among many in the globalized, specialized or arthouse film sector. Standing out in this crowd can be difficult, particularly in places like the United Kingdom and elsewhere in Europe where exhibitors are offered significant financial incentives to screen independent films produced in the European Union over titles from further afield (see Europa Cinemas 2012).

Charlie & Boots (Dean Murphy, 2009)

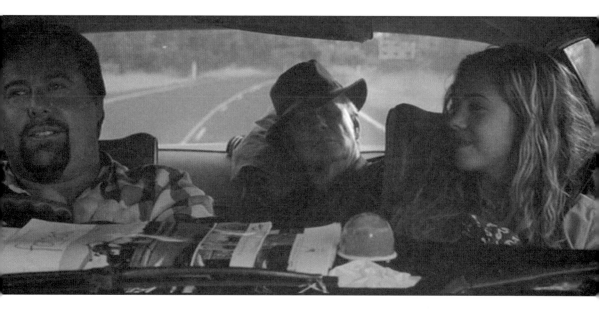

Charlie & Boots was exhibited in the United Kingdom as part of the line-up for the 16th London Australian Film Festival in 2010 and released commercially by StudioCanal (formerly Optimum Releasing), although only on DVD. At a rudimentary level, *Charlie & Boots* shares commonalities with other Australian titles that have done relatively well in the United Kingdom. Rural and bush landscapes are a prominent feature of both the mise-en-scène and the narrative, and this echoes films like *The Adventures of Priscilla: Queen of the Desert* (Stephan Elliot, 1994), *Wolf Creek* (Greg McLean, 2005), and more recently *Red Dog* (Kriv Stenders, 2011) and *The Hunter* (Daniel Nettheim, 2011). The deliberate signposting of the trip to Cape York, mostly by the character Boots, provides guidance for geographically challenged audiences, and it is easy to speculate that the producers may well have had international audiences in mind when building this into the story. Australian humour has also proved capable of striking a chord with UK audiences as far back as the Crocodile Dundee films through to *Muriel's Wedding* (PJ Hogan, 1994) and *Kenny*.

Paul Hogan's name was perceived by the organizers of the London Australian Film Festival as being a genuine hook for its marketing. As Festival Programmer at the 16th London Australian Film Festival, Moira McVean, explained, 'a generalisation I know, but if you quizzed the average UK person on their knowledge of Australian cinema back then [2010], Paul Hogan in *Crocodile Dundee* was usually their first thought!' (McVean, personal communication, 16 August 2012). However, while Hogan may have been well known, neither he nor Jacobson were perceived by the film's commercial distributor, StudioCanal, as big enough stars to carry it into a theatrical release. The story, characterizations and comedic elements were also not seen as sufficiently engaging for a cinema audience unlikely to be swept along by the nostalgia of hits like *Crocodile Dundee* and *Kenny* (Candy Vincent-Smith [UK Catalogue Consultant at StudioCanal], personal communication, 25 September 2012).

The film was a relatively small release for StudioCanal and has performed modestly in terms of rental and retail sales in the United Kingdom. However, by way of contrast, it was one of the standout successes at the London Australian Film Festival in 2010. Moira McVean recalls it as being one of the fastest selling films of the festival and was very positively received by audiences. It screened as part of the 'LAFF out loud' strand, as opposed to the festival's 'Dark Side of Down Under' strand, targeting viewers looking for a lighter style of entertainment. In terms of audience composition, the festival typically attracts a mixed audience – approximately 60 per cent UK nationals to 40 per cent Australian. McVean understood that for many of their repeat attendees as well as for ex-pats both Hogan and Jacobson would be highly recognizable faces. Dean Murphy's *Strange Bedfellows* had played at the 2005 festival and done well. *Kenny* had also performed respectably in its UK theatrical release and McVean believed Jacobson's new film would be 'eagerly anticipated'. Australian Film Institute Awards (AFI) nominations and a solid performance at the Australian box office also played into the decision to program the film and were important in its promotion within the festival (McVean, personal communication, 9 October 2012).

The success of *Charlie & Boots* at the festival, as opposed to its mainstream DVD release, attests to the importance of the context of viewing as much as the content that is viewed (Harbord 2002). However, at the same time, it also highlights the difficulties Australian films can face in making inroads in overseas markets outside specialized or supported/subsidized situations. Some local movies are able to break through the mainstream industry's commercial and structural barriers, though many more are not, as *Charlie & Boots* illustrates. But the story does not have to end there. The film did find an enthusiastic audience – insignificant in economic terms but an audience nonetheless. It attracted viewers who came along not just to experience Australian cinema but to experience a bit of Australia – for example via tie-ins with the Australia Shop in London which supplied audiences with local food 'staples' such as Tim Tams, Twisties, Violet

Crumbles, Cherry Ripes, Caramello Koalas and Minties. Whether for ex-pat or UK national patrons, these cross-cultural encounters play a part in building awareness and positivity around Australian films. Situated as special events, the context of such screenings can significantly enhance their perceived sociocultural value, and in turn perhaps even enhance the reception of the film consumed (Harbord 2002: 38–59). The fortunes of *Charlie & Boots* in the United Kingdom underscore the fact that places do exist for Australian movies overseas, but that it may not always be possible to measure success in terms of box office returns.

Karina Aveyard

References

Aveyard, Karina (2011) 'Australian films at the cinema: Rethinking the role of distribution and exhibition', *Media International Australia*, 138, pp. 36–45.

BFI (British Film Institute) (2012) *Statistical Yearbook 2011*, http://statisticalyearbook11. ry.com/?id=82760. Accessed 13 October 2012.

Europa Cinemas (2012) 'Europa Cinemas', http://www.europa-cinemas.org/en/. Accessed 18 October 2012.

Harbord, Janet (2002) *Film Cultures*, London: Sage.

MPAA (Motion Picture Association of America) (2012) 'Theatrical Market Statistics 2011' [industry report], http://www.mpaa.org/resources/5bec4ac9-a95e-443b-987b-bff6fb5455a9.pdf. Accessed 13 October 2012.

Roach, Vicky (2009) 'Charlie & Boots' blokes of a feather', *Daily Telegraph*, 2 September, http://www.dailytelegraph.com.au/entertainment/charlie-boots-blokes-of-a-feather/story-e6frewyr-1225768880754. Accessed 12 October 2012.

Screen Australia (2010a) 'Australian films at the local box office in 2009', Media Release, http://www.screenaustralia.gov.au/news_and_events/Media-Release-documents/2010/mr_100121_boxoffice.pdf. Accessed 8 October 2012.

Screen Australia (2010b) 'Australian Film Showcase set for US', Media Release, 10 May, http://www.screenaustralia.gov.au/news_and_events/Media-Release-documents/2010/mr_100510_showcase.pdf. Accessed 15 October 2012.

Screen Australia (2012) 'Number of Australian and overseas films released in Australian cinemas 1984–2011', http://www.screenaustralia.gov.au/research/statistics/wcfilmxcountry.asp. Accessed 13 October 2012.

Swift, Brendan (2009) 'Box Office: Charlie & Boots breaks $800K', *IF Magazine*, 7 September, http://if.com.au/2009/09/07/article/LLRPTCPDTJ.html. Accessed 14 October 2012.

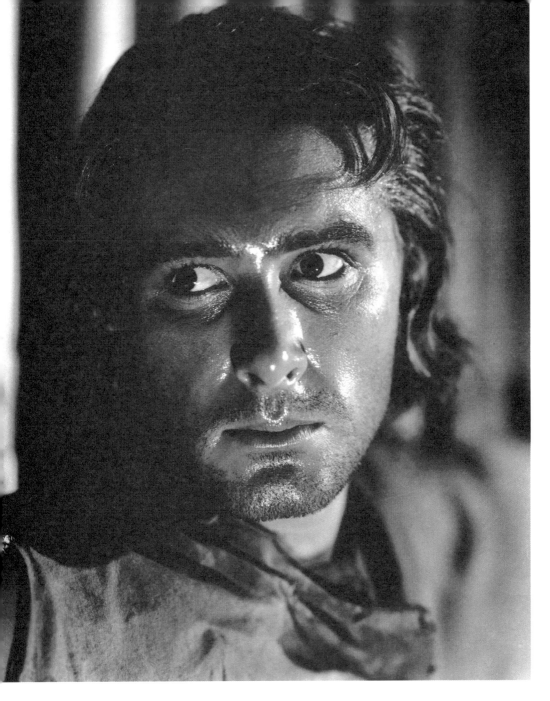

Errol Flynn in *Captain Blood*
(Michael Curtiz, 1935).
© Kobal Collection

STAR STUDY
ERROL FLYNN (1909–1959)

Errol Flynn was one of the most popular and bankable Hollywood stars of the 1930s and 1940s. A mercurial and often unmanageable persona, Flynn's peak of stardom only lasted for a relatively short period of time, and by the late 1940s he started to appear in a generally lacklustre series of films that mostly copied or parodied such earlier triumphs as *Captain Blood* (Michael Curtiz, 1935), *The Adventures of Robin Hood* (Michael Curtiz and William Keighley, 1938) and *They Died with Their Boots On* (Raoul Walsh, 1941). Largely shunned by his studio, and by then a somewhat lethargic and slightly bloated presence, he experienced something of a late career revival with close-to-the-bone performances as alcoholics in *The Sun Also Rises* (Henry King, 1957) and *Too Much, Too Soon* (Art Napoleon, 1958), before a bizarre final venture to Castro's Cuba and his inevitable early death at the age of 50 in 1959.

Despite the fact that he was born in Tasmania, and lived in Hobart and Sydney for most of the first twenty or so years of his life, Flynn has not been widely celebrated or discussed within Australia. Even in Hobart, and despite the efforts of an enthusiastic local appreciation society, the markers of his formative years are not generally highlighted, with only a nondescript seashore park and an isolated star outside the Theatre Royal noticeably trading on his name. This is partly to do with the fact that Flynn never again set foot in Australia after leaving for Britain in 1933. He seldom played roles that highlighted his background despite an often noticeable Antipodean accent, and commonly featured in films that emphasized his heroic contribution to the war effort despite his own reluctance to serve. He was widely promoted by his studio Warner Bros. as being of Irish nationality and descent. Even when Flynn did play identifiably Australian characters, such as Flight Lieutenant Terry Forbes in Raoul Walsh's *Desperate Journey* (1942), the initial attempts of the film to signify stereotypical nationality ('Waltzing Matilda' on the soundtrack, playful references to kangaroos, etc.) quickly became conflated within a pan-British identity.

Flynn provides an important example of the common fate of Australian performers in Hollywood and is inarguably the principal Australian actor to succeed there before the 1980s. He is also a figure who has maintained a significant star persona and notoriety long after his demise, and is still one of the most written about and discussed of classical Hollywood actors. But much of this discussion is dependent upon the legend and myth of his star persona, and often revolves around his salacious sexual exploits (bolstered by the catchphrase 'In like Flynn'), particular repeated anecdotes, his largely negative attitudes towards film acting, and such fanciful claims as his alleged Nazi sympathies (largely levelled at Flynn by the controversial author and biographer Charles Higham). As a result of this, Flynn's significance as a particular kind of romantic action star, as well as the quality of many of his performances and the films in which he starred, have been undervalued.

Although Flynn seems to have led a breezy, somewhat adventurous and fairly comfortable life in Australia in the 1910s and 1920s before decamping to New Guinea in the early 1930s, he only appeared in one film prior to leaving Australia, Charles Chauvel's *In the Wake of the Bounty* (1933). There is a fascinating and revealing screen test of Flynn shot by Chauvel for this somewhat creaky and at times unconvincing film, with its striking and extensive location footage shot by Tasman Higgins in the Pitcairn Islands. As is evident from this test, and from Flynn's performance in the subsequent film, he had very little acting experience in front of the camera and was not adequately supported by Chauvel's direction (though his performance is in keeping with many others elsewhere in Chauvel's ambitious, but highly artificial, often mannered cinema). Other than the roughness and raw magnetism of the actor (still evident beneath an appalling wig and frankly stilted, glowering delivery), the most interesting aspect of this test is Chauvel's direction:

'I want you to forget you're Errol Flynn' (Chauvel 1938). Although this is a common instruction to untrained actors trying to embody a fictional character – in this case Fletcher Christian – it resonates across Flynn's subsequent career, and with the difficulties he encountered breaking free from particular types of roles and specific ways of reading the relation between the star and the characters he played.

Flynn's astonishing and almost immediate rise to stardom was both a blessing and a curse. He had featured, woodenly, in Chauvel's film, a couple of British films made at Warner Bros.' Teddington studio, and had small roles in several films at Warners in America (one in the not exactly featured role of a corpse). His prominence in films that featured the actor in period costume, in 'tights', in artificial and carefully modulated environments, and in films that played upon generalized notions of his gentlemanly British/Irish ancestry, made it difficult for Warner Bros. to conceive of Flynn outside of these established and highly restrictive frameworks. This straightjacketing was not loosened by the fact that many of the Flynn films made outside of the swashbuckling, western and broader adventure genres were considerably less successful at the box office than their action-centred counterparts. Even Jack Warner, who obviously stood to benefit considerably from more flexible and malleable star personas, admitted, 'Flynn in modern clothes just doesn't seem to go over' (included in a memo from Jack Warner to producer Hal Wallis, see Behlmer [1986: 174]). Flynn himself became increasingly dismissive of his film career – for example, his infamous but highly readable late career autobiography *My Wicked, Wicked Ways* (1959) has little to say about his movies – bristling particularly against the efforts of the studio to cast him in westerns where his accent and manner often required further, somewhat tortured explanation.

Flynn had pretensions as a writer and adventurer beyond the movies, but was also cocooned by the physical comforts and distractions offered by stardom. Nevertheless, it is the period that covers his initial seven-year contract with Warners, and the first half of the second, that incorporates most of his key films and performances – the ones that we largely remember him for today. Flynn was essentially a quixotic actor whose physical prowess and ultimate psychological and bodily frailty meant that the peak of his career lasted only ten years (Flynn had physical difficulties on numerous films, including a minor heart attack during the making of *Gentleman Jim* in 1942 and recurring malaria on *Objective Burma!* in 1945, both directed by Walsh). The loosening of studio controls on talent in the late 1940s and 1950s, circumstances that proved highly beneficial to figures like James Stewart and Kirk Douglas, was more problematic for Flynn. Although he had long wanted to break free from studio interference and its deadening work ethic, he actually needed the structure and protection of such systems to control his physical environment and public persona, particularly once his health started to significantly deteriorate.

Despite Flynn's legendary rabble-rousing, unreliability, alcoholism and reactions against the studio system, his career is marked by sustained collaborations with two vastly different Hollywood directors, figures who were deemed able to control his often distracted and self-destructive approach to making movies. Flynn's screen persona has tended to be defined by the eleven films he made with the notoriously authoritarian Michael Curtiz (a figure he came to loathe) in the first phase of his Hollywood career for Warner Bros., often starring alongside Olivia de Havilland. This prejudice is unsurprising considering the quality and iconicity of the films that best represent these partnerships and collaborations: *Captain Blood*, *The Charge of the Light Brigade* (1936), *The Adventures of Robin Hood*, *Dodge City* (1939) and *The Private Lives of Elizabeth and Essex* (1940). These films made in the short period between 1935 and 1940 – alongside the Flynn-only *The Sea Hawk* (Michael Curtiz, 1940) – work to define Flynn's dominant and inescapable screen persona: a star image that projected a seemingly effortless physicality, balletic athleticism, good humour, anti-authoritarianism, 'mock overconfidence' (Farber 1998), a 'fabulous smile – one that both charms and cons' (Basinger 2007), beauty and grace, and was marked by Flynn's reliance upon Hollywoodized affectations and stereotypes of particular historical periods and a broadly configured Britishness.

But I would argue that it is a second group of seven films directed by Raoul Walsh between 1941 and 1948 that consolidate and further define, even complicate Flynn's persona – including *Gentleman Jim*, *Uncertain Glory* (1944) and *Objective Burma!*. The Flynn-Walsh films are marked by a malleability, indistinctness and questioning of identity, ethnicity and nationality in relation to their central characters, as well as a degree of self-consciousness in terms of how they present Flynn on-screen. They are even more fascinating in this regard when one recognizes that they coincide with a broader interrogation of Flynn's loyalty, heroism and even nationality by certain parts of the critical fraternity and the popular press. But by the time of 1948's *Silver River*, Flynn's final collaboration with close friend Walsh, it was clear that the actor's persona and career had become somewhat ossified. Despite the relatively brief peak of his career, and failure to reflect upon his Australian origins until late in his life (he wrote extensively of his Hobart upbringing in his autobiography), Flynn remains a salient and formative example of the fate that still awaits many Antipodean actors in the murky waters of international cinema.

Adrian Danks

References

Basinger, Janine (2007) *The Star Machine*, New York: Alfred A. Knopf.

Behlmer, Rudy (1986) *Inside Warner Bros. (1935–1951)*, London: Weidenfeld and Nicolson.

Chauvel, Charles (1938) *Screen tests for Errol Flynn and Mary Maguire and the grooming for stardom of Betty Pike and Patricia Firth*, Sydney: Expeditionary Films, http://www.nfsa.gov.au/site_media/uploads/file/2011/12/05/NFSA_Charles_Chauvel_amended.pdf. Accessed 3 January 2013.

Farber, Manny (1998) *Negative Space*, New York: Da Capo Press.

DIRECTORS

JANE CAMPION (b.1954)

Almost before her career had begun Jane Campion was enthusiastically hailed as an auteur-in-the-making. On the basis of a series of accomplished short films (in particular, *Peel* [1982], *Passionless Moments* [1983] and *A Girl's Own Story* [1984]) she earned early success at the Cannes Film Festival, winning the 1986 Short Film Palme d'Or with her Australian Film, Television and Radio School student work *Peel*. While her most prominent career success to date remains the breakout 'artbuster', *The Piano* (1993), a 'cross-over' film that won her the Palme d'Or at Cannes and catapulted her into mainstream cinemas, the ongoing importance of film festivals to Campion's career is evident.

Jane Campion has been a steadfast presence on the festival circuit, relying on a range of festivals to launch her films. The Venice Film Festival, for example, premiered *An Angel at My Table* (1990), *Portrait of a Lady* (closing-night film, 1996) and *Holy Smoke* (1999). Her more clearly generic titles have opened on the more apposite North American festival circuit: *In the Cut* (Toronto 2003) and *Top of the Lake* (Sundance 2013). Her first feature film after a significant break from film-making, *Bright Star* (2009), returned her resolutely to the scene of her earliest success (Cannes).

The importance of the Cannes Film Festival throughout Campion's career cannot be underestimated. Following her precocious success there, her feature debut *Sweetie* (1989) also competed at Cannes. Then, after completing *An Angel at My Table*, she secured a second Palme d'Or in 1993 with *The Piano*, which also earned Holly Hunter a Best Actress Award and anticipated its wider success, most notably at the Academy Awards. The film won three Academy Awards (including Best Original Screenplay for Campion herself), and was nominated for five others including Best Picture, Best Director, and Best Cinematography.

Whichever way it is examined, this has been a relationship of mutual benefit for both Campion and Cannes. For example, Campion has described in detail the value of her association with the Cannes Film Festival to the financing of *The Piano* (Verhoeven 2009: 186–89). Conversely, in 2007, she was the only woman in a list of 35 auteurs selected to participate in the Cannes fiftieth anniversary celebrations.

In 2013, Campion was selected to lead the prestigious Cinéfondation and Short Film Jury for the 66th Festival de Cannes. The Festival President, Gilles Jacob, described with some sense of rhapsody and romance, the longstanding relationship between Campion and Cannes:

> Jane is a child of Cannes. I know this as it was I who selected her first three short films for the festival, because I liked her style and consistency [...] I am delighted that the love story between Lady Jane and the festival continues today as she takes on the role of president. (Keslassy 2013)

Jacob's observation that the key attributes for auteurist appreciation are formal style and consistency is especially interesting and points to the importance of the constants in Campion's career rather than the contradictions.

Although Campion's career has spanned a period of rapid industrial change and her fortunes have waxed and waned in correspondence with it, it is the perception of her personal ability to span these vicissitudes that gives power to her auteur persona. Campion in this sense is best understood as an expansive figure, able to traverse boundaries of many kinds: geopolitical (her dual status as a New Zealander and Australian); generic (working across a multitude of genres – arthouse, comedy, period drama, thriller); format (moving repeatedly between feature film, short film and television); scope (working locally and internationally, often simultaneously); and scale (working variously with low, medium and high budgets).

Similarly, her preference for returning to key cast members and crew from film to film lends coherence to her eclectic production choices despite the otherwise evident differences between projects: Holly Hunter stars in both *The Piano* and *Top of the Lake*; Nicole Kidman stars in *Portrait* but had a producer role in *In the Cut*; Jan Chapman produced *Bright Star*, *Holy Smoke* and *The Piano*; Gerard Lee co-wrote *Sweetie* and *Top of the Lake* with Campion. And so on.

The Piano (Jane Campion, 1993). © Kobal Collection

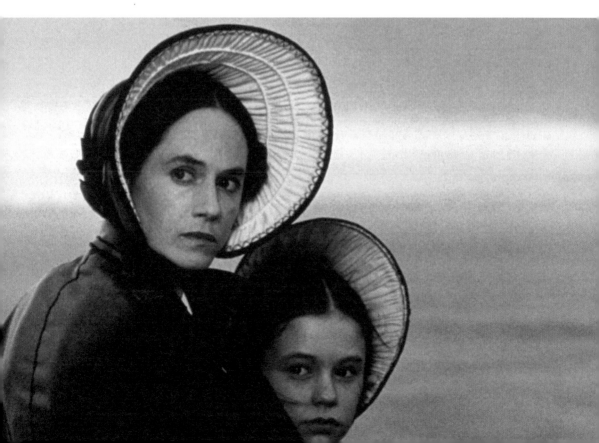

Campion's cinema has also been the subject of remarkable academic and critical interest with the same film title at once provoking swooning appreciation *and* columns of complaint. Despite this diagnostic division over individual films, critical efforts to stabilize Campion's point of difference as an auteur are mostly manifest through the conjuring of thematic returns across her work. Gilles Jacob for example, attempts a summary: 'Naively perverse young girls, teens closed in around their solitude, and women mulling over desires and regrets: Jane's is a passionate universe that she firmly holds in check as she draws these intricate group portraits' (Knegt 2013). Campion herself, reflecting in 2005 on her work to date, noted: 'I've only just started to realize how common my motifs are to myself. I think I've been very preoccupied with the idea of who a woman is in the world and love and sex' (Verhoeven 2009: 190). In support of these observed preoccupations is a vast body of critical and scholarly literature centred on Campion's distinctive visual flair, what Gilles Jacob referred to in his pithy assessment of her auteur credentials, as 'style' (Knegt 2013).

Campion leapt into global prominence with her graphically striking feature film *The Piano*. But stylistic quirks and hallmarks were features of her earliest work and figure prominently in initial assessments of her auteurist promise. Citations for her student films at the 1984 Melbourne Film Festival, for example, noted her 'compelling stylistic innovation'.

Recalling Roland Barthes (1981) observation of the *punctum*, Campion's work often provides opportunity for incidental details to trigger intense and sometimes traumatic opportunities for recognition in the viewer. Vivian Sobchack (2004: 53–84) has written on the visceral impact of Campion's imagery on her own viewing of *The Piano*, describing the phenomenological force of Campion's visual choices in purely physical terms. These provocative signature images may be drawn from Campion's own personal repertoire, (such as the ceramic horse figurines that appear in *Sweetie*), or story-related details such as the close-ups of buttons in *Bright Star*. Typically, they are intensely visual images that are not necessarily intended to provoke meanings beyond their status as an image. They may however dwell on their history *as an image*, such as the surrealist talking beans in *Portrait of a Lady*, or the travel brochure images of outback Australia in *Holy Smoke*. Kathleen McHugh (2007: 129) has further identified how specific image-motifs return throughout Campion's films, skipping from title to title, like the ever-present images of shoes in *Sweetie* and *In the Cut* for example, or the close-ups of fingers in *The Piano* and *Portrait*.

As if to underscore this idea of the image as *punctum*, as the cause for a traumatic disruption of personal spectatorship, many of Campion's characters are also depicted as engaging with images on this basis. Scenes of traumatic voyeurism and partial viewing are critical to the narrative momentum of films such as *The Piano* and *In the Cut*. In the opening scenes of *In the Cut* for instance, Meg Ryan's character glimpses something that she cannot quite 'name' despite her evident skill as a wordsmith and which eventually becomes her undoing.

Campion herself has spoken about the significance of visual style to her own workflow. Commenting on her most recent work, the made-for-TV mini-series *Top of the Lake* she noted: 'I can't but have to deliver something I think is gorgeous. Because otherwise I don't want to go there. It's just insulting' (The Hollywood Reporter 2013).

Unapologetically ambitious in vision, Campion's work has inspired generations of film-makers and academics alike. The para-textual setting for Campion's cinema (through media commentary, academic works and other films) has been instrumental in providing a receptive context for her work, even when she has withdrawn from the production of films themselves for periods of time.

Her popularity amongst academics is especially notable. As early as 1999 a collection of interviews with Campion (some translated from French) was published as part of a Conversations with Filmmakers series by the University Press of Mississippi. Two years later Dana Polan published his critical assessment of her career in the British Film Institute's World Directors series. Three years later Sue Gillett's appreciation of *The Films Of Jane Campion* was released. And then in 2007, a monograph, *Jane Campion* by Kathleen McHugh, was included in the Contemporary Film Directors series by University of Illinois Press. More recently in 2011 Alistair Fox contributed to the field of academic analysis of Jane Campion's work with his *Jane Campion: Authorship & Personal Cinema*. Critical debate on individual titles, particularly *The Piano* is an entire academic industry alone (see Verhoeven 2009: 147–82).

These scholarly works provide yet another facet to the prism of authorship that defines Jane Campion's singular career. If Campion is any guide, the path to success as a contemporary auteur involves navigating volatile industrial and aesthetic expectations under the uncompromising glare of many eyes. That Campion has somehow forged a signature cinema, despite her own misgivings and evident ambivalences along the way, is perhaps the best evidence we have of her remarkable talents as a contemporary auteur: 'As I get older I certainly don't take a particularly serious view of life. It's kind of best lived lightly. I'm not even interested in myself much; the story of me as I developed it; I'm over it' (quoted in Verhoeven 2009: 201).

Deb Verhoeven

References

Barthes, Roland (1981) *Camera Lucida*, New York: Hill and Wang.
Keslassy, Elsa (2013) 'Campion to head Cannes short film juries', *Variety*, 5 February, http://www.variety.com/article/VR1118065669/. Accessed 28 September 2013.
Knegt, Peter (2013) 'Jane Campion to Head Cannes Cinéfondation and Short Film Jury', *IndieWire*, 5 February, http://www.indiewire.com/article/jane-campion-to-head-cannes-cinefondation-and-short-film-jury. Accessed 28 September 2013.
McHugh, Kathleen (2007) *Jane Campion*, Urbana and Chicago: University of Illinois Press.
Sobchack, Vivian (2004) *Carnal Thoughts: Embodiment and Moving Image Culture*, Los Angeles: University of California Press.
The Hollywood Reporter (2013) Jane Campion's "Top of the Lake"' [interview], http://www.youtube.com/watch?v=IMjNeD8Ec8k. Accessed 28 September 2013.
Verhoeven, Deb (2009) *Jane Campion*, London: Routledge.

ARTHUR CANTRILL (b.1938) and CORINNE CANTRILL (b.1928)

Arthur and Corinne Cantrill started their extraordinary collaborative film-making careers in 1960, and remain two of the most significant and productive figures in the history of international experimental cinema. Their work is an intimate, highly formal, and remarkably cinematic exploration of the Australian landscape (as well as, on occasion, various international locations such as Ubud in Bali and Berlin), their immediate domestic and working environments, the material qualities of the cinema, the relationship between image and sound, the conditions of film exhibition, and key artistic influences on their work and life. It also ranges across a wide array of audio-visual forms and genres including documentary, experimental film, performance art, expanded cinema, and sound art. In fact, defining and categorizing the Cantrills' work in such a way makes little sense of the shared and shifting frameworks that characterize their work.

Initially making documentaries in Brisbane for the Children's Library and Crafts Movement, some of Arthur and Corinne Cantrill's most significant contributions to Australian film culture include: their groundbreaking expanded cinema works of the early 1970s including *Concert for Electric Jugs* (1971); Corinne's monumental autobiographical performance and film, *In This Life's Body* (1985); the series of films they made with other artists including the Dutch mime Will Spoor, *Moving Statics* (1969), and poet and activist *Harry Hooton* (1970); the couple's materialist but expressively organic work in the field of three-colour separation; and *Cantrills Filmnotes*, one of the most significant, long-running and groundbreaking publications devoted to 'independent film and video' published anywhere in the world. Their pre-eminent position as mentors and collaborators, and the legacy of their 50-year journey through the medium of film, register them as two of the most significant figures in the history of Australian cinema, a position that is only somewhat marginalized by their insistent work in less mainstream and often uncompromising forms of materialist film practice. Arthur and Corinne Cantrill's often artisanal and challenging work across film-making, exhibition, publishing, writing, distribution and other forms of artistic and cultural practice demonstrates a tireless, sometimes relentless and lifelong commitment to cinema.

The Cantrills' voluminous work also maintains a preoccupation with place, time and situation, and often reflects their immediate physical, experiential and cultural environments (it is generally less direct in its political or immediate social engagement). In this regard their work can also be considered as an important contribution to what might be called 'environmental cinema', a documentary and experimental film practice shared by contemporaries and colleagues such Pat O'Neill, Stan Brakhage and Rose Lowder, and that explores the relationship between cinematic materiality, place and ecology. Most remarkable in this regard are a series of expanded cinema and performance works that explore and bear witness to domestic, urban and regional environments such as *Projected Light* (1988) – a paean to the ontology of cinema and the nature of light shot in their Brunswick home – *The Berlin Apartment* (1986) and *The Becak Driver: A Story from Yogyakarta* (1998), as well as a remarkable series of films exploring the bush, coastal and desert landscapes of Australia: *At Uluru* (1977), *Meteor*

Crater: Gosse Bluff (1978), *Wilpena* (1981), *Tidal River* (1996), and numerous others. Some of the films in this last series also highlight an intermittent preoccupation with the specificity and legacy of Indigenous culture further explored in such works as *Two Women* (1980), which combines footage of a trip to the MacDonnell Ranges with a song cycle performed by Pitjanjatjara women.

In essence, the Cantrills' artistic practice and essential work within film culture is local and international, rigorously specific and 'cosmic', restless and continuously returning to a series of preoccupations and practices. Although they have seldom worked within the realm of what is commonly called found-footage cinema (a series of works exploring the ethnographic films and images of Walter Baldwin Spencer are a notable exception), their films and performances often also rework and represent earlier images. The temporal specificity and materiality of the film screening itself (on 16 mm or 8 mm) – a form of exhibition they have always insisted upon, controlling much of the distribution of their films and not allowing it to be transferred to video or DVD – is central to any understanding of their work. Although their creations are only occasionally directly autobiographical, and rarely address audiences in a conventionally expository fashion, the presence of the Cantrills around their work – often presenting it at screenings, providing voices and sounds of accompaniment, operating projectors and other 'technologies' in their multi-screen and expanded cinema presentations, writing within the pages of *Cantrills Filmnotes* and so on – is central to its circulation, reception and understanding.

Although the Cantrills started their film work in 1960, it is not really until the late 1960s and early 1970s that their contribution to Australian film culture becomes truly significant with the first publication of *Cantrills Filmnotes*, a landmark series of expanded cinema performances, and a string of important short and longer films. This coincides with their return to Australia after a period in Britain. The earlier work, initially created in Brisbane and then the United Kingdom, is still fascinating for the hints it gives of the forms and practices they would subsequently develop and follow. A fair amount of this early work is devoted to images of children – the Cantrills themselves had two children, both of whom feature significantly in their work and, in the case of Ivor, became important collaborators – and such artists and artisans as Charles Lloyd and Robert Klippel. The series of films they made about Klippel's creations, or 'junk sculptures', explore the sculptural dimensions of the artist's work, combining often high contrast, almost abstract imagery with equally 'modernist' music and sound. Although these films do mimic some of the conventions of the art documentary, they strive to create forms and experiences that transcend these boundaries.

The expansive but uncompromising qualities of the Cantrills' singular contribution to Australian film culture is perhaps best exemplified by their remarkably resilient publication, *Cantrills Filmnotes*. Running from 1971 until the end of the millennium, this irregular journal published 100 issues (though this was enabled by a final edition that incorporated the last eight installments). It contains a vast array of material covering the experimental film scene in Australia, expanded cinema and sound performance, contributions and reports by a vast array of international figures, marginalized film history (early cinema technologies, home movies, etc.), important discussions of developments in emergent areas such as Super 8 and video, and people whose contributions and activities may have gone largely undocumented – and that would definitely have been less meticulously recorded – without the intercession of the journal. *Cantrills Filmnotes* also provides a significant record and archive of often-ephemeral films and practices, its high level of illustration reflecting the sobering reality that many of the works it discussed and championed may now only be accessible (and even 'exist', in some cases) within the pages of the journal.

The Cantrills were quite explicit from the start that their actions in editing and publishing the journal were to some extent political, an attempt to question and rethink the dominant priorities of mainstream film practice and governmental policy (though, somewhat ironically, the journal did receive some institutional support). But the journal is now most valuable as a kind of archive, documenting and recording ephemeral practices, films, cultural contexts and modes of thought in a manner that allows us to attain some understanding of the flows and activities of a now troublingly distant moment in time.

Although some of the Cantrills' films do contain elements of story and narrative, their work is generally marked by a conscious resistance to such forms, even within the looser framework of experimental cinema. In this regard, their work consistently examines and explores the dimensions of time, space and place. In a film such as *Waterfall* (1984), three separate 'moments' are placed over one another to create a wondrous and strange re-presentation of colour – each of the strips of film uses a different coloured filter and is then combined to create a composite 'single' image in projection – and to register the shifts in time between each of these elements. Although all of the strips of film were shot from the same camera position, and in fairly close temporal proximity, they still record the changes and differences between these three elements and moments. In the hands of other film-makers this approach might have overstated the broader physical, materialist and reflexive properties of the cinema, but the Cantrills also give time and priority to the documentation and representation of this particular place – it is both a site of cinema *and* geography. In the process, *Waterfall* records the contrasting temporalities of cinematic, everyday and geological time.

This practice of three-colour separation is one of a series of devices the Cantrills utilized to interrogate the specificity of the cinema, to examine its various constitutive elements and explore its ontology. But this technique also points towards an overriding concern with film history and the technologies associated with both early- and pre-cinema. For Arthur and Corinne Cantrill, the cinema is an endlessly shifting and developing medium but also one defined by a continuity of practices and material qualities. It is therefore unsurprising that their 50-year career largely coincides with the rise of independent film culture and the ultimate demise of analogue forms of film-making. An overwhelming preoccupation of their work is the specific and sometimes mercurial qualities of celluloid and projected light, and their often overpowering but measured work stands as a testament to a life lived in and with film.

Adrian Danks

KEN G HALL (1901–1994)

Ken G Hall was the producer and principal director for Australia's most prolific film studio, Cinesound Productions, from the 1930s to the 1950s. A self-styled showman with a background in publicity, his work encapsulates a period in which Australian film-making placed overt emphasis on market-driven, Hollywood-inspired entertainment. His feature films, produced in the 1930s and 1940s, juxtapose Australian subject matter with an embrace of modern capitalism and artifice, a combination fuelled by the need to compete with American cinema. While expressing overt admiration for Hollywood, however, Hall retained a commitment to local content; he produced the Australian newsreel, *Cinesound Review*, from 1932 to 1956. His films' juxtaposing of imported and local elements envisages a modern, urban Australia; their spectacles and local glamour present optimistic views of interwar and mid-century Australia.

After starting his career as a cadet reporter, Hall became a publicist in 1917 for Union Theatres/Australasian Films and eventually progressed to the position of national publicity director. In 1924, he moved to publicity for the local branch of American company First National Pictures, for which he was also asked to direct a partial remake of a German film for local release; the result is *The Exploits of the Emden* (1928). Hall returned to Union Theatres/Australasian Films, becoming the assistant to managing director Stuart Doyle in 1931. It was Hall who drew Doyle's attention to Arthur Smith's locally invented sound-on-film recording system, a less expensive alternative to American sound equipment. Smith's system was put to use when Doyle decided to commence producing talking films as a solution to the company's near bankruptcy. Hall was asked to direct *On Our Selection* (1932), an adaptation of the successful stage show, and to create the newsreel *Cinesound Review* (which ran from 1931–70), from which the Cinesound studio derived its name in 1932. When approached by Twentieth Century Fox to produce its rival local newsreel, *Fox Movietone News* (1929-70), Hall opted to remain with Cinesound and became the company's only film director.

Although not in financial control of the studio, Hall exerted more direct influence over its productions than did any other individual. He was involved in the production schedule, scriptwriting, filming, publicity and releases. He directed all but one of Cinesound's feature films and was a spokesperson for the company's commitment to 'continuous production', a Hollywood-inspired model that aimed to provide steady employment to local personnel. The one Cinesound feature film that he did not direct, William Freshman's *Ants in His Pants* (aka *Come Up Smiling* [1939]), was conceived, produced and supervised by Hall. After the studio stopped making feature films in 1940 because of the Second World War, Ken G Hall directed only one more feature, *Smithy* (1946), for American company Columbia Pictures.

Hall's work for Cinesound after 1940 centred on newsreels. He produced and edited the first Australian film to win an Academy Award, a Cinesound newsreel entitled *Kokoda Front Line!* (1942), which features the work of cameraman Damien Parer. The film shared the 1942 Oscar for Best Documentary. Representing a crucial phase of Australia's involvement in the war, *Kokoda Front Line!* exemplifies the challenges of wartime reporting in a context in which heavy censorship prevailed, as Neil McDonald's history of the production reveals (McDonald 2002). Hall left Cinesound in 1956 to become general manager for television station TCN-9, from which he retired in 1966.

In subsequent years, Hall continued to be an observer of Australian film-making. However, his showman's ethos created tension with a new generation who shaped the revival of the local film industry in the 1970s. Whereas Hall retained admiration for Hollywood, many of the new Australian film-makers drew inspiration from European cinema. Hall's 1977 autobiography took a pessimistic view of the industry's revival as another short-lived peak that reflected a failure to learn from earlier film-makers. In turn, he was criticized by such figures as Albie Thoms, who accused Hall of promoting monopoly capitalism, failing to lobby for local film-makers and refusing to consider alternatives to Hollywood's mass-market orientation. While Hall's disagreements with contemporary commentators came close to overshadowing his work, television revivals of Cinesound films in 1971 attracted considerable public interest.

Hall's modelling of himself on major Hollywood producers obscured the fact that Cinesound's operation was on a scale more akin to companies at the periphery of the American studio system. One of few similarities with Hollywood's major studios was that Cinesound was part of a vertically integrated organization; its films were guaranteed release through Greater Union. The fact that the only American actors Cinesound could attract, however, were struggling or second-tier players, such as Helen Twelvetrees and Lloyd Hughes, is redolent of American independent production companies. Although Cinesound's films were among the most prestigious Australian productions and were often supported in their local releases by American 'B' films, Hall's features display affinities with Randall Clark's definition of 'B' films as having low budgets, a market orientation and genres that mirror more expensively made films (Clark 1995: 32–34). Viewed today, when low-budget movies are camp, often highly valued by film buffs and can attract cult audiences, Hall's work may be appreciated for presenting Australian variations on Hollywood genres and styles.

Hall's feature films reflect a context in which learning from Hollywood had become necessary for film industries to compete, even for local audiences. These films embrace Hollywood cinema as a 'global vernacular', a set of conventions through which local experiences of modernity could be expressed (Hansen 1999: 68). For instance, Hall's films emulate American genres, spectacles and techniques. Most of his films are situated within international genres, such as melodrama (*The Silence of Dean Maitland* [1934], *The Broken Melody* [1938], *The Squatter's Daughter* [1933], *Tall Timbers* [1937], *Lovers and Luggers* [1937]); comedian comedy (*Strike Me Lucky* [1934], *Let George Do It* [1938], *Gone to the Dogs* [1939], *Ants in His Pants*); comedy of manners (*It Isn't Done* [1937]); animal stories (*Orphan of the Wilderness* [1936]); and the biopic (*Smithy*). Whereas Richard Fotheringham notes that some of the films derive plots from Hollywood (Fotheringham 1995: 178–79), Hall combined these elements with Australian subject matter, settings and characters.

Cinesound's embrace of the distinctively Australian has its most sustained expression in the series of Dad and Dave films that star Bert Bailey as Dad Rudd. Having originally viewed as old-fashioned Doyle's decision to adapt *On Our Selection* to the screen, Hall responded to the film's record success by producing three more films that display progressively more tenuous links to Steele Rudd's work. The films in this series – *On Our Selection*, *Grandad Rudd* (1935), *Dad and Dave Come to Town* (1938) and *Dad Rudd, M. P.* (1940) – are central to the subgenre of back-blocks comedy, an Australian variety of rural comedy. Ironically, the Dad and Dave films highlight, more than most Cinesound films, the demise of the bush legend and the emergence of a modern Australia. As the series progresses, it increasingly emphasizes the stereotypical aspects of Dad and Dave by juxtaposing these characters with the artifice of modern life. The films derive humour from their encounters with such entities as clothing mannequins and a modern bathroom (in *Dad and Dave Come to Town*) and a gas stove (in *Dad Rudd, M. P.*). The Dad and Dave series exemplifies Hall's paradoxical embrace of international styles and local subject matter by updating the Rudds for contemporary audiences and responding to the influences of modern capitalism and radio, particularly the serial *Dad and Dave from Snake Gully* (1937–53) (Fotheringham 1995: 177–78).

More conspicuously than those of his local contemporaries, Hall's films feature spectacles that centre on large settings, stunts, elaborate performance numbers and technological gimmickry. Deb Verhoeven observes that the Australian rural setting of *The Squatter's Daughter* provides motivation for patriotic spectacles involving sheep (Verhoeven 2006: 62), a theme that has a musical echo in *Ants in His Pants*. Spectacle is emphasized in climactic outdoor action sequences in *The Squatter's Daughter*, *Tall Timbers*, *Lovers and Luggers* and *Let George Do It*. From *Strike Me Lucky* onwards, when Hall worked more independently of Stuart Doyle, his films often feature displays of Hollywood-style glamour in local settings. Examples are the musical numbers in *Strike Me Lucky*, *The Broken Melody* and *Gone to the Dogs* and the costumes designed by Mavis Ripper for *Thoroughbred* (1936), *It Isn't Done*, *Lovers and Luggers*, *Dad and Dave Come to Town* and *Smithy*. The artifice of technological spectacle is evident in the use of rear projection in Hall's films from *Thoroughbred* onwards, a technique that he adopted after a visit to Hollywood.

Hall's direction reflects a flair for comedy, a genre that encompasses the majority of his films. This strength emerged from his collaboration with Bert Bailey, whom Hall credited as a major influence on his films. Hall's experience with comedy was furthered by the challenge of working alone in directing *Strike Me Lucky*, a highly-anticipated and ambitious vehicle for the vaudeville comedian Roy Rene that was ultimately a relative financial failure. After going on to work with Bailey again on *Grandad Rudd*, Hall's subsequent films display increasing confidence with a range of comedic material, from slapstick in the George Wallace vehicles to double entendres in *Dad and Dave Come to Town* and comedy of manners in *It Isn't Done*. Comedic moments also punctuate Cinesound films of other genres, including *The Squatter's Daughter*, *The Silence of Dean Maitland*, *Thoroughbred*, *Tall Timbers* and *Lovers and Luggers*. Hall's work as a comedy director is central to Cinesound's prolificacy during the 1930s, a decade in which Australian feature film production was in numerical decline. Cinesound was the only local studio in operation at the end of the decade.

A capacity to invoke buoyant optimism at moments of potential gloom is also evident in Hall's films. When Sir Charles Kingsford Smith (Ron Randell) faces death in *Smithy*, for example, the final shot effects a transition from a sense of foreboding to symbolic continuity. Darkness gives way to a dreamlike, cloud-filled sky into which Smithy's plane is shown to be followed by later generations of aviators. In *The Silence of Dean Maitland*, the embodiment of hope in a blind boy (Bill Kerr) at the moment of his father's death reflects Hall's ability to balance melodrama with a gentle tone. Even when humour is the prevailing mode in Hall's films, it can serve to enhance serious concerns. For example, *Mr Chedworth Steps Out* (1939) centres on a timid man (Cecil Kellaway) who loses his job and embarks on a series of risky financial ventures in an effort to fulfil his wife's upwardly mobile social aspirations. While the film's array of plotlines is designed to entertain, it also explores concerns associated with modern, Australian life, including the stifling effects of middle-class identity, suburban conformity and financial struggle.

Ken G Hall's feature films encapsulate the optimism of interwar Australian popular culture. They bring together lingering attachments to the bush and

Britain with a forward-looking embrace of American capitalism and Hollywood styles. *Cinesound Review* extends this optimism by offering confident and unified responses to news events. Viewed in a larger context, Hall's films contribute to the development of Australia's increasingly international view of itself after the Second World War.

Lesley Speed

References

Clark, Randall (1995) *At a Theater or Drive-in Near You: The History, Culture, and Politics of the American Exploitation Film*, New York and London: Garland.

Fotheringham, Richard (1995) *In Search of Steele Rudd: Author of the classic Dad and Dave stories*, St Lucia: University of Queensland Press.

Hansen, Miriam Bratu (1999) 'The Mass Production of the Senses: Classical Cinema as Vernacular Modernism', *Modernism/Modernity*, 6: 2, pp. 59–77.

McDonald, Neil (2002) 'Getting It Right – Damien Parer, Osmar White and Chester Wilmot on The Kokoda Track', *Sydney Papers*, 14: 2, pp. 96–1109.

Verhoeven, Deb (2006) *Sheep and the Australian Cinema*, Carlton: Melbourne University Press.

BRIAN TRENCHARD-SMITH (b. 1946)

Brian Trenchard-Smith is one of Australia's most prolific directors; with 42 films and television series as well as a series of advertisements, trailers and 'making of' documentaries under his belt. Born in England in 1946, but with an Australian father, Trenchard-Smith started making films as a teenager, drawing inspiration from works such as Alfred Hitchcock's *Vertigo* (1958). According to Trenchard-Smith, his initial attempts to enter the British film industry were 'thwarted' by the 'closed shop' policy of the Association of Cinematograph, Television and Allied Technicians (the dominant union for film and television technicians at the time) so he migrated to Australia in 1965 in the hope of pursuing his ambitions as a film-maker (Mitchell 2010). Most of Trenchard-Smith's better-known films were produced in the 1970s and 1980s, including *The Man from Hong Kong* (1975), *Deathcheaters* (1976), *Stunt Rock* (1980), *Turkey Shoot* (1982), *BMX Bandits* (1983) – in which Nicole Kidman made her screen debut – and *Dead End Drive-In* (1986).

Rather than locating himself and his work within the Australian national cinema paradigm, Trenchard-Smith has aligned himself firmly to transnational forms of film-making that unashamedly revolve around strongly commercial and generic traditions, notably that of the action film. As the director himself explains in Mark Hartley's film *Not Quite Hollywood* (2008), 'it became clear to me that action was the universal currency of the movie market […] and transcended all language barriers.' In 2003, Quentin Tarantino, a long-time admirer of Trenchard-Smith's work, dedicated *Kill Bill Volume 1* (2003) to the director at its Australian premiere during the Sydney International Film Festival. Five years later, Trenchard-Smith's often schlocky, sensational techniques guaranteed him a place in the documentary *Not Quite Hollywood*, which reframed Australian genre cinema under the umbrella

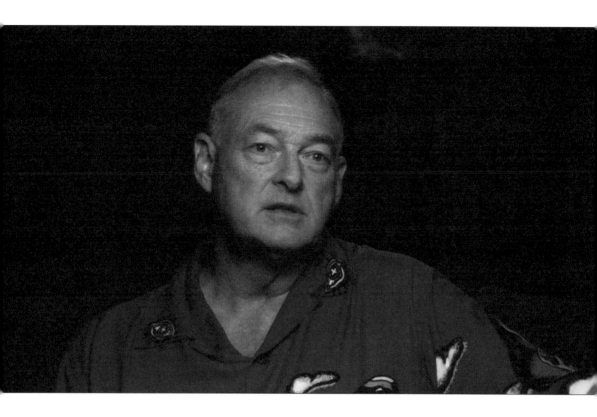

Brian Trenchard-Smith. A still from the motion
picture *Not Quite Hollywood: The Wild, Untold
Story of Ozploitation!* (Mark Hartley, 2008)

of 'Ozploitation'. In many respects much of Trenchard-Smith's work is perhaps
best considered and evaluated within this context, as, unlike a number of other
Australian directors of genre cinema whose work has been celebrated under this
banner (such as Richard Franklin), much of Trenchard-Smith's work displays the
necessary sensationalism of higher end exploitation cinema (Thomas 2009: 90–95).

The Man from Hong Kong (MFHK) launched Trenchard-Smith's career, and
is his most successful film to date. Made on the relatively generous budget
of AU$900,000, the film was part funded by the Australian Film Development
Corporation (the predecessor of the Australian Film Commission) and was one of
Australia's first unofficial co-productions with an Asian film company (Becchio 2006:
175). MFHK situated itself in a global market cycle at the time in kung fu movies,
most famously exemplified by those of the master himself, Bruce Lee. (Golden
Harvest, the Hong Kong co-producer of MFHK, had also been responsible for the
successful Bruce Lee vehicle, Enter the Dragon [Robert Clouse, 1973].) However,
as Trenchard-Smith himself notes in the DVD commentary, MFHK also configures
itself as a kind of 'James Bond-like spoof' crammed with the director's signature
visual and verbal gags.

MFHK's plot revolves around Inspector Fang (played by Asia's 'Steve McQueen',
successful Hong Kong star, Jimmi Wang Yu) from the Hong Kong Special Branch,

who is sent on a mission to Australia to help extradite drug smuggler, Win Chan (Sammo Hung). However, Fang is really intent on pursuing the head of the dope ring, Jack Wilton (George Lazenby), which leads him into a series of misadventures in which he has the opportunity to floor a host of opponents by his mastery over kung fu, winning the hearts of several local girls along the way. The film was developed in an environment in which 'the message was that Australian films, regardless of their fiscal success internationally, could create an awareness of Australia in Europe and America that would, if maintained, benefit tourism and encourage export opportunities' (Becchio 2006: 174). This may explain the series of helicopter shots showcasing Australian national landmarks such as Uluru (then known as Ayers Rock) and various Sydney locations such as the harbour and Opera House. *MFHK* also trades in the 'laughs and gasps' style cultivated by Trenchard-Smith. The action sequences include the director's signature trademarks, such as sensational stunts (most performed by Australian extreme stuntman Grant Page), lengthy and intricate car chases, hyperbolic smash-ups, real-life fire stunts, and 'corny dialogue and visual jokes' (Goldsmith 2010: 246).

The film also treads a sometimes uneasy path between multicultural acceptance and politically incorrect racism largely intended, the director later claimed, as a satirical gesture to mock Australian stereotypes (Becchio 2006: 174). The local cops, Grosse and Taylor, act as comic foils for the Asian hero. The film comes down firmly on Fang's side as he almost singlehandedly defeats the villainous Wilton, while seducing and satisfying the opposite sex in a series of 'groundbreaking' interracial love scenes with white women (Goldsmith 2010: 247).

Turkey Shoot, a marriage of producer, Anthony Ginnane and Brian Trenchard-Smith, was beset by budget cuts which ensured the film transitioned from its original more serious Orwellian premise to an exploitation 'high-camp splatter movie' (Verhoeven 2010: 74), in spite of the presence of its relatively high profile international stars Steve Railsback and Olivia Hussey. Set in a totalitarian future of prison camps designed to 're-educate' people deemed social deviants, three inmates make a deal with Thatcher, the camp head. In exchange for their freedom, they will participate in a 'Turkey Shoot' where they are hunted as unarmed human prey.

An examination of the critical reception of the film at the time of its release in 1983 to its more recent revival as 'Ozploitation' reveals the way in which *Turkey Shoot* exemplifies latter-day transitions in Australian cinema that revolve around discourses of cultural value, pleasure and cult entertainment. Condemned for the way it 'relies almost completely on mutilation, torture and killing' (Mayer 1983: 71), with noted critic Phillip Adams reputedly claiming that it was the worst film he had ever seen (Mayer 1983: 69), *Turkey Shoot* has over the passage of time been celebrated by 'bad film' aficionados, who revel in its hyper-aware camp excess, gory mutilations, grotesque characters, cheesy dialogue and gratuitous attempts at sexual innuendo and titillation.

Like *Turkey Shoot*, *Dead End Drive-In* is set in a dystopian near future. On the face of it, the film appears as a somewhat uneven, 'B' grade *Mad Max* (George Miller, 1979) exploiting over-the-top punk styling and extreme vehicular stunts, including a then-world-record truck jump of 160 feet by stuntman, Guy Norris. However, it is actually a relatively faithful adaptation, bar the ending, of the short story, *Crabs* (1974), by Australian literary luminary Peter Carey. *Dead End Drive-In* tells the story of a young tow-truck driver Crabs, and his girlfriend Carmen, who unwittingly become interned in a drive-in, which the government has converted into a detention camp for unemployed young adults. Towards the end of the film, Crabs seizes an opportunity to escape when a busload of Asian migrant detainees also arrive, resulting in violent opposition from the young people intent on jealously guarding their prison terrain. Intended as a critique of the xenophobia which accompanied the wave of immigration by Vietnamese 'boat' people around the time the film was made, this somewhat clunky storyline also provides a discomforting 'phobic narrative' in the latter-day context of ongoing debates in Australia about border protection, asylum seekers and migrant detention facilities (Johinke 2009: 309).

Twenty-five years later, Trenchard-Smith, now based in Los Angeles, is still making and releasing films. He has no pretentions about his work; as he reveals in *Not Quite Hollywood*, 'I could be oddball but I could also be glossy. Sometimes in the land of low budget it is hard to be both.' However, his ongoing enthusiasm for the film industry and his playful comprehension of the generic requirements of the action film, and its ability to generate entertainment for global audiences, is indisputable.

Deborah J Thomas

References

Becchio, Penny (2006) 'Interview with Brian Trenchard-Smith', *Metro*, 149, pp. 174–77.

Goldsmith, Ben (2010) 'The Man from Hong Kong', in Ben Goldsmith and Geoff Lealand (eds), *Directory of World Cinema: Australia and New Zealand*, Bristol and Chicago: Intellect.

Johinke, Rebecca (2009) 'Not Quite Mad Max: Brian Trenchard-Smith's Dead End Drive-In', *Studies in Australasian Cinema*, 3: 3, pp. 309–18.

Mayer, Geoff (1983) 'Turkey Shoot', *Cinema Papers*, 42, pp. 69–71.

Mitchell, Robert (2010) 'My Interview with Brian Trenchard-Smith', http://soldierofcinema.blogspot.com.au/2010/12/my-interview-with-brian-trenchard-smith.html. Accessed 17 October 2012.

Thomas, Deborah (2009) 'Tarantino's Two-Thumbs up: Ozploitation and the Reframing of the Aussie Genre Film', *Metro*, 161, pp. 90–95.

Verhoeven, Deb (2010) 'It was an experience that totally blew up in my face: Steve Railsback and Turkey Shoot', *Studies in Australasian Cinema*, 4: 1, pp. 73–79.

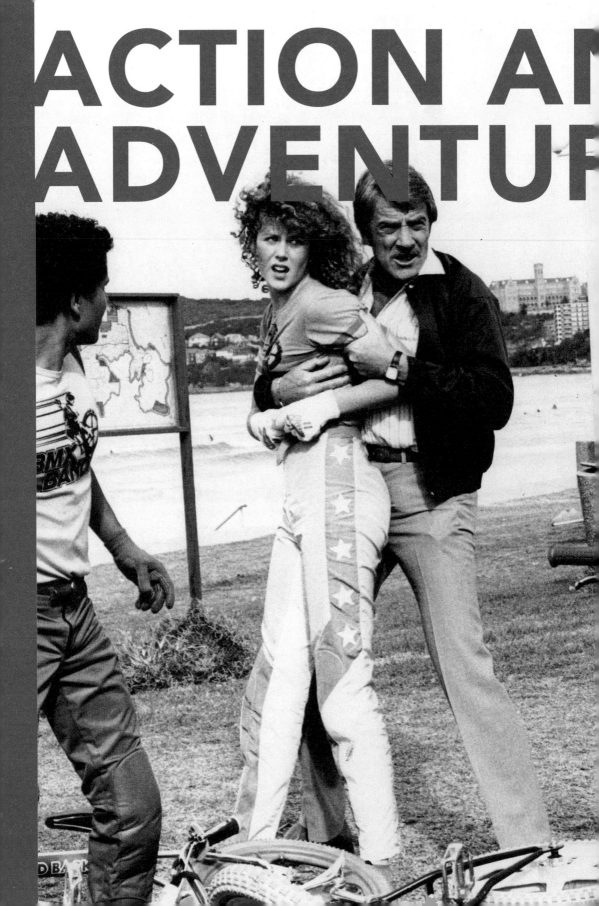

ACTION AN
ADVENTUR

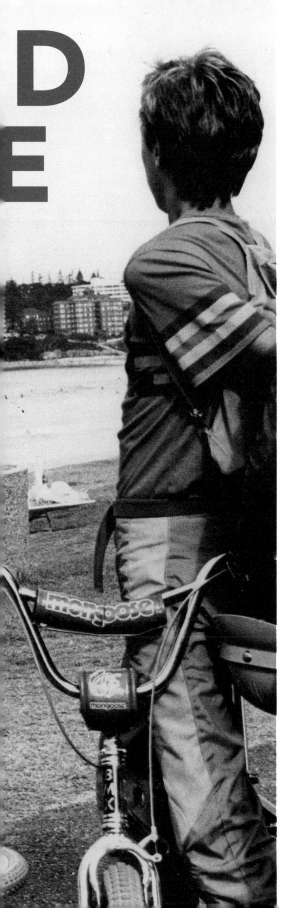

D
E

BMX Bandits (Brian
Trenchard-Smith, 1983).
© Kobal Collection

Action is the very essence of cinema. As the
director's universal instruction that initiates
filming, and as the 'motion' in motion pictures,
action literally both precedes and defines film.
Adventure, action's constant companion, is
the beating heart of narrative film. The 'action-
adventure film', however, is a loose category
in contemporary cinema. Together, action and
adventure exceed genre; as Yvonne Tasker
reminds us, 'the terms "action" and "adventure"
never referred to secure generic objects' (Tasker
2004: 3). Action sequences and dramatic quests
can be located at all points on the cinematic
spectrum, while action and adventure films
adopt settings and scenarios from a wide array
of (sub)genres. It is this hybridity, or fluidity,
that has in part contributed to the questions
of whether action and adventure constitute a
genre at all, and what the codes, conventions
and characteristics of action and adventure films
might be.

From the very earliest days, film's capacity to
capture motion, movement, people and things
in action set it apart from photography and
painting. The recording of action and activity
were cinema's principal attractions for its first
audiences. The earliest films – the *actualités* –
depicted ordinary people doing ordinary
things: workers leaving a factory (*La Sortie des
Usines Lumière à Lyon* [Louis Lumière, 1895]),

travellers disembarking a boat (*Passengers Alighting from the Ferry 'Brighton'* *at Manly* [Marius Sestier, 1896]). While the 'action film' may have since taken on so much baggage as to render it virtually unrecognizable from these early documents, there are other more resilient links back to this early period. The spectacular visual and physical special effects that we now associate with the form have their origins in the alternative tradition of the trick film most closely associated with Georges Méliès (for example, *Le Voyage dans la Lune/Voyage* *to the Moon* [1902] and *Voyage à Travers L'impossible/The Impossible Voyage* [1904]). These films brought action and adventure together with spectacle and storytelling, and this combination would define the earliest feature-length narrative films.

In recent times, what Larry Gross (2000 [1995]: 3) has called 'the Big Loud Action Movie' with an emphasis on stunts, spectacle and visceral thrills over narrative development, has come to define contemporary Hollywood, at least in its blockbuster form. The popularity of these films among audiences has typically not generally been shared by many critics, for whom these films have 'failed to meet the markers of aesthetic and cultural value typically applied within contemporary film culture' (Tasker 2004: 2). It should be noted, however, that these 'markers of aesthetic and cultural value' have typically been laid down by the selfsame film critics who deride action films and their large and appreciative audiences.

Summarizing a survey of action and adventure films produced in the first decade of the new Australian cinema, Susan Dermody attempts to identify some of the features of the action-adventure film both as a general form, and in its particular Australian guise. She notes the 'articulation of ideals through plots based on adventure into difficult or unknown terrain, with action sequences as the crux of the adventure, putting to test the ideals and the hero' (Dermody 1980: 79). Dermody locates the action-adventure film in the 'quest-romance' tradition, in which 'the quest is fulfilled through a series of physical challenges in unfamiliar territory, and the governing motivation of the hero is idealist rather than comic, tragic, or satiric and pessimistic' (79). And importantly Dermody argues that in Australian action-adventure films, 'the natural (as opposed to the man-made) landscape is an important repository of traditional, even conservative, values, while the city is seen as a sterile wasteland in which those values wither' (79). This raises the long-standing dichotomy in Australian cultural representation between the city and the bush, in which from the late nineteenth century onwards the bush was positioned as the repository of 'authentic' or 'distinctive' Australian values and way of life, while the city was negatively associated with imported cultures and characteristics. The dichotomy was given new life in Australian cinema in the 1970s, since cultural nationalism in general, and its late nineteenth century expressions in novels, poetry and short stories in particular, were important touchstones for film-makers. Importantly, this cinematic nostalgia was laced with guilt over the colonial legacy and the treatment of Aboriginal people. These factors distinguish Australian action-adventure films of this period (and indeed, Australian cinema as a whole) from American and international counterparts, and complicate at least one of Tasker's (admittedly broadbrush) generic groupings of the contemporary action film, 'crime and urban action' (Tasker 2004: 4). (Tasker's other groupings are 'fantasy, e.g. science fiction or horror; and war or military movies' [4]).

While action and adventure films do not define Australian cinema in quite the same way as they define contemporary Hollywood cinema, many examples can be identified, dating back to the very early days of film-making in this country. Charles Tait's *The Story of the Kelly Gang* (1906) presented what were described at the time as 'sensation scenes' depicting events leading up to the last stand of the notorious Kelly gang in country Victoria in 1880. Tait's film is the most celebrated of the bushranging cycle of films made before 1912, when screenings were banned in New South Wales and Victoria. These films typically featured elements recognizable in contemporary action films including chases, fights and occasionally rudimentary special effects. They also showcased the prowess of early stunt performers, as Pike and Cooper note: 'Bushrangers [i.e. bushranging films] usually included at least one daring leap in their adventures, whether alone or on horseback, from a cliff into the ocean or from a bridge into a flooded river' (Pike and Cooper 1998 [1980]: 2).

Expert horsemanship and stunt work were characteristics that propelled the film career of multi-talented sportsman and Olympic medallist, Reginald 'Snowy' Baker, who made action and adventure films both in Australia and in Hollywood. Snowy Baker was the first in a long line of Australian actors known for their work in local and international action-adventure films. Others include Errol Flynn (*Captain Blood* [Michael Curtiz, 1935]; *The Sea Hawk* [Michael Curtiz, 1940], see Adrian Danks essay in this volume); Chips Rafferty (*Forty Thousand Horsemen* [Charles Chauvel, 1940]; *Walk into Paradise* [Lee Robinson, 1957]; *Mutiny on the Bounty* [Lewis Milestone, 1962]); Rod Taylor (*King of the Coral Sea* [Lee Robinson, 1954]; *Dark of the Sun* aka *The Mercenaries* [Jack Cardiff, 1968]); Mel Gibson (the Mad Max trilogy [George Miller, 1979, 1981, 1985]); Russell Crowe (*Proof of Life* [Taylor Hackford, 2000]; *Body of Lies* [Ridley Scott, 2008]); and Hugh Jackman (*Swordfish* [Dominic Sena, 2001]; *Real Steel* [Shawn Levy, 2011]).

The prominence of these international Australian stars points up one of the criticisms that has often been levelled at action-adventure films in general: 'the "hero" of the action-adventure is usually literally that, and not a heroine' (Dermody 1980: 81). This is largely true of the 1970s Australian action-adventure films that Susan Dermody was writing about, and to some extent it remains true of Australian action films. It has not always been the case, however, and it is certainly not true of Australian cinema before the 1950s, or of many children's adventure films made in Australia in recent years.

Prior to the Second World War, a number of Australian action-adventure films depicted active (rather than reactive and passive) female characters either at the centre of action sequences, or forced to deal with physical challenges. The figure of the 'independent leading woman' (Routt 1989: 31) featured particularly prominently in films set in the outback, in the common character of 'the bush woman' (see Tulloch 1981; Routt 1989), the 'squatter's daughter' or 'the girl of the bush' (Pike and Cooper 1998 [1980]: 2). Examples include the characters played by Olive Wilton in Bert Bailey's 1910 version of *The Squatter's Daughter*, Lottie Lyell in Raymond Longford's *'Neath Austral Skies* (1913), Brownie Vernon in *Silks and Saddles* (John K Wells, 1921), Jocelyn Howarth in Ken G Hall's 1933 version of *The Squatter's Daughter* and Daphne Campbell in *The Overlanders* (Harry Watt, 1946). Mention must also be made of *Jewelled Nights* (Louise Lovely and Wilton Welch, 1925), about a young Australian woman who jilts a man she does not love at the altar and, dressed as a man, goes prospecting in Tasmania. *Jewelled Nights* was Louise Lovely's last film; she made several films in Australia as Louise Carbasse before venturing to Hollywood where Carl Laemmle renamed her and where she spent the best part of a largely unsatisfying decade.

Among the small but growing band of children's films made in Australia are many which feature stories oriented around the exploits or adventures of girls or young women. Yoram Gross has made many animated feature films for children, but is perhaps best known for the series of films about the adventures of a girl named Dot, beginning with *Dot and the Kangaroo* (1977) (see Caputo 1995 and Chris Carter's essay on animated films in this volume). Brian Trenchard-Smith's teen action film *BMX Bandits* (1983) features Nicole Kidman in her first major role, though her character is largely a witness to, rather than an agent of, action. In the same year, another popular Australian actress, Claudia Karvan starred in her first feature film, *Molly* (Ned Lander, 1983), the story of the adventures of a young girl and a singing dog. In Donald Crombie's time travel adventure yarn *Playing Beattie Bow* (1986), 17-year-old Abigail (Imogen Annesley) is transported back to nineteenth-century Sydney where she is kidnapped and narrowly avoids being sold into prostitution, before rescuing a young invalid from a fire. Mario Andreacchio's *The Dragon Pearl* (2010) about an Australian boy and a Chinese girl's adventures after the discovery of a golden dragon, is also noteworthy as the first film produced under the official Australia-China coproduction agreement. A band of teenage guerrillas led by Ellie (Caitlin Stasey) fight against an invading army in the first film based on John Marsden's series of books (1993-99), *Tomorrow, When the War Began* (Stuart Beattie, 2010). In *Nim's Island* (Jennifer Flackett and Mark Levin, 2008), a young girl enlists an agoraphobic author of children's adventure novels to help find her missing father. The sequel, *Return to Nim's Island* (Brendan Maher, 2013) stars Bindi Irwin as the title character who tries to protect her island home from property developers. Bindi is the daughter of one of Australia's best loved, and sorely missed, adventurers: the Crocodile Hunter, Steve Irwin.

In addition to these children's films, Australia has hosted the production (and postproduction) of a number of 'big, loud' action and adventure films in recent years, many of which have been attracted by the range of financial and other incentives on offer from federal and state governments. Major international action and adventure films shot in Australia include *Killer Elite* (Gary McKendry, 2011), *Ghost Rider* (Mark Steven Johnson, 2007) and *Knowing* directed by Australian Alex Proyas (2009), all of which were shot in and around Melbourne; *Stealth* (Rob Cohen, 2005) and *The Wolverine* (James Mangold, 2013), which were shot in or around Sydney; and *Nim's Island*, *Return to Nim's Island* and *The Chronicles of Narnia: Voyage of the Dawn Treader* (Michael Apted, 2010), which were shot on the Gold Coast, Queensland. In addition, a growing number of international action and adventure films that were shot in other countries have employed Australian visual effects and postproduction companies. Examples include *300* (Zack Snyder, 2006), for which the Sydney-based firm Animal Logic produced several hundred VFX shots, and for which the firm's Grant Freckleton was credited as Visual Effects Art Director, and *Journey 2: The Mysterious Island* (Brad Peyton, 2012), for which Adelaide-based firm Rising Sun Pictures produced VFX for a chase scene through a tropical forest.

Ben Goldsmith

References

Caputo, Raffaele (1995) 'The Animated Features of Yoram Gross', in Scott Murray (ed.), *Australian Film 1978–1994*, Melbourne: Oxford University Press, pp. 398–400.

Dermody, Susan (1980) 'Action and Adventure', in Scott Murray (ed.), *The New Australian Cinema*, West Melbourne: Thomas Nelson Australia, pp. 79–95.

Gross, Larry (2000 [1995]) 'Big and Loud', in José Arroyo (ed.), *Action/Spectacle Cinema*, London: BFI, pp. 3–9.

Pike, Andrew and Cooper, Ross (1998 [1980]) *Australian Film, 1900–1977: A Guide to Feature Film Production*, Melbourne: Oxford University Press.

Routt, William D (1989) 'The Fairest Child of the Motherland: Colonialism and Family in Australian Films of the 1920s and 1930s', in Albert Moran and Tom O'Regan (eds), *The Australian Screen*, Ringwood: Penguin, pp. 28–52.

Tasker, Yvonne (2004) 'Introduction: Action and Adventure Cinema', in Yvonne Tasker (ed.), *Action and Adventure Cinema*, London and New York: Routledge, pp. 1–13.

Tulloch, John (1981) *Legends on the Screen: The Australian Narrative Cinema 1919–1929*, Sydney: Currency Press, Australian Film Institute.

BMX Bandits

Country of Origin:

Australia

Studio/Distributor:

Nilsen Premiere

Director:

Brian Trenchard-Smith

Producers:

Paul Davies
Tom Broadbridge

Screenwriters:

Patrick Edgeworth
Russell Hagg

Cinematographer:

John Seale

Production Designer:

Ross Major

Composer:

Colin Stead
Frank Strangio

Editor:

Alan Lake

Duration:

87 minutes

Genres:

Children's
Action

Cast:

Nicole Kidman
David Argue
John Ley
Angelo D'Angelo
James Lugton
Bryan Marshall

Format:

35 mm

Year:

1983

Synopsis

A gang of masked men rob a Sydney bank. Their getaway car narrowly misses two BMXers, Goose and PJ, forcing the BMXers to ride through a shopping mall, where they crash in to a line of supermarket trolleys being collected by Judy. Despite her protestations that she needs the job to save up and buy a BMX bike, Judy's boss fires her. Meanwhile, the gang meet at a warehouse to divide their haul. The Boss tells them about another job in two days time for which they will need specially adapted walkie-talkies. Goose, PJ and Judy find the walkie-talkies before two members of the gang, Whitey and Moustache, arrive to collect them. The kids test the walkie-talkies before selling most of them, without realizing that they are tuned to frequencies used by the police. Goose, PJ and Judy are chased through a cemetery by Whitey and Moustache, but manage to escape. The next day, Goose, Judy and PJ use the earnings from sales of the walkie-talkies to buy new BMX bikes. Judy is cornered by Whitey and Moustache, but manages to escape. Another chase ensues; the kids on their bikes are trailed by Whitey and Moustache in a car over a sports field, through a shopping mall, into an empty warehouse, and eventually into a quarry where the car crashes. Discovering that there is a reward for catching the gang, Goose, PJ and Judy hatch a plan involving all the local BMXers, before the final showdown with the gang.

Critique

Hoping to capitalize on a craze of the early 1980s, producer Tom Broadbridge suggested revising writer Russell Hagg's original screenplay about the adventures of a trio of young children on bicycles. The youngsters became teenagers, and the nondescript bikes became BMXs – extremely popular off-road racing bicycles that could also be used for stunts and trick riding. In the process, *BMX Bandits* became – according to the film's own publicity – the first 'BMX film'. Although a BMX had appeared on-screen the previous year in Steven Spielberg's *E.T. The Extra-Terrestrial* (1982), that film did not feature the extended stunt sequences that could be said to define this niche subgenre. Aside from the BMX documentary film culture that continues to thrive on DVD and online, there have been very few other features. Examples include two American features, *Rad* (Hal Needham, 1986), and *Heroes of Dirt* (Eric Bugbee, 2013), and the 1987 New Zealand television series *Steel Riders* that was released as a film in the United States under the title *Young Detectives on Wheels* (Wayne Tourell, 1987).

    BMX Bandits is perhaps better known for its other claim to primacy, as Nicole Kidman's first film. It shares this accolade with Henri Safran's *Bush Christmas* (1983); both films were released in Australia on the same day, just before Christmas 1983. Both *BMX Bandits*'s director, Brian Trenchard-Smith and Australian critic David Stratton (a reviewer for *Variety*), forecast the star potential of the then-16-year-old schoolgirl.

    Broadbridge and his producing partner Paul Davies approached Trenchard-Smith to direct *BMX Bandits* on the strength of the action scenes in his previous film, the critically reviled *Turkey Shoot* (1982;

released as *Escape 2000* in the United States, and *Blood Camp Thatcher* in the United Kingdom). Trenchard-Smith convinced the producers to relocate the film from its original setting in the Melbourne bayside suburb of Williamstown to Manly and the northern beaches of Sydney. The director made use of many of the same locations that had featured in his earlier film *Deathcheaters* (1976), including the Warringah Mall, which hosted another destructive chase sequence. Both *BMX Bandits* and *Deathcheaters* are also notable for the tendency for key scenes to be shot against spectacular backdrops of Sydney harbour and the city's northern beachside suburbs.

One reviewer described the film on release as '*Mad Max* on pushbikes'. While this is clearly hyperbole given the differences in storylines, settings and address between the two films, *BMX Bandits* does share a number of connections to George Miller's seminal action film. Both are packed with inventive and novel stunts, many of which are shot with cameras mounted on speeding bikes or cars. Actor John Ley who plays Moustache in *BMX Bandits* had a small role in *Mad Max* (George Miller, 1979), while *Bandits* producer Tom Broadbridge was both a production assistant and an extra on Miller's film. Chris Murray, special effects co-supervisor on *Bandits* and now one of Australia's most experienced physical special effects practitioners, made his feature debut as SFX supervisor on *Mad Max*. And yet despite these points of connection, the action film comparison with *Mad Max* is somewhat unfair on *Bandits*'s director Brian Trenchard-Smith who already had a well-established reputation as director of stunt-filled action movies through his work on films like *The Man from Hong Kong* (1975) and *Deathcheaters*.

Alongside its action credentials, *BMX Bandits* also works as a children's film. The three main teenage characters not only outsmart the bad guys, they also manage to stay one step ahead of the police and ultimately claim the reward for the gang's capture, which they use to benefit all the local BMXers. Despite the gunplay in the opening bank-robbery scene, the kids are never in any serious danger; Whitey and Moustache are slapstick villains who pose more threat to each other than to Goose, PJ and Judy, while the unwitting hotline to the police ultimately assures their safety.

BMX Bandits was released on 50 screens around Australia on 22 December 1983. The many inventive local promotions included a parade of 370 young BMXers at the premiere in Hobart. The film was also successful in the United Kingdom and Japan, although it had only a limited release in the United States. *BMX Bandits* received four Australian Film Institute Awards (AFI) nominations: David Argue (Whitey) for Best Supporting Actor, Patrick Edgeworth for Best Adapted Screenplay, Alan Lake for Best Editing, and Andrew Steuart, John Patterson, Robyn Judge, Phil Judd and Gethin Craig for Best Sound. None were successful.

Ben Goldsmith

Deathcheaters

Country of Origin:

Australia

Studio/Distributor:

Nine Network

DL Taffner

Trenchard Productions

Director:

Brian Trenchard-Smith

Producer:

Brian Trenchard-Smith

Screenwriter:

Michael Cove

Director of Photography:

John Seale

Production Designer:

Darrell Lass

Editor:

Ron Williams

Duration:

93 minutes

Genre:

Action

Cast:

John Hargreaves

Grant Page

Margaret Gerard

Noel Ferrier

Judith Woodroffe

Ralph Cotterill

Format:

35 mm

Year:

1976

Synopsis

Stuntmen and Vietnam veterans Steve and Rod work together on the filming of a large-scale re-enactment of an eleventh-century battle, before moving on to a commercial for an automobile product. During the commercial shoot, they witness a police car being shot at and forced from the road. Steve and Rod give chase, following the gunmen's car through a shopping centre and eventually capturing them. A police sergeant tells them that the men have robbed a bank and locked a number of people in a vault where the air supply is rapidly running out. Rod and Steve immediately offer their services. Rod is taken at gunpoint from his home to an empty building, where Steve is already being held. They are taken to meet spymaster Culpepper who reveals that the car chase and the bank job were hoaxes designed to test Steve and Rod's suitability for a special mission. At a secret location, Culpepper shows them a clandestinely shot film of a factory complex in the Philippines, controlled by an enemy of the state named Agustin Hernandez. The Philippines government has asked the Australian secret service to help obtain secret papers from Hernandez's complex. Unwilling to take on the job themselves, the Australians have decided to hire Steve and Rod as mercenaries who can be disowned if the mission fails. After a brief period of training, Steve and Rod are taken by submarine to the Philippines, where they attempt to complete their mission.

Critique

Deathcheaters was Brian Trenchard-Smith's follow-up to his successful and influential second feature, *The Man from Hong Kong* (1975). Trenchard-Smith (here credited as Brian Trenchard Smith) deploys similar technique and style in *Deathcheaters* as in *The Man*, including a well-developed grasp of both the demands of the action genre and the value of incorporating in his feature films imagery and backdrops typically used to promote tourism. *The Man from Hong Kong*, for example, opens with a spectacular fight and chase on and around Uluru, with the opening credits that follow showcasing Hong Kong from the air as a hang-glider descends into the city. *Deathcheaters* opens with a large-scale battle involving horses, swordplay and hand-to-hand combat, followed by a car chase through Sydney's northern beaches and around the harbour, ending in the Warringah Mall. A later scene in which Steve and Rod meet Culpepper for the first time takes place at Vaucluse Bowls Club, with the Sydney Harbour Bridge framed prominently in the background.

    Deathcheaters's structure resembles that of the soft-core and sex-themed films common in the early years of the revival such as *Fantasm* (Richard Franklin, 1976) and Trenchard-Smith's own *The Love Epidemic* (1975); a flimsy plot is barely stretched across a series of action sequences and stunts that are bookended by terrible puns and comic one-liners. But it is really more of a showcase of the stuntman's art than a narrative feature, and represents a further expansion of the director's preoccupation with spectacular action and its cinematic manufacture evident in both *The Man from Hong Kong* and Trenchard-Smith's award-winning television documentary *The Stuntmen* (aka *Dare Devils* [1973]). *Deathcheaters* is built around the prowess of Australia's leading and best-known stuntman, Grant Page, who had already formed a productive partnership with the director, starring in *The Stuntmen*, playing himself in both Trenchard-Smith's television documentary *Kung Fu Killers* (1974) and the 'semi-documentary' *The Love Epidemic* (1975), and coordinating the action sequences in *The Man from Hong Kong* (Pike and Cooper 1998 [1980]: 284). By the time Page starred (as himself) in two further Trenchard-Smith productions (the feature *Stunt Rock* [1980] and the documentary *Dangerfreaks* [1989]), he had established an international reputation for his work as the stunt coordinator on *Mad Max* (George Miller, 1979).

The decision to locate the climactic mission in the Philippines is noteworthy. It prefigured the series of action films made in the Philippines in the late 1980s by Australian producer Anthony I Ginnane's company Eastern Film Management Corporation, which included the 1989 feature *The Siege of Firebase Gloria*, directed by Brian Trenchard-Smith. Ginnane had previously produced Trenchard-Smith's *Turkey Shoot* (1982), and the pair would work together again almost thirty years later on *Arctic Blast* (Brian Trenchard-Smith, 2010). The decision to frame the stuntmen's mission as a clandestine response by the Australian government to a request from Filipino President Ferdinand Marcos's regime to act against an opponent and potential revolutionary insurgent, can be read as an uncharacteristically strong political statement in itself. While Rod and Steve are just doing their jobs like good soldiers or employees, and do not concern themselves with the larger question of why the Australian secret service is contracting out intelligence work in another country, the film does indicate a preferred reading. In the scene in which Rod and Steve are briefed about the mission, the walls of the briefing room are adorned with portraits of dictators: Napoleon, Hitler, Idi Amin. The last image in the sequence is that of Australia's then-Prime Minister, Malcolm Fraser. This uncharacteristic and none-too-subtle political joke references Trenchard-Smith's strongly held views about the ousting of the Whitlam Labor government in late 1975, which occurred in the early stages of the film's production. By the time Ginnane and Trenchard-Smith went to work in the Philippines, the state of martial law that existed in that country at the time of the filming of *Deathcheaters* was long past, and the Marcos regime had finally been ousted.

Ben Goldsmith

References

Pike, Andrew and Cooper, Ross (1998 [1980]) *Australian Film, 1900–1977: A Guide to Feature Film Production*, Melbourne: Oxford University Press.

Tomorrow, When the War Began

Country of Origin:

Australia

Studio/Distributor:

Ambience Entertainment
Paramount Worldwide

Director:

Stuart Beattie

Producers:

Andrew Mason
Michael Boughen

Screenwriter:

Stuart Beattie, from the novel
Tomorrow, When the War
Began by John Marsden (1993)

Director of Photography:

Ben Nott

Production Designer:

Robert Webb

Synopsis

In a video diary, teenager Ellie recounts the story of the previous few weeks after she and six friends who all live in and around the small rural town of Wirrawee went camping over the Australia Day long weekend. Ellie, Corrie, Kevin, Homer, Fi, Lee and Robyn spend three nights at an isolated local beauty spot, Hell. On the second night, they are awoken by a large number of aeroplanes overhead. Returning home, they discover their houses are all deserted. Ellie, Corrie and Kevin make their way to the town's showgrounds, to find it being used as a holding camp for the town's population who are guarded by heavily armed soldiers. The trio are spotted and chased by soldiers through the town. They make their way back to Corrie's house, only narrowly escaping when it is destroyed by an airstrike. The group decides to make their base at Hell. On the way they stop to rest at the house of local stoner Chris who has managed to avoid being captured. Reaching Hell, they hear a radio report about the invasion by a coalition of neighbouring countries. They resolve to disrupt the invasion in whatever ways they can. In the video diary, Ellie says, 'A month ago, we were teenagers. Now we're soldiers, fighting behind enemy lines. We won't give up until the war is won.'

Critique

John Marsden's enormously popular series of teen fiction novels about a group of young Australians who become resistance fighters following a surprise invasion by an unnamed Asian country, was an obvious candidate for adaptation to the screen. With a strong

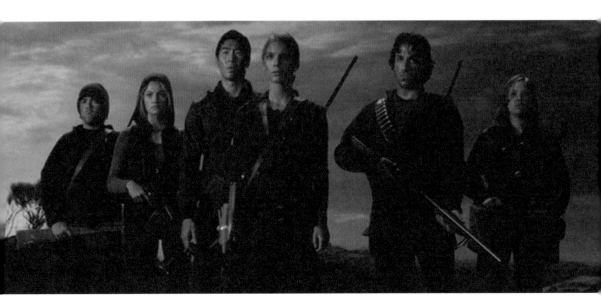

Tomorrow, When the War Began
(Stuart Beattie, 2010)

Composer:

Reinhold Heil

Johnny Klimek

Editor:

Marcus D'Arcy

Duration:

103 minutes

Genres:

Action

Adventure

Cast:

Caitlin Stasey

Rachel Hurd-Wood

Lincoln Lewis

Deniz Akdeniz

Pheobe Tonkin

Chris Pang

Ashleigh Cummings

Andy Ryan

Colin Friels

Format:

35mm

Year:

2010

narrative thread running through the seven novels, multiple action set-pieces, and a virtually guaranteed audience who had grown up with the teenage heroes, on paper the prospect of turning the books into a blockbuster film (and potentially a lucrative franchise) appeared strong. And yet, both blockbusters and action films are rare in Australian cinema, not least because of budget requirements and the consequent virtual necessity of overseas success to ensure sufficient returns. The film's estimated AU$27 million budget – enormous by Australian standards – was co-funded by the Omnilab Media group and Paramount Worldwide following development investment from Screen Australia. It earned over AU$13.5 million at the Australian box office, sold well on DVD and was the best performing Australian film of 2010 but it was less successful outside Australia. The film was released in the United States simultaneously in cinemas, Video on Demand on iTunes and on Facebook in February 2012, but did not repeat its local success. For a number of reasons including the gaoling on unrelated tax fraud charges of one of its producers (Lamont 2012), and the blossoming Hollywood career of director Stuart Beattie, the first proposed sequel has been delayed indefinitely.

Although *Tomorrow* was Beattie's first film as a director, he had already established a reputation in Australia and in Hollywood as a scriptwriter, with writing and co-writing credits including the four Pirates of the Caribbean films, *Collateral* (Michael Mann, 2004) and *Australia* (Baz Luhrmann, 2008). Beattie won the 2010 Australian Film Institute (AFI) Award for Best Adapted Screenplay for *Tomorrow* (one of the film's two awards from nine nominations), and the 2010 Inside Film (IF) Award for Best Script. The film won three further IF Awards including Best Film, and Best Actress for Caitlin Stasey (Ellie). Stasey was already well known to Australian television audiences through her long-term role in the soap *Neighbours* (Grundy Television, Seven Network 1985-86; Network Ten 1986-), while Lincoln Lewis (Kevin) had appeared in almost 550 episodes of the other leading Australian soap, *Home and Away* (Seven Network, 1988-). Ashleigh Cummings (Robyn) and Pheobe Tonkin (Fi) had also appeared in several episodes of the latter serial, though Tonkin was also familiar to *Tomorrow*'s target teenage audience through her lead role as mermaid Cleo in the children's television drama *H2O: Just Add Water* (Jonathan M. Shiff Productions, Network Ten, 2006-10). She has since played roles in the American cable television series *The Secret Circle* (Warner Bros. Television/CBS Television Studios/Alloy Entertainment/Outerbanks Entertainment, The CW, 2011-12) and *The Vampire Diaries* (Warner Bros. Television/CBS Television Studios/Alloy Entertainment/Outerbanks Entertainment, The CW, 2009-).

The film, like the books on which it is based, has been criticized for tapping into deep-seated and long-standing xenophobic and isolationist Australian attitudes that have found regular expression in narratives involving invasion by an Asian force seeking to exploit Australia's natural resources and wide open spaces (Bartlett 2010; Kevin 2010; Ross 2009). Catriona Ross identifies 30 Australian novels on this theme, beginning with *White or Yellow? A Story of the Race-*

War of AD 1908 (1888) by William Lane, a radical journalist, trade unionist and utopian who left Australia in 1893 to found a communal settlement, New Australia, in Paraguay (Ross 2009). China was initially the principal antagonist of such novels, before the rise of Japan in the early twentieth century shifted the locus of fear eastwards. After the Second World War, the threat was perceived to come from those Asian nations that had embraced Communism, primarily China, although Indonesia was also increasingly portrayed as a danger in more recent fiction of this type. In both the book and film versions of *Tomorrow*, the invading country is not specifically identified; in the film it is a coalition of Australia's regional neighbours, driven by over-population and under-resourcing in their homelands. Like the books, the film deploys Australian national(ist) symbolism throughout: many homesteads fly Australian flags, while the invasion occurs as the town of Wirrawee celebrates the Australia Day long weekend. The racist undertones of the narrative are only partly undercut by the presence of two non-Anglo characters (Greek Australian Homer, and unspecified Asian Australian Lee). In an intriguing moment in the film as the characters prepare to rescue Lee, Ellie finds herself staring at a mural commemorating the 1788 landing of the First Fleet. Her gaze is drawn to two Indigenous men in the background, recognizing perhaps the fact of invasion that founded modern Australia and aligning the young guerrillas with Indigenous resistance to colonial rule. The connection is however only implied; there are no Indigenous teenage characters to make the point more explicitly, or the film perhaps more interesting as a result.

Ben Goldsmith

References

Bartlett, Myke (2010) 'Sex, Violence and Cultural Anxiety: Tomorrow when the War Began', *Screen Education*, 60, pp. 113–18.

Kevin, Tony (2010) 'Australian Invasion Anxiety in Adolescent Fantasy', *Eureka Street*, 20: 17, pp. 8–9.

Lamont, Leonie (2012) 'Prison for Offenders as Courts get Tough on Tax Evasion', *Sydney Morning Herald*, 17 May, p. 3.

Ross, Catriona (2009) 'Paranoid Projections: Australian Novels of Asian Invasion', *Antipodes*, 23: 1, pp. 11–16.

Turkey Shoot (aka Escape 2000 [US], Blood Camp Thatcher [UK])

Country of Origin:

Australia

Studio/Distributor:

Filmco Limited
Hemdale Films
FGH

Director:

Brian Trenchard-Smith

Producers:

William Fayman
Anthony I Ginnane

Screenwriters:

Jon George
Neill Hicks

Director of Photography:

John McLean

Synopsis

Set in a dystopian future, suspected misfits of an oppressive society are sent to behavioural modification camps to become 'normal' productive citizens. But the detention system has become severely overcrowded and the immoral prison warden Thatcher, who rules with sadistic malice, has devised a novel way of dealing with the problem. Wealthy members of society are invited to hunt prisoners of their choosing on a 'turkey shoot' over a 24-hour period. The prisoners, in exchange for their participation, are offered a chance for freedom if they survive the hunt. Enter the movie's protagonists and newcomers to the prison: the political activist and escape artist Paul Anders; suspected prostitute Rita Daniels; and the innocent citizen, caught in the wrong place at the wrong time, Chris Walters. The protagonists soon discover that they are about to battle for not only their freedom, but for free will and the sanctity of the human spirit.

Critique

Like so many 'Ozploitation' films, *Turkey Shoot* can easily be viewed as mindless violence and misogynist trash. On the DVD cover of the uncut collector's edition – released by Umbrella Entertainment – Hussey is armed with a machine gun, prisoners are splattered in blood, and the grotesque animalistic mutant Alph features prominently with blood streaming from one eye. A quote from film critic David Stratton sums up the general critical attitude to the film: 'A sadistic … ultra-violent … futuristic bloodbath. A catalogue of sickening horrors.' The movie's accompanying documentary, 'Blood

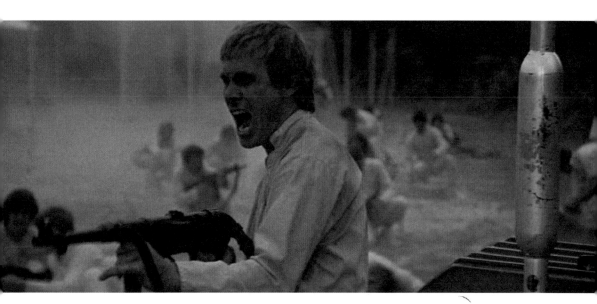

Turkey Shoot
(Brian Trenchard-Smith, 1982)

Production Designer:

Bernard Hides

Composer:

Brian May

Editor:

Alan Lake

Duration:

93 mins

Genre:

Action

Horror

Cast:

Steve Railsback

Olivia Hussey

Michael Craig

Carmen Duncan

Lynda Stoner

Michael Petrovitch

Steve Rackman

Noel Ferrier

Format:

35mm

Year:

1982

and Thunder Memories: 2003', includes an interview with actress Lynda Stoner who fervently dismisses the film as trash.

The movie features high levels of gore, with prisoners and guards being dispatched in the most gruesome of ways. Limbs are chopped off, multiple arrows pierce flesh, and there are several attempted rapes. The women are portrayed as either fragile creatures who need to use their bodies to survive, liabilities who need a man to save them or as aggressive and murderous as the most violent male character (a trope common in exploitation films). It is only when Chris lowers herself to the level of her male counterparts that she has any chance of rising above the stereotype of the downtrodden innocent, and surviving. The promiscuous heroine, Rita, is violently mutilated as punishment, it is suggested, for her unashamed sexual confidence.

Budget constraints played a major role in distracting critics from some of the movie's central themes. As outlined in the DVD's accompanying documentary, last-minute cuts forced the removal of the first twelve to fifteen pages of the script. This may explain why the film opens with the protagonists en route to the camp, and why the narrative is mostly limited to life in the camp with only the briefest glimpses of the oppressive society that sanctioned these institutions. Aside from Anders' revolutionary diatribes about the totalitarian society, our only view into the culture of this dystopian future is via the three wealthy hunters who attend the hunt: the obese hedonist Secretary Mallory (Noel Ferrier); the campy Eurotrash Tito (Michael Petrovitch) and his mutant primate Alph (Steve Rackman) (who has a penchant for human flesh and wrestling moves); and the sadistic lesbian Jennifer, mischievously portrayed by Carmen Duncan. This lack of detail about life outside the camp hinders the overall impact of the movie's narrative.

Although not an original story – it is a retelling of *The Most Dangerous Game* (Irving Pichel and Ernest B. Schoedsack, 1932) – and a low-brow exploitation movie, *Turkey Shoot* at some level explores complex themes. In particular, it delves into the dark side of the human psyche, and the extent to which masculinity is defined by sexual prowess – although these themes are unfortunately presented in stereotypical ways. Characters are represented in terms of the binaries of good and evil, and civilized and primitive. Anders is a stereotypical example of a strong alpha male. He is a shining example of the power of the human spirit, personified by his 'you can't break me' attitude. Antagonists are presented as sadists who perpetrate every violent act with elation, particularly against women. Misogynistic violence can be seen to relate to a lack of sexual prowess. Mallory is a flaccid specimen, fat, unappealing and sweaty, while Thatcher is sexually repressed or impotent. (Jennifer makes quips about his inability to sexually satisfy her and his repressed homosexuality.) Then there is Tito. He is a stereotypically feminine homosexual character but arguably attempts to compensate for this through his control of the grotesquely masculine primate slave/man-servant Alph. All three male antagonists revert to primitive demonstrations of dominance through violence to reaffirm a lack of (traditionally defined) masculinity. Alph, dressed in a respectable, old fashioned Victorian-era hunting costume, personifies the movie's central theme that deep down, we are simply well-dressed beasts.

Sharn Treloar

Walk into Paradise (aka Walk into Hell)

Country of Origin:

Australia/France

Studio/Distributor:

Discifilm
Southern International

Director:

Lee Robinson

Producer:

Chips Rafferty

Screenwriter:

Rex Reinits, from an original story by Lee Robinson and Chips Rafferty

Cinematographer:

Carl Kayser

Composer:

Georges Auric

Editor:

Alex Ezard

Duration:

93 minutes

Genre:

Adventure

Cast:

Chips Rafferty
Reginald Lye
Françoise Christophe
Pierre Cressoy
Somu
Fred Kaad

Synopsis

'Sharkeye' Kelly discovers oil in the remote and uncharted New Guinean highlands. He returns to the town of Madang, where District Officer Fred Kaad convinces him to return to the site in an expedition led by Patrol Officer Steve McAllister. The patrol will scout locations for an airstrip near the oil strike, which the Department of District Services and Native Affairs wants to build in order to 'open up' the country for mining. Twelve New Guinean policemen accompany them, under the command of McAllister's wartime buddy Sergeant Towalaka. Reluctantly, McAllister agrees to take UN malaria expert and French doctor Louise Demarchet to the village of Yamu. The group travel for several days by boat, overland by foot and then by canoe, but when they arrive they find the village deserted, apart from a delirious and dishevelled crocodile hunter, Jeff Clayton. The group is ambushed by the villagers. McAllister and Towalaka negotiate their way out without violence. Several days later, the group arrives at Paradise Valley, where Kelly found oil. The whole village is grieving; the chief's two sons are on the verge of death. McAllister convinces the chief that Clayton is a doctor and can help them, knowing that the village will not accept a woman with medical powers. The policemen build a hut for Demarchet to treat the boys without being seen, but the village witchdoctor witnesses her at work. The villagers attack the group, testing McAllister's resolve to avoid violence, and threatening the success of the mission.

Critique

The theme of partnership runs through *Walk into Paradise*, the third feature collaboration between director Lee Robinson and producer/star, Chips Rafferty. From bit parts in Ken G Hall's Cinesound films *Come Up Smiling* (aka *Ants in His Pants* [William Freshman, 1939]) and *Dad Rudd, M.P.* (1940), Rafferty had become a major star through his work in *Forty Thousand Horsemen* (Charles Chauvel, 1940), *The Rats of Tobruk* (Charles Chauvel, 1944) and Harry Watt's *The Overlanders* (1946), not least because of his ability to personify a popular ideal of 'Australianness'. Born John William Pilbean Goffage, Rafferty had worked as an ironmoulder, drover, shearer, deckhand and ice cream vendor before turning to acting in the late 1930s. Robinson had worked as a documentary film-maker with the Department of the Interior, where his work included a profile of Aboriginal Australian artist Albert Namatjira, *Namatjira the Painter*

Format:

35mm

Year:

1957

(1947). He began writing for radio, and met Rafferty while writing for the latter's serial, *Chips: A Story of the Outback*. In 1952, Rafferty and Robinson separately sought funding for feature film projects, but were both stymied by the post-war restrictions on capital investment, which limited film financing to £10,000. They pooled their talents and made their first feature *The Phantom Stockman* (Lee Robinson, 1953) for just over the financing limit. In a strategy that for the most part would serve them well in later ventures, Rafferty and Robinson earned enough from international sales to put the film in profit even before its Australian release. These funds enabled the production of the first film under the banner of their production company Southern International, *King of the Coral Sea* (Lee Robinson, 1954), which was shot in the Torres Strait Islands and north Queensland. International sales of *King* were channelled in to the production of their next film, *Walk into Paradise*.

During preproduction of *Walk into Paradise*, Southern International was approached by French producer Paul-Edmond Decharme to partner with his company Discifilm on a series of co-productions. Two French actors (Françoise Christophe and Pierre Cressoy) were given leading roles, and with the assistance of French dialogue coach Marcel Pagliero (who was given a director credit on the French release of the film) Robinson shot each scene twice, first in English and then in French. The final film was a great success, particularly in the United States (where it was retitled *Walk into Hell*). Robinson later claimed in an interview included on the DVD release that it earned AU$6 million in its first twelve months and was the highest grossing Australian film to that date. The film-makers received none of the profits, however, having sold the American rights to Joseph E Levine of MGM for £60,000 to finance Southern International-Discifilm's next venture, *The Stowaway* (Lee Robinson and Ralph Habib, 1958). Like the third and final co-production, *The Restless and the Damned* (Yves Allégret, 1959), *The Stowaway* was shot in Tahiti, but neither was as successful as *Walk into Paradise*.

The final shot of *Walk into Paradise* is reminiscent of the equivalent shot in *Casablanca* (Michael Curtiz, 1942): McAllister and Towalaka watch the plane take off, turn to each other smiling at a job well done, then head off away from the camera to continue their beautiful friendship. Just as McAllister/Rafferty personifies 'Australianness' – the 'heroic' Patrol Officer of the 1950s represents 'a sort of new-styled colonial digger, a militarily derived and matured Australian masculinity' (Landman 2006: 212) – so too does Towalaka/Somu stand in for Papua New Guinea. The wartime connection between the two characters evokes the close relationship between Australia and the then-British colonies of Papua and New Guinea during the Second World War, while the role that Towalaka and his troops take as protectors of the group evokes the Australian sense of the importance of PNG to Australia's defence in the post-war period. Rafferty towers over Somu, but in the spirit of the film and of Australian post-war colonialism, they are partners working together for mutual advantage. And, as Jane Landman argues in her book on Australian Pacific colonialism and the cinema, the 'buddy' structure of the film (referring less to the McAllister–Towalaka axis, and more to McAllister–Kelly) is underpinned by the partnership of commerce and government in the quest to drill for oil and 'open up' the country (Landman 2006: 194).

In addition to his work in Australian films, Rafferty's international profile was forged on Hollywood features including *Mutiny on the Bounty* (Lewis Milestone, 1962), and through his many guest appearances in 1960s UK and US television series including *Emergency Ward 10* (ATV, ITV, 1957-67), *Tarzan* (Banner Productions, NBC, 1966-69) and *The Monkees* (NBC/Raybert Productions/ Screen Gems Television, NBC 1966, CBS 1969-72, ABC 1972-73). But even though he frequently worked in the United States and elsewhere, and unlike his contemporaries Rod Taylor and Peter Finch, he remained based in Australia and was a staunch advocate for the Australian film industry during its lean period in the 1950s and 1960s.

Ben Goldsmith

Reference

Landman, Jane (2006) *The Tread of a White Man's Foot: Australian Pacific Colonialism and the Cinema, 1925–1962*, Canberra: Pandanus Books.

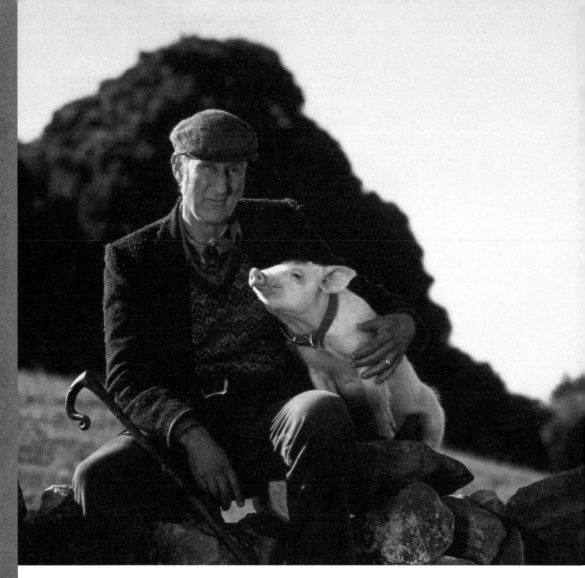

Babe (Chris Noonan, 1995).
© Kobal Collection

AUSTRALIAN
ANIMATED
FEATURE
FILMS

Australian animated films can be traced back to as early as the short-form work of cartoonist Harry Julius in 1912. Despite these early beginnings, however, it was the introduction of television that possibly had the greatest influence on the development of a local workforce capable of animating a feature film.

Eric Porter is arguably the most significant animator in Australia's pre-television history (Bradbury 2001: 209). Porter had been producing animated shorts from the 1930s, but it was his move into animated television-series production under contract from major American animation companies that established his Sydney studio as a viable option for animating a feature-length film. Porter oversaw offshore US productions while working for Australian animation studio Artransa, however the first television series that Porter's own studio (Eric Porter Studios) worked on was a Hanna-Barbera production, *Abbot and Costello* (1967–68). According to Porter (1976), the production of content for television coupled with the financial support of an American investor provided him with enough money to move into feature film production. Porter produced Australia's first animated feature film, *Marco Polo Jnr Versus the Red Dragon* (Eric Porter, 1972).

Marco Polo Jnr Versus the Red Dragon was produced for as much as AU$650,000 with investment from Porter himself, the Australian Film Development Corporation and American comic-book artist and collaborator Sheldon Moldoff's company Animation International (Pike and Cooper 1998 [1980]: 343). *Marco Polo Jnr* is significant to animation in Australia because Porter adopted assembly line production methods and merchandizing strategies that had been developed in the American studio system (Bradbury 2001: 216). The film won the 1973 Australian Film Institute (AFI) Gold Award, with Porter himself winning an AFI for Best Achievement in Direction. However, despite this critical acclaim, *Marco Polo Jnr* was a financial failure. Although Porter considered the film a personal achievement, it ultimately resulted in the closure of his studio.

As Eric Porter's experience indicates, television provided new opportunities for the production of animated content in Australia, and led to the development of a local feature animation industry. Television program standards, first introduced in 1960, restricted foreign content in advertising and effectively required Australian television stations to broadcast locally produced advertisements. This led in part to the growth of a local animation workforce. Animation proved to be an affordable and effective tool for television advertising, and for local animation studios, the regularity of the work provided a stable source of income (Bradbury 2001: 212). A similar business model continues to dominate the contemporary Australian animation industry, where production houses spread their income-generating activity across a range of sectors including television advertising, postproduction and visual effects services for other businesses (Screen Australia 2011: 38).

Australian animation studios such as Eric Porter Studios and Air Programs International (API) had been producing animated programs for the American market from as early as the 1950s, but by the early 1970s, expertise in animation production and lower labour costs made Australia an attractive offshore location for American animation production. Hanna-Barbera Productions, a leading independent animation studio and creators of well-known animated children's series such as *The Yogi Bear Show* (ABC [USA], 1961–62) and *The Flintstones* (ABC [USA] 1960–66), worked in collaboration with Southern Star Entertainment (now one of Australia's largest independent film production companies) to establish a local presence in 1972, making Australia the first country to host a major offshore US animation company (Bradbury 2001: 240). In Australia, Hanna-Barbera produced animation predominantly for television, before the studio was eventually sold to Walt Disney Television Australia in 1989. The presence of Hanna-Barbera and Disney, two major global animation companies, had both positive and negative implications for Australian animation.

On the one hand, Hanna-Barbera and Disney had well-established production workflows and the volume of work generated employment opportunities that helped establish a local workforce capable of animating feature-length films. However, perhaps the most significant negative impact for the local industry was the drain of talent away from local independent production (Bradbury 2001: 215). Moreover, a long-term effect of Hanna-Barbera and Disney's presence in Australia throughout the 1970s and 1980s was the adoption of a visual aesthetic that overshadowed the development of a distinctively Australian style. Local animators trained in the production methods and art styles of the American studios-produced animation that could be considered derivative of the dominant Hollywood animation aesthetic.

A key exception was the animation of Yoram Gross. Originally an experimental film-maker, Polish-born Gross immigrated to Sydney from Israel in 1968, and continued to produce award-winning experimental films. By 1977, Gross and his wife had established an animation studio in Sydney. The studio's first feature film, *Dot and the Kangaroo* (Yoram Gross, 1977), established what would become a signature style: cel animated characters and animals matted onto live-action backgrounds of the Australian bush. The use of live-action backgrounds was not the standard practice for feature animation at the time. While it was undoubtedly cheaper to produce live-action backgrounds than fully animated scenery, Gross later claimed that the backgrounds remained live action because he felt the scenery of the Blue Mountains was so beautiful that there was no need to transfer them to drawings (Rutherford 2003: 257).

Alexander Stitt was another influential local animator and feature film-maker. Stitt began production on his first feature film in 1975; *Grendel Grendel Grendel* (Alexander Stitt, 1981) was based on the well-known Scandinavian poem *Beowulf*. Unlike conventional cel animated films of the time, which featured a black line to delineate character detail and colour, *Grendel Grendel Grendel* featured no line at all. The absence of the black line in *Grendel Grendel Grendel* resulted in a film that 'achieved a certain status of dimensional believability' (Torre and Torre 2009: 119). The lack of lines prevented the imagery from appearing flattened, and allowed the figures to blend with the backgrounds. Despite a conventional linear narrative and visually interesting aesthetics, *Grendel Grendel Grendel* was not a financial success and Stitt's second animated feature, *Abra Cadabra* (1983), brought him close to financial ruin. The financial failure of Stitt's productions would have a lasting impact on investment in Australian animation production.

Strangely, it was an insurance company that would back one of Australia's most recognizable animated features. *FernGully: The Last Rainforest* (Bill Kroyer, 1992) was an American/Australian co-production produced by Kroyer Films and FAI Films. The movie was adapted from a book of the same title by Diana Young, and based on a nature reserve at the foot of Mount Warning, near the northern New South Wales coast. The film illuminates environmental issues of concern for the local communities surrounding the Night Cap National Park – Nimbin, The Channon, Lismore, Byron Bay and Murwillumbah.

FernGully was an innovative production that relied upon emerging digital technologies. As many as 40,000 frames were computer animated, including elements such as flocking birds and running animals. This effectively halved the production time typical for animated features at the time (Rickitt 2000: 147). Unfortunately, despite the film's Australian story, setting and characters, there is a notable lack of an Australian accent. The film was clearly developed to appeal first to the US market. The choice of cartoon imagery, musical score and the use of the voices of well-known American actors (Robin Williams and Christian Slater among others) are derivative of the Disney style. As a consequence, the film seems disjointed from its Australian roots, although this approach is likely to have played a significant part in the film's moderate box office success internationally (earning over US$30 million).

The impact of digital technologies on film-making has made it increasingly difficult to delineate animated films from their live action counterparts. Furniss (1998: 5) explains that when discussing animation and live-action films it is helpful to think of them existing on a continuum of aesthetic possibilities as opposed to existing in separate spheres. Films that sit at the intersection of animation and live action, such as *Babe* (Chris Noonan, 1995), can complicate any discussion on animation. *Babe* combined live-action, animatronics and CG animation within the same frame to create the illusion of talking animals. To further complicate the discussion on Australian animation, early productions such as *FernGully* and *Babe* had to turn to companies in the United States to meet their digital production needs. For example, the animation technique used in *Babe*, to map CG heads onto live action animals, was pioneered by US studio Rhythm and Hues (Rhythm & Hues Studios 2013). The technique earned them their first Academy Award for Achievement in Visual Effects, which was shared with the Australian company John Cox's Creature Workshop.

Transnational films such as *Babe* have played significant roles in establishing Australia's current technologically capable animation workforce. Studios such as Sydney's Animal Logic and Adelaide-based Rising Sun Pictures have developed a substantial body of work in the area of visual effects. Consequently, Australia now has a relatively vibrant visual effects industry servicing high-end international movies, including both films produced in Australia such as *The Matrix* (Andy and Lana Wachowski, 1999) and *X-Men Origins: Wolverine* (Gavin Hood, 2009), and films made elsewhere, including the Harry Potter series. As a result, local artists are given the opportunity to work on big-budget projects that require them to adapt to continually advancing digital technologies and processes.

In recent years, a number of Australian film-makers have adopted the clay animation (or claymation) method. Melbourne-based animator Adam Elliot won an Academy Award in 2004 for his short claymation film *Harvie Krumpet*. This success enabled him to make the claymation feature film *Mary and Max* (Adam Elliot, 2009). While *$9.99* (Tatia Rosenthal, 2009) was Australia's first claymation feature film, *Mary and Max* is Australia's most prominent stop-motion feature film. In keeping with Elliot's earlier work, *Mary and Max* features a very limited range of character movement. The film is partially set in New York, and Philip Seymour Hoffman provides the voice for Max Jerry Horowitz. Unlike *FernGully*, Elliot used Australian actors for Australian characters including – possibly in an attempt to ensure international appeal – the refined, pseudo British accent of Barry Humphries as narrator. This trend of avoiding the Australian accent in animated production is also evident in recent 3D CG feature films.

Animal Logic's success in television commercials and visual effects provided a foundation for the production of Australia's first fully-digitally animated feature film, *Happy Feet* (George Miller, 2006). While talking and singing animals are staples of Disney films, *Happy Feet* departs from this approach in an important way. At the time of writing, Disney and Pixar do not use motion capture to create character movement and their characters and environments are 3D interpretations of cartoon-style imagery. *Happy Feet* on the other hand features photorealistic representations of animals and the environment together with naturalistic performances derived from both motion capture and highly skilled animators. This approach proved to be engaging for audiences (earning over US$380 million at the box office worldwide) and won *Happy Feet* multiple awards including the 2007 Academy Award for Best Animated Feature, and an Academy Award nomination for Best Picture. The international success of *Happy Feet* proved that Animal Logic and its team of artists and technicians were capable of producing world-class CG animated feature films.

Animal Logic's growing expertise in animated feature film production secured their second feature *Legend of the Guardians: The Owls of Ga'Hoole* (Zack Snyder, 2010). Backed by Warner Bros. Pictures and Village Roadshow Pictures, the movie is based upon the first three (of fifteen) books in a series written by American author Kathryn Lasky. Directed by American Zack Snyder, *Legend of the Guardians* built upon the photorealistic characteristics of *Happy Feet* to produce some of the most visually stunning CG animation ever seen.

Even though the visuals are superior, *Legend of the Guardians* did not repeat *Happy Feet*'s extraordinary international success, although it managed a respectable box office take of US$140 million worldwide. Nevertheless, through Animal Logic's success in the international marketplace, and the development of an ongoing slate of projects, the company is helping create stable employment opportunities for local animators. Through projects such as *Happy Feet* and *Legend of the Guardians*, Animal Logic has managed to further strengthen the local industry. This was not to be the case for *Happy Feet's* director George Miller in his attempt to establish his own animation and visual effects studio.

Dr D Studios was established by George Miller and Doug Mitchell in partnership with the Omnilab Media Group in 2008. Their first animated feature production was *Happy Feet Two* (George Miller, 2011). *Happy Feet Two* was released with only 45 per cent of the attendance figures of its predecessor *Happy Feet* and earned US$150 million at the box office (Baker 2011: 8). With no other animated film in production to provide continuity of employment, as many as 600 employees subsequently lost their jobs. The impact of such dramatic layoffs was amplified by the strong Australian dollar and subsequent loss of 'service work' in the visual effects industry. Artists that may once have been able to find employment working in visual effects found they had few employment options.

Australia's animation industry has successfully made the transition to digital animation technologies and the continuation of fee-for-service work for an increasingly global digital effects industry has developed a highly skilled animation workforce. The increasing emphasis placed on the production of higher-budget movies and local blockbusters since 2007 has been a valuable boost for the production of local animated features. However, comparatively low investment in Australian animation continues to stunt the growth of the feature animation industry, and prevents the development of an identifiable Australian animation style.

Chris Carter

References

Baker, Leo (2011) *The Winston Churchill Memorial Trust of Australia: Report*, Victoria, Australia: The Churchill Fellows' Association of Victoria.

Bradbury, Keith (2001) 'Australian and New Zealand Animation', in Lent, J. (ed.), *Animation in Asia and the Pacific*, Bloomington: Indiana University Press.

Furniss, Maureen (1998) *Art in Motion: Animation Aesthetics*, Sydney: John Libbey.

Pike, Andrew and Cooper, Ross (1998 [1980]) *Australian Film, 1900–1977: A Guide to Feature Film Production*, Melbourne: Oxford University Press.

Porter, Eric and Edmondson, Ray (1976) 'Eric Porter interviewed by Ray Edmondson' [sound recording], Australia: National Library Australia.

Rhythm & Hues Studios (2013) 'Babe', http://www.rhythm.com/features/credits/babe/. Accessed 22 March 2013.

Rickitt, Richard (2000) *Special Effects: The History and Technique*, New York: Billboard Books.

Rutherford, Leonie (2003) 'Australian Animation Aesthetics', *The Lion and the Unicorn*, 27: 2, p. 251–51.

Screen Australia (2011) *Convergence 2011: Australian Content State of Play: Informing Debate*, Sydney: Screen Australia.

Torre, Dan and Torre, Lienors (2009) 'Recording Australian Animation History', *Animation Studies–Animated Dialogues 2007*, pp. 115–24. http://journal.animationstudies.org/dan-lienors-torre-recording-australian-animation-history/ Accessed 28 September 2013.

Babe

Country of Origin:

Australia/USA

Director:

Chris Noonan

Screenwriters:

George Miller
Chris Noonan, based on the
novel *The Sheep-Pig* by Dick
King-Smith (1983)

Producers:

George Miller
Bill Miller
Doug Mitchell

Director of Photography:

Andrew Lesnie

Production Designer:

Roger Ford

Composer:

Nigel Westlake

Editors:

Marcus D'Arcy
Jay Friedkin

Duration:

89 minutes

Genres:

Family film
Animation

Cast:

James Cromwell
Magda Szubanski
voices by Roscoe Lee Browne,
Christine Cavanaugh, Miriam
Margolyes and Hugo Weaving

Format:

35mm

Year:

1995

Synopsis

From a grim beginning at an industrial pig farm, piglet Babe is chosen to be a giveaway at a local carnival. Not one to raise pigs, taciturn Farmer Hoggett nevertheless forms a strange connection with Babe, guessing his weight and winning him as a prize. Back on the farm, Border Collie Fly takes in Babe as one of her own, but her mate and former sheepdog champion, Rex, is cold toward the new arrival. After an unfortunate incident with a duck, a cat and paint, Babe is scolded by Rex for not knowing his place within the farm order. Yet the young pig refuses to become prejudiced and continues to gently flout convention, making friends with all sorts of creatures, even the lowly sheep. Although initially intending to someday butcher Babe for meat, Hoggett becomes increasingly fond of the pig and notices that he has an aptitude for sheepherding, with the ability to communicate gently with the sheep rather than instilling fear in them. Despite the ludicrousness of the idea, Hoggett enters 'Pig' in the local Sheepdog Trials.

Critique

Based on Dick King-Smith's novel *The Sheep-Pig* (first published in 1983), *Babe* was a labour of love for writer/producer George Miller, known for the Mad Max trilogy (1979, 1981, 1985, as distinct from George Miller, director of *The Man from Snowy River* [1982], who had previously made children's films involving a seal [*Andre* (1994)] and talking creatures [*The Neverending Story II: The Next Chapter* (1990)]). What sets *Babe* apart from other talking animal films popular at the time, such as Disney's *Homeward Bound: The Incredible Journey* (Duwayne Dunham, 1993) and the same studio's inferior talking-pig film released the same year, *Gordy* (Mark Lewis, 1995), was not only its timeless tale, one enjoyed by children and adults alike, but also the groundbreaking digital effects and robotic animals (a special effects technique known as animatronics). The Australian company responsible for the animatronics, John Cox's Creature Workshop, deservedly shared the 1996 Academy Award for Best Visual Effects with the American companies Rhythm and Hues and Jim Henson's Creature Shop. *Babe* was nominated for six other Academy Awards: Directing, Best Picture, Writing (Screenplay Based on Material Previously Produced or Published), Film Editing, Art Direction, and Actor in a Supporting Role (James Cromwell). Veteran television actor Cromwell's performance in *Babe* led to a wealth of subsequent Hollywood roles from the corrupt police captain in *L.A. Confidential* (Curtis Hanson, 1997) to President George HW Bush in *W.* (Oliver Stone, 2008).

The storybook opening sets up *Babe* as a fairy tale ('This is a tale about an unprejudiced heart, and how it changed our valley forever'). A chorus of three mice, who are primarily extra-diegetic even though they have a limited diegetic presence, announce the film's 'chapters'. This endearing tale of overcoming prejudice and friendship without borders exhibits a certain cine-literacy, such as the use of the archaic iris shot or the scene in which Babe arrives on the farm that recalls the orange skies of the Tara plantation in *Gone with the Wind* (Victor Fleming, 1939).

Babe was a box office success, making over US$250 million worldwide, and came to be regarded as one of the more inspirational films of the decade, a *Rocky* (John G Avildsen, 1976) for the talking-animal genre. While almost as magical but not nearly as successful with audiences, *Babe: Pig in the City*, directed, written and produced by Miller, followed in 1998. *Chicago Tribune* film critic Gene Siskel named the sequel as his choice for the best film of the year. But there is no better praise than that from Hoggett himself in *Babe*'s last line: 'That'll do, Pig. That'll do.'

Zachary Ingle

FernGully: The Last Rainforest

Country of Origin:

Australia/USA

Studio/Distributor:

Twentieth Century Fox

Director:

Bill Kroyer

Producers:

Peter Faiman

Wayne Young

Screenwriter:

Jim Cox, based on the book *FernGully: The Last Rainforest* by Diana Young (1992).

Production Designer:

Ralph Eggleston

Victoria Jenson

Composer:

Alan Silvestri

Editor:

Gillian Hutshing

Duration:

76 minutes

Genres:

Animation

Children's

Cast (Voices):

Tim Curry

Synopsis

FernGully is a remote rainforest that is protected and nurtured by a race of fairies. The fairies believe humans to be extinct until they are forewarned by a demented flying fox who has had experience with humans as evident by the wires and antennas fused to his head. On investigating disturbances in the outer reaches of the rainforest, young fairy Crysta discovers trees destroyed, and the human, Zak Young, an advance scout of a logging crew who has become separated from his team. Shrinking him to her size to save him from a falling tree Crysta introduces him to the immersive delights of a rainforest environment. Now more environmentally aware, Zak with fairies Crysta and Pips and wildlife friends – Batty Koda and the Beetle boys – strives to save the rainforest from logging and the world from the pollutant effects that the malevolent spirit Hexxus unleashes when an ancient baobab tree is destroyed by logging activity.

Critique

Inspired by the children's books written by Diana Young (1992), *FernGully: The Last Rainforest* has been identified by Nicole Starosielski (2011: 147) as exemplary in its depiction of nature as an 'elastic, potentially interactive space' in line with contemporary Gaian notions of nature as a living, dynamic force. Starosielski suggests that the animated feature served as an important metaphor and parable for the environmental movement, becoming the first feature film to be screened at the UN General Assembly Hall on Earth Day 1992. It was also shown at the UN Earth Summit in Rio de Janeiro two months later. Certainly parallels were drawn at the time with the anti-logging campaigns in the forests of the Amazon and in the high-profile campaigns of Malaysian Borneo during the late 1980s. But the story was inspired by Diana Young's own attachment to the rainforest habitats found on the family's rural property in northern New South Wales, and by her husband Wayne Young's involvement in non-violent protests against the logging of nearby Gondwana Rainforests of Terania Creek.

'Place' however, has inspired the production in other ways. Co-producer Peter Faiman (director of *Crocodile Dundee* [1986]) led

Samantha Mathis
Christian Slater
Jonathan Ward
Robin Williams

Format:

35mm

Year:

1992

a party of sound recordists and fifteen animators on a four-week excursion into Australian heritage-listed rainforests on the New South Wales/Queensland border. The outcome is a lush and luxuriant backdrop rendered in traditional painted cel techniques that is clearly inspired by Australian subtropical rainforests, such as the shady glades of strangler figs, tall timbers festooned with staghorn and bird's-nest ferns, diverse fungi including luminescent varieties, vocalizing frogs with billowing throat membranes, and a particularly malevolent depiction of the leeches encountered 'during one day-long trek […] in pouring rain' (Ryan 1992). The film also incorporates other locational markers: Zak's wallet identifies him as a resident of Byron Bay (northern New South Wales), and the Mount Warning in the story is drawn to resemble prominent local mountain, Mt Warning.

FernGully: the Last Rainforest is an unofficial Australian/US co-production. Young's book was adapted to animation by veteran Disney scriptwriter, Jim Cox, and realized visually by ex-Disney director Bill Kroyer. To Australian eyes, the jarring elements of this film are what one reviewer describes as the 'Saturday morning cartoon aesthetics' inspired by Disneyesque characters and story themes (Maslin 1992). The charm in this film is in the realist depiction of a rainforest environment that is recognizably a place in Australia.

Susan Ward

References

Maslin, Janet (1992) 'Children's Animated Tale with Political Messages', *New York Times*, 10 April. http://www.nytimes.com/1992/04/10/movies/review-film-children-s-animated-tale-with-political-messages.html Accessed 28 September 2013.

Ryan, James (1992) 'Save the Rain Forest, He Says, Animatedly', *San Diego Union-Tribune*, 11 April, p. E6.

Starosielski, Nicole (2011) '"Movements that are Drawn": A History of Environmental Animation from *The Lorax* to *FernGully* to *Avatar*', *International Communication Gazette*, 73: 1–2, pp. 145–63.

Legend of the Guardians: The Owls of Ga'Hoole

Country of Origin:

Australia/USA

Studio/Distributor:

Animal Logic
Warner Bros.
Village Roadshow

Synopsis

Two brother owlets, Soren and Kludd, are kidnapped by an evil clan of owls known as the Pure Ones. Led by Metal Beak, the arch enemy of the Owls of Ga'Hoole – guardians of the owl kingdom – the clan kidnap, brainwash and train young Tyto owls to become soldiers for a secret army. Escaping in the hope of rescuing his brother and freeing the owls from captivity, Soren begins a journey in search of the guardians. Meeting various creatures along the way, including Twilight (Anthony LaPaglia, a great grey owl) and Digger (David Wenham, a burrowing owl), and reuniting with the family nanny Mrs P (Miriam Margolyes, a nest-maid snake), they travel across a vast ocean to reach the Great Tree of Ga'Hoole. After convincing the Guardians' council of the uprising, they prepare for the final epic battle against the Pure Ones.

Director:

Zack Snyder

Producer:

Zareh Nalbandian

Screenwriters:

John Orloff
Emil Stern

Production Designer:

Simon Whiteley

Composer:

David Hirschfelder

Editor:

David Burrows

Duration:

83 minutes

Genres:

Animation
Fantasy

Cast (Voices):

Jim Sturgess
Hugo Weaving
Emily Barclay
Joel Edgerton
Anthony LaPaglia
Ryan Kwanten
Miriam Margolyes
David Wenham

Format:

35 mm, Technicolor 3D.

Year:

2010

Critique

Director Zack Snyder's first animated feature film *Legend of the Guardians: The Owls of Ga'Hoole* was an unofficial American/ Australian co-production, produced by Animal Logic's founder Zareh Nalbandian. The film had a modest production budget estimated at US$80 million which is comparatively low when considered on a world scale against other films produced using similar techniques of 3D CG animation. For example, films such as *Kung Fu Panda 2* (Jennifer Yuh, 2011), produced by Dreamworks Animation, can have budgets that exceed US$150 million. Despite the comparatively low budget, *Legend of the Guardians* did earn US$140 million worldwide after a somewhat disappointing initial release in the United States. The PG rating along with the darker themes could have contributed to its underperformance as parents may have hesitated to take younger children to see the film.

Legend of the Guardians is a visually stunning animated feature and a technical milestone for photorealistic computer animation. The film deservedly won the Australian Academy of Cinema and Television Arts (AACTA) 2011 Award for Best Visual Effects. However, rarely does visual style and animation technique save a bad story, and *Legends of the Guardians* is no exception. The movie attempts to pack an epic adventure into an 83-minute narrative but fails to develop engaging characters or empathy for their plight. While the journey (and its associated trials and tribulations) is an established, some may say a critical, generic component of the epic adventure movie, what should have been a long and treacherous journey to discover the Guardians – as memories of the Owls of Ga'Hoole are fading and only live on through children's fables in the movie's narrative – takes less than 13 minutes of screen time. As a result, there is little sense that the journey challenges or transforms the protagonists, as is typical in the genre. Moreover, the representation of the Guardians and the Pure Ones is little more than a contrast between good and evil. As a result, character motivation and narrative conflict is shallow and underdeveloped.

The decision to render the imagery in a photorealistic style is well-suited to both the epic genre, and the serious tone of the story. However, the notion that owls are capable of crafting ornate helmets, weapons, buildings and other objects, pushes plausibility to the limit. In other words, the photorealism is so good in this film that it leaves nothing to the imagination. Perhaps a more stylized fantasy-based aesthetic would have allowed the audience to become more engaged and help build empathy for the large ensemble of characters. That said, Animal Logic have done an excellent job in adapting such an epic tale into such a short movie. *Legend of the Guardians* is a stunning piece of animation and is well worth seeing for the visual feast alone.

Chris Carter

Mary and Max

Country of Origin:

Australia

Studio/Distributor:

Melodrama Pictures

Director:

Adam Elliot

Producer:

Melanie Coombs

Screenwriter:

Adam Elliot

Cinematographer:

Gerald Thompson

Production Designer:

Adam Elliot

Composer:

Dale Cornelius

Editor:

Bill Murphy

Duration:

92 minutes

Genres:

Animation
Comedy
Drama

Cast:

Toni Collette
Philip Seymour Hoffman
Eric Bana
Barry Humphries

Format:

35mm

Year:

2009

Synopsis

To escape from her dysfunctional family and the trials of growing up, 8 years, 3 months and 9 days old Mary Daisy Dinkle finds solace in her written correspondence with an unlikely pen pal. Looking through names in a New York phonebook, Mary wonders where American babies come from. She decides to find out by writing a letter to someone chosen randomly – Max Horovitz, an overweight middle-aged New Yorker with Asperger's syndrome. Mary's letter sends Max into a panic attack, but after eighteen hours of staring out of a window he decides to write back. Their correspondence begins a long-distance friendship that lasts for almost twenty years until Mary finally travels to New York to meet her friend for the first time in person.

Critique

Mary and Max displays director Adam Elliot's distinctive and deceptively simple visual style: stop-motion claymation, a muted colour palette, limited character movement and irregular shapes and model surfaces. The sepia tones of Mary's world are reminiscent of 1970s colour photographic processing in Australia, while the colour scheme of Max's New York is dominated by blacks, whites and greys. *Mary and Max* is Elliot's fifth animated narrative film, and his first at feature length. While his four previous short films – *Uncle* (1996), *Cousin* (1998), *Brother* (1999), *Harvie Krumpet* (2003) – each revolve around an eccentric central character defined by physical or psychological disabilities, *Mary and Max* explores the biography of two main characters. The film is narrated by Barry Humphries and, unlike Elliot's earlier films which use a single omniscient narrator, the lead characters Mary (Toni Collette) and Max (Philip Seymour Hoffman) also contribute to the movie's narration through the dictation of letters.

Mary and Max is an intriguing film, and for the most part, Elliot delivers an engaging balance of humour and melancholy. However, the lack of action and movement is a limitation. While at times a dialogue-heavy plot and limited character movement accompanied by sound effects is quaint, this style struggles to carry a feature-length narrative, and the movie's second act becomes somewhat laboured. The film's budget, relatively low when compared to independent animated features of a similar ilk overseas, may have been a factor. *Mary and Max* was produced for just AU$8 million, while the popular claymation *Wallace & Gromit: The Curse of the Were-Rabbit* (Steve Box and Nick Park, 2005) cost almost US$30 million to make.

Mary and Max has won multiple international awards including the 2009 Ottawa International Animation Festival's Grand Prize for Best Animated Feature. And yet despite widespread critical acclaim, *Mary and Max* underperformed at the box office. The film seems destined to follow in the important but unprofitable footsteps of early Australian feature animation such as *Marco Polo Jnr Versus the Red Dragon* (Eric Porter, 1972) and *Grendel Grendel Grendel* (Alexander Stitt, 1981).

With copulating dogs, alcoholism, depression-driven suicide, mental illness, toilet humour and interesting ideas on procreation, *Mary and Max* is a film targeted at a mature audience. Nonetheless, the film deserves a place alongside other influential independent animated features such as Sylvain Chomet's *Les Triplettes de Belleville/The Triplets of Belleville* (2003). Both films depart from the conventional narrative forms popular in Hollywood animated features, and the visual styles typical of the dominant Disney aesthetic. *Mary and Max* takes animation to new ground while still managing to tell a compelling story about average people that has meaning and appeal for a wide audience.

Chris Carter

SPLASH DOWN

COMEDIAN
COMEDY

Kenny (Clayton
Jacobson, 2006).
© Kobal Collection

One of the most prominent subgenres of Australian comedy film, comedian comedy has proliferated during periods of change in the local film industry. At its peaks, this subgenre has been exceptionally popular and includes some of the most financially successful Australian films. Defined by Steve Seidman (1979: 2) as a film featuring a comedian who began their career in another entertainment medium, comedian comedy has a history in Australia that parallels, but exists independently of, the American tradition of film vehicles for established comedic performers. The distinctiveness of Australian comedian comedies derives from a local entertainment landscape that encompasses film, television, theatre and radio.

The comedian comedy film appeals to an existing audience by centring on a character who displays elements of the performer's established persona (Seidman 1979: 3). Examples of characteristic traits of Australian comedians are Paul Hogan's colloquial disdain for social niceties; Mick Molloy's slovenly yet articulate demeanour; Nick Giannopoulos's combining of diverse cultural references with musical performance; Jane Turner's and Gina Riley's chameleon-like abilities to imitate distinct female social types; and Judith Lucy's laconic and self-deprecating style of speech. In a comedian comedy film, a disjunction typically exists between the performer's existing persona and the narrative's positioning of him or her as a character confronting situations in the plot (Seidman 1979: 3). In Australian examples, this disjunction is frequently associated with a 'fish out of water' plot, in which the protagonist encounters an environment in which s/he is out of place or lacks skills to function effectively. Early examples are the social displacement of Australian soldiers in Europe in Pat Hanna's Diggers films (*Diggers* [FW Thring, 1931]; *Diggers in Blighty* [Pat Hanna, 1933]); the naivety of rural migrants to the city in George Wallace's comedies (*His Royal Highness* [FW Thring, 1932]; *Harmony Row* [FW Thring, 1933]; *A Ticket in Tatts* [FW Thring, 1934]; *Let George Do It* [Ken G Hall, 1938]; *Gone to the Dogs* [Ken G Hall, 1939]). More recent examples include *Crocodile Dundee*'s (Peter Faiman, 1986) encounters with modern, urban American lifestyles; a loafer's infiltration of a bowling club in *Crackerjack* (Paul Moloney, 2002); the outback adventures of Irish immigrants in *The Craic* (Ted Emery, 1999); and the positioning of Greek Australian Steve Karamitsis as a cultural outsider in the Wog Boy films (*The Wog Boy* [Aleksi Vellis, 2000]; *Wog Boy 2: Kings of Mykonos* [Peter Andrikidis, 2010]). In these narratives of displacement, comedian comedy contributes to what Tom O'Regan terms the 'othering' of the Australian, a local storytelling tradition that expresses 'ambivalence' towards that which is considered to be distinctively Australian (O'Regan 1996: 250).

Australian comedian comedy reached an early peak in the 1930s, when local studios Efftee and Cinesound developed films as vehicles for vaudeville performers such as Pat Hanna, George Wallace, Roy Rene and Will Mahoney. These comedies were conceived as local alternatives to Hollywood productions.

The most prominent comedic performer in local films at this time was George Wallace, who starred in five feature films in the 1930s that remain the most sustained series of Australian comedian comedies. By contrast, this subgenre virtually disappeared from Australian film during the subsequent decades, when local feature film production diminished in general. In the meantime, radio and television provided opportunities for a new generation of comedians who became influential in the 1970s and 1980s.

Australian comedian comedy returned to prominence with the success of Peter Faiman's *Crocodile Dundee* (1986). Described by Ben Goldsmith in the first volume of this Directory as 'the real monster of Australian comedy' (Goldsmith 2010: 15) in relation to the local industry's small size, the film is credited by Felicity Collins with drawing Australian audiences back to local films (cited in McFarlane, Mayer and Bertrand 1999: 74). *Crocodile Dundee* links the 'ocker' humour of the 1970s, particularly television's *The Paul Hogan Show* (Seven Network,1973–77, Nine Network 1978-84), to 1980s tax incentives for investment in Australian screen production, upon which this film capitalized spectacularly. As well as forming a model for Hogan's three subsequent films, *Crocodile Dundee* established a precedent for a wider range of contemporary Australian comedian comedies. Screen Australia's statistics indicate that ten of the top fifty local films of all time are comedian comedies, all dating from this period onwards: *Crocodile Dundee*, *Crocodile Dundee II* (John Cornell, 1988), *The Wog Boy*, *Crackerjack*, *The Man Who Sued God* (Mark Joffe, 2001), *Kenny* (Clayton Jacobson, 2006), *Crocodile Dundee in Los Angeles* (Simon Wincer, 2001), *Lightning Jack* (Simon Wincer, 2004), *The Craic* and *Wog Boy 2: Kings of Mykonos*. Domestically and abroad, comedian comedy has served to define both Australia and its humour and to highlight the work of prominent comedians, many of them Australian. Beyond the success of Paul Hogan's films, however, relatively few of these films centre on a single performer. The films starring Hogan, Billy Connolly (*The Man Who Sued God*) and Shane Jacobson (*Kenny*) constitute an elite subcategory of Australian comedies rather than typifying this subgenre.

Ensemble humour is more characteristic of Australian comedian comedy. Although top billing is likely to be given to one performer, close examination reveals that many Australian comedies feature two or more central comedic characters. These films depart from the convention of pairing a central comedian with a 'straight' or non-comedic character. For instance, Mick Molloy's films *Bad Eggs* (Tony Martin, 2003) and *Crackerjack* feature the comedian Judith Lucy in significant supporting roles. Equally, the Wog Boy films position Nick Giannopoulos and Vince Colosimo as a comedic duo. Other ensemble comedian comedies include *Charlie & Boots* (Dean Murphy, 2009), *Fat Pizza* (Paul Fenech, 2003) and *Kath & Kimderella* (Ted Emery, 2012). Deriving from traditions of stage and television performance, these ensembles have a local antecedent in the 1930s Diggers films, which centre on comedic interaction between Pat Hanna, George Moon and Joe Valli. The ensemble form in Australian comedian comedy reflects both the abundance of local talent and the small size of the local production industry, in which casting more than one prominent comedian in a film is considered to maximize its audience appeal.

In terms of ethnicity and gender, Australian comedian comedy displays imbalances that are consistent with the male dominance of the genre internationally. The exceptions, however, reflect distinctive aspects of Australian society. Roy Rene's film *Strike Me Lucky* (Ken G Hall, 1934) is unusual because it centres on a Jewish performer and includes ethnic humour, whereas Australia has not had a continuous tradition of Jewish comedians. Even today, film displays less diversity than contemporary stand-up comedy in terms of gender, ethnicity and physical abilities. An exception is the box office success of the Wog Boy films, which centre on Greek and Italo Australian characters. *Fat Pizza* contributes further ethnic diversity to Australian comedian comedy. Whereas these films continue the tradition of male dominance, however, *Kath & Kimderella* is unusual among Australian films for centring on two female comedians. Television is key in this context. The fact that both *Kath & Kimderella* and *Fat Pizza* are spin-offs of television series reflects that a more diverse range of comedic talent can be found on the small screen, with its generally lower production budgets and concomitant capacity to take greater risks. A tendency for female comedic performers to achieve greater prominence in television than film is evident in the television series *Acropolis Now* (Seven Network, 1989–92), *Full Frontal* (Seven Network, 1993–97), *Laid* (ABC [Australia] 2011) and *After the Beep* (ABC [Australia] 1996), as well as *Kath & Kim* (Riley Turner Productions, ABC [Australia] 2002–07, Seven Network 2008-). Similarly, television's inclusion of comedians of ethnic backgrounds who are less often seen in local films is evident in the series *Lawrence Leung's Choose Your Own Adventure* (Chaser Broadcasting, ABC [Australia] 2008) and *Lawrence Leung's Unbelievable* (ABC [Australia], 2011), as well as *Pizza* (SBS, 2000–07).

Indeed, a full understanding of comedian comedy encompasses various media. Just as the stars of comedian comedy films established their careers in television, radio or theatre, some comedians are very successful in these media without having starred, or even appearing, in a film. The importance of various media is nowhere more evident than in the careers of two of Australia's most celebrated performers, Graham Kennedy and Barry Humphries. Although both achieved great success, neither of these comedians is the star of a film that has achieved a degree of popularity or acclaim comparable to their work in television, theatre or radio. From one point of view, their careers exist at the periphery of comedian comedy because their most significant comedic film performances are in supporting parts, such as Humphries's portrayals of Edna Everage in the Barry McKenzie films (*The Adventures of Barry McKenzie* [Bruce Beresford, 1972]; *Barry McKenzie Holds His Own* [Bruce Beresford, 1974]) and Kennedy's roles in the ensemble films *Don's Party* (Bruce Beresford, 1976) and *The Odd Angry Shot* (Tom M Jeffrey, 1979). From another point of view, however, the careers of Kennedy and Humphries reveal that comedian comedy is limited neither to cinema nor to works that are vehicles for a single performer. Indeed, some of the most important film contributions by prominent humourists are behind the scenes of Australian comedian comedies: examples are John Clarke's screenplay for *The Man Who Sued God* and Tony Martin's work as director and writer of *Bad Eggs*. In these ways, Australian comedian comedy both derives from and is reflected in a wide media landscape.

Lesley Speed

References

Goldsmith, Ben (2010) 'Introduction: Australian Cinema', in Ben Goldsmith and Geoff Lealand (eds), *Directory of World Cinema: Australia and New Zealand*, Bristol: Intellect, pp. 9–21.

McFarlane, Brian, Mayer, Geoff and Bertrand, Ina (eds) (1999) *The Oxford Companion to Australian Film*, Melbourne and New York: Oxford University Press.

O'Regan, Tom (1996) *Australian National Cinema*, London and New York: Routledge.

Seidman, Steve (1979) *Comedian Comedy: A Tradition in Hollywood Film*, Ann Arbor, MI: UMI Research.

Bad Eggs

Country of Origin:

Australia

Studio/Distributor:

A Million Monkeys
Double Yolker Films
Roadshow Films

Director:

Tony Martin

Producers:

Stephen Luby
Tony Martin
Greg Sitch

Screenwriter:

Tony Martin

Director of Photography:

Graeme Wood

Production Designers:

Carrie Kennedy
Ben Morieson

Composers:

David Graney
Clare Moore

Editor:

Peter Carrodus

Duration:

96 minutes

Genres:

Comedian comedy
Thriller

Cast:

Mick Molloy
Bob Franklin
Judith Lucy
Shaun Micallef
Bill Hunter
Alan Brough
Robyn Nevin
Marshall Napier
Chris Peters

Format:

35mm

Year:

2003

Synopsis

A magistrate, Rodney Poulgrain, gasses himself in his car after receiving an envelope containing photographs of his visits to a brothel. As he falls unconscious, he knocks the car into gear. It careens down the road and into a shopping centre. Two undercover detectives, Ben and Mike, chase the now-dead Poulgrain, and shoot the corpse numerous times. They are subsequently removed from a major corruption case they are investigating, and demoted to uniform duties. Sent to Poulgrain's house to tidy up, they accidentally burn the house down. The officers who take over the corruption case, Wicks and Pendlebury, arrest a journalist, Julie, alleging she was blackmailing Poulgrain. Ben realizes that Julie has been set up, and convinces police computer technician Northey to help them discover evidence of police corruption. It soon becomes clear that the cover up not only involves high-ranking police officers, but reaches to the very pinnacle of the political establishment.

Critique

Bad Eggs represents a change of direction for first-time writer-director Tony Martin and his collaborators (Mick Molloy, Judith Lucy and Bob Franklin) away from the straight-out comedy work in radio, television and film that made their names, into the subgenre of the political thriller. While Martin dutifully incorporates many of the genre's key conventions and semantic elements – low-level innocents discover a network of corruption involving the police, politicians and casino operators, only to be threatened by the conspirators, and framed for the misdeeds of their colleagues and superiors – these are overshadowed by the comedians and the comedy. To its credit, the film never quite tips over into parody, but the serious and somewhat convoluted plot about police graft and political corruption is undercut not only by the use of actors more familiar as comedians in the lead roles, but also by the fact that the actors play thinly veiled versions of themselves. The characters played by Mick Molloy (Mike) and Judith Lucy (Julie) in particular are almost indistinguishable from their carefully honed comedian personas; the former slovenly, careworn and blokily incompetent, the latter mordant, sardonic and icily bitter. Their acting styles are examples of what Barry King terms 'personification', in which an actor plays a role that is close to their own personality or image (King 1991: 130). Personification is perhaps most common in film comedies in which established comedians are cast precisely in order to reproduce the personality or image familiar from their prior comedy work. But while the mode works well in comedy, it is less successful in films like *Bad Eggs* that straddle genres (comedy-thriller) and require the comedian-actors to play more rounded characters and to go beyond a purely comic role.

Given the backgrounds and connections between the key cast and crew, it should come as no surprise that the banter between characters and the elaborate comic set pieces (which include cinema's slowest car chase) are the real strengths of the film. Although this was Tony Martin's first feature as writer-director, he and several of the film's other leading lights – particularly Molloy but also Lucy and Franklin, Shaun Micallef and Gina Riley (who appears in a minor role) had a history of collaboration prior to *Bad Eggs*. All are long-standing members of the loose collective of comedians based in Melbourne that grew out of, or spun off from *The D-Generation*, an ABC/Seven Network television series (1986–89) and breakfast radio show (1986–92). The collective – which also includes key Australian comedy figures in Rob Sitch, Santo Cilauro, Tom Gleisner, Jane Kennedy, Jane Turner, Michael Veitch and Magda Szubanski – would, in various combinations, go on to produce some of the highest profile and most popular films, radio and television comedy series over the last three decades, including *The Castle* (Rob Sitch, 1997), *Fast Forward* (Artist Services, Seven Network,1989–92), *Full Frontal* (Seven Network, 1993–97), *The Late Show* (D-Generation Productions, ABC [Australia] 1992–93), *Big Girls Blouse* (Artist Services, Seven Network, 1994), *Frontline* (Frontline Television Productions/Working Dog, ABC [Australia], 1994–97), *Kath & Kim* (Riley Turner Productions, ABC [Australia] 2002–07) and *Thank God You're Here* (Global Television Services/Working Dog, Network Ten, 2006–09). Martin and Molloy began their collaboration as writers and later as performers on *The D-Generation*, before going on to become core members of the ABC television sketch comedy series *The Late Show* in the early 1990s. They returned to commercial radio in the highly successful *Martin/ Molloy* show (1995–98), before working again in television on the *Mick Molloy Show* (Radiant Industries, Nine Network, 1999), which also featured *Bad Eggs* collaborators Judith Lucy and Bob Franklin. Unfortunately the attempt to reproduce the radio show's loose mix of sketch comedy, chat and music for Saturday night television did not appeal to executives at the Nine Network, and the series was cancelled after only eight episodes. Martin later had small roles in the feature films *Crackerjack* (Paul Moloney, 2002) and *BoyTown* (Kevin Carlin, 2006), both of which were co-written by and starred Molloy, although the two reportedly fell out over the non-inclusion on the *BoyTown* DVD of a mockumentary, directed by Martin, about the film's fictional band.

Ben Goldsmith

Reference

King, Barry (1991) 'Articulating Stardom', in in Jeremy G. Butler, (ed.), *Star Texts: Image and Performance in Film and Television*, Detroit: Wayne State University, pp. 125–54.

The Craic

Country of Origin:

Australia

Studio/Distributor:

The Crack

Foster Gracie

Synopsis

In 1988, Fergus and Wesley travel to Australia after an altercation in Belfast with prominent terrorist Colin. The altercation leads to Colin's arrest by British SAS soldiers, Barry and Bob. In Sydney, Wesley and Fergus outstay their tourist visas. Realizing that he could stay if he is in a de facto relationship with an Australian, Fergus becomes a contestant on a television dating show. Just after Fergus leaves

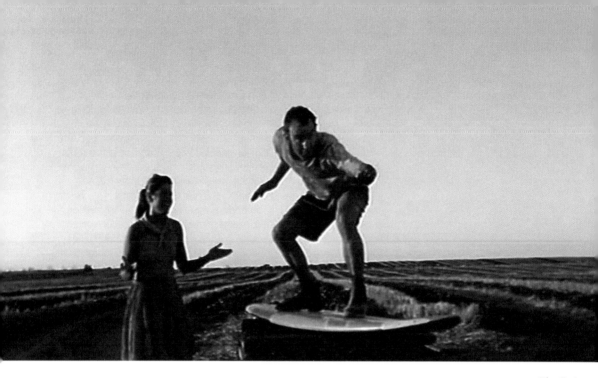

The Craic
(Ted Emery, 1999)

Village Roadshow
Director:
Ted Emery
Producers:
David Foster
Marc Gracie
Jimeoin McKeown
Screenwriter:
Jimeoin McKeown
Cinematographer:
John Wheeler
Production Designer:
Penny Southgate
Composer:
Ricky Edwards
Editor:
Michael Collins
Duration:
89 minutes
Genre:
Comedian comedy
Cast:
Jimeoin

Sydney to travel to the Gold Coast to film the dating part of the show, immigration agents raid his house. Wesley narrowly escapes, wearing only his underpants. Meanwhile, unbeknownst to the boys, Colin has become a supergrass, and has been brought to Queensland under Barry and Bob's protection. He soon escapes from his safe house and starts to follow Fergus and Wesley. After the boys' van breaks down in the outback, Colin appears, and chases them across the desert. The boys end up in the small town of Mundi Mundi, where they decide to surrender to the authorities in order to return to Belfast. Colin appears in town just as the immigration agents arrive to arrest the boys, with the SAS soldiers also hot on the trail.

Critique

Northern Irish stand-up comedian Jimeoin was already a familiar face on Australian television when he wrote and starred in his first feature film, *The Craic*, in 1999. He first came to Australia in the late 1980s, initially working in the building industry before breaking into comedy. Before he became a household name, he appeared on the long-running Australian television dating show *The Perfect Match* (Network Ten, 1984–89), on which the show in *The Craic* is clearly modelled. Greg Evans, host of three seasons of *The Perfect Match*, performs the same role in the film.

Jimeoin's appearances in the early 1990s on the variety show *Hey Hey It's Saturday* (Somers Carroll Productions, Nine Network, 1971–2010) and the daytime talk show *Good Morning Australia* (Network Ten, 1992–2005) with Bert Newton, along with a role as a convict in the series *Bligh* (Artist Services, Seven Network, 1992) and guest spots

Alan McKee
Robert Morgan
Colin Hay
Bob Franklin
Kate Gorman
Geoff Paine
Kyle Morrison

Format:

35mm

Year:

1999

in the sketch comedy series *Full Frontal* (Seven Network, 1993–97), earned him his own show, *Jimeoin* (Artist Services, Seven Network, 1994–96), which ran for three series. Regular cast members included Bob Franklin (who co-stars in *The Craic* as an SAS soldier obsessed with *Neighbours* [Grundy Television, Seven Network 1985–86; Network Ten 1986–]), and the show's directors included Marc Gracie and Ted Emery, respectively producer and director of *The Craic*. Although *The Craic* was Emery's first feature film, he was already a well-established and successful director of television comedy, with credits including pivotal Australian shows such as *Acropolis Now* (Seven Network, 1989–92), *The D-Generation* (ABC [Australia] 1986-89), *Fast Forward* (Artist Services, Seven Network, 1989–92) and *Full Frontal*. Emery is perhaps best known now for his television work with Gina Riley and Jane Turner on *Kath & Kim* (Riley Turner Productions, ABC [Australia] 2002–07, Seven Network 2008–); he also directed the feature film spin-off, *Kath & Kimderella* in 2012.

With such a well-credentialled and much loved creative team and strong backing from one of Australia's largest and most diverse media companies, Village Roadshow, it now seems entirely predictable that *The Craic* should have immediately struck a chord with Australian audiences. At the time of its release in April 1999, however, Australian films had struggled for success for several years, and few expected *The Craic* to record the third highest opening weekend for an Australian film to that date. Jimeoin earned further publicity for the film when, wearing a safari suit rather than the required black tie, he tried to gatecrash a screening at the Cannes Film Festival. The film went on to earn over AU$5 million at the Australian box office, and remains one of the top fifty domestic films of all time.

Much of the film's appeal lies in the likeable, charming character of Jimeoin/Fergus, and in the familiar comic trope of the outsider's experience of Australia. This places *The Craic* in a line of Australian film comedy that runs from *They're a Weird Mob* (Michael Powell, 1966), and *Sunstruck* (James Gilbert, 1972), to *Crocodile Dundee* (Peter Faiman, 1986) and beyond. On the surface, *The Craic* appears to tread well-worn ground with its jokes about surfing, sunburn, incomprehensible accents and deadly wildlife, but it is Jimeoin and his compatriots who are as much the butt of the jokes as their Australian counterparts. One running joke has Fergus and Wesley's accent repeatedly misidentified as Scottish, while it is the tourists and locals who are a threat to Australian fauna rather than the other way around; the toll at the end of the film includes several cockroaches, two cane toads, a kangaroo, a snake, and a murder of crows. The kangaroo is run over by Wesley and Fergus's fried out Kombie – a sly reference to a line in the unofficial Australian national anthem, Men at Work's 'Down Under' (first released in 1981), which was written and sung by Colin Hay, who plays the second SAS soldier, Barry. An acoustic version of the song plays over the end credits, rounding out a carefully chosen and highly evocative soundtrack of hits from the 1980s.

Ben Goldsmith

A Few Best Men

Country of Origin:

Australia/UK

Studio/Distributor:

Parabolic Pictures
Stable Way Entertainment
Production

Director:

Stephan Elliott

Producers:

Antonia Barnard
Gary Hamilton
Laurence Malkin
Share Stallings

Screenwriter:

Dean Craig

Cinematographer:

Stephen F. Windon

Production Designer:

George Liddle

Composer:

Guy Gross

Editor:

Sue Blainey

Duration:

97 minutes

Genre:

Comedy

Cast:

Laura Brent
Xavier Samuel
Kris Marshall
Kevin Bishop
Tim Draxl
Olivia Newton-John
Rebel Wilson
Steve Le Marquand
Jonathan Biggins

Format:

35mm

Year:

2012

Synopsis

Englishman David Locking travels to the remote Pacific island of Tuvalu where he meets the Australian, Mia. It is love at first sight, and they decide to marry. David returns to London to ask the friends who have been his only family for most of his life to be his best men. Tom is an immature, easy-going prankster who never takes anything seriously, Graham is a whiny hypochondriac with a cheese allergy, and Luke is suicidal after his girlfriend leaves him. Although not entirely happy about the prospect of losing their friend, all agree to be best men and travel with David to Australia for the wedding. Upon arrival, the best men make a detour to buy marijuana from Ray, a drug dealer they found on the Internet. Meanwhile, at Mia's parent's house, David is introduced to Mia's bored cocaine-snorting mother, Barbara, Mia's pretend-lesbian sister, Daphne, and her father Jim, a conservative politician whose prize ram, Ramsey, is the son he never had. After the best men organize an alcohol fuelled 'buck's night' for David, a series of drug-fuelled mishaps and bad behaviour threaten to derail the wedding. Then Ray arrives with a shotgun, and what remains of the reception descends into chaos.

Critique

Like most of Stephan Elliott's movies, *A Few Best Men* is difficult to discuss without focusing on the director himself. A wedding-gone-wrong comedy, *A Few Best Men* is Elliott's first Australian feature film in fifteen years. After directing the low-budget crime-thriller *Frauds* (1993), Elliott achieved worldwide success as writer-director of the Oscar-winning road movie *The Adventures of Priscilla, Queen of the Desert* (1994). A quirky and visually striking film about two drag-queens and a transsexual's journey across the harsh Australian outback in a bus named Priscilla, the movie earned over US$70 million at the international box office and became an instant Australian classic. Elliott's career, however, self-destructed soon after. As one commentator observed, 'in the giddy aftermath of Priscilla's success' indiscretions 'became de rigueur as Elliott cut a swath through the media, shooting his mouth off at Ray Martin, Baz Luhrmann and anyone else he fancied taking a potshot at' (Guilliatt 2012). As Elliott later conceded, 'Post-*Priscilla* I had a lot of microphones in my face and said what I thought. I had some journalists turn on me, entire networks turn on me. How dare I say our most popular television host is a dick? [referring to Ray Martin]' (Guilliatt 2012).

His follow-up Australian movie, the grotesque and absurd comedy *Welcome To Woop Woop* (1997) about an American con man kidnapped by a nymphomaniac and forced to live in a degenerate 'outback' town ruled by a patriarch named Daddy-O, was critically savaged and failed dismally at the box office. His next film, the Canadian/UK co-production *Eye of the Beholder* (1999), 'descended into chaos after the producers went belly-up and Elliott almost bankrupted himself trying to complete it' (Guilliatt 2012). To make matters worse, the movie's costume designer and Elliott's close

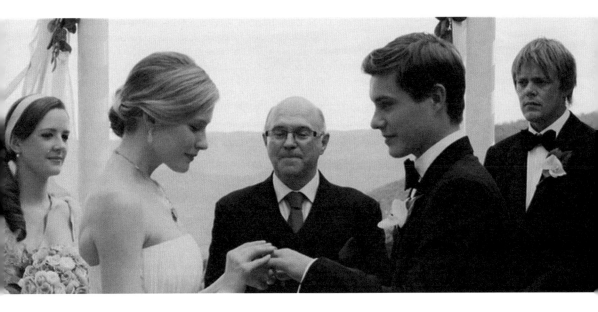

A Few Best Men
(Stephan Elliott, 2012)

friend, Lizzy Gardiner, filmed a making-of documentary entitled
'Killing Priscilla' which 'captured the director staggering from on-set
chaos to angst-ridden psychotherapy sessions to bruising meetings
with his producers like a man choreographing his own downfall'
(Guilliatt 2012). Following the movie's release, Elliott's film-making
career stalled. In 2004 he suffered a horrific skiing accident in the
French Alps that almost ended his life. However, after a long and
painful recovery, Elliott returned to film-making with the Canadian/
UK period drama *Easy Virtue* (2008) starring Colin Firth and Jessica
Biel. Receiving positive critical reviews and earning over US$18
million at the box-office, *Easy Virtue* rekindled Elliott's career. *A Few
Best Men* would be his next movie.

A Few Best Men was written by Dean Craig (who also wrote
the twice-filmed *Death at a Funeral* [Frank Oz, 2007; Neil LaBute,
2010]). It features a relatively strong cast including up-and-coming
Australian actor Xavier Samuel best known for his role as Riley in
The Twilight Saga: Eclipse (David Slade, 2010), English actor Kris
Marshall from *Death at a Funeral* fame, Australian singer and cultural
icon Olivia Newton-John and Australian comedian and actress
Rebel Wilson, a rising star following her roles in the Hollywood
movies *Pitch Perfect* (Jason Moore, 2011) and *Bridesmaids* (Paul
Feig, 2011). With a budget of AU$14 million, *A Few Best Men* is
one of the highest-budget Australian comedies produced in the
last decade. Although the movie did not live up to expectations, it
performed moderately well at the box office earning AU$5.6 million
in Australia and a total of AU$14 million worldwide. The movie ranks

as one of the most popular local comedies at the Australian box office in the last decade alongside *Red Dog* (Kriv Stenders, 2011), which earned over AU$21 million at the Australian box office; *The Sapphires* (Wayne Blair, 2012), over AU$14 million; *Bran Nue Dae* (Rachel Perkins, 2009), AU$7.6 million; *Kenny* (Clayton Jacobson, 2006), AU$7.6 million, and *Strange Bedfellows* (Dean Murphy, 2004), AU$4.8 million. Nonetheless, the critical reception was poor. Controversial Australian reviewer Jim Schembri gave the movie no stars and labelled it 'unreleasable [...] a witless, brainless, gormless, senseless, tasteless and – worst of all – laughless comedy about a country wedding reception gone wrong' (Schembri 2012). Although not always as severe in their assessments, international critics shared these sentiments. Phelim O'Neill in *The Guardian* concluded that 'what must have seemed at some point in production to be charming and hilarious arrives on-screen as neither of those things' (O'Neill 2012), while a reviewer for the *Hollywood Reporter* described the film as a 'scatological Australian comedy' that 'makes *The Hangover* look highbrow' (Wood 2011).

An over-the-top farce, the movie is a conscious attempt to cash-in on a recent cycle of wedding comedies in the vein of *The Hangover* (Todd Phillips, 2009) and *Bridesmaids*. But rather than bringing a novel perspective to this cycle, the narrative is highly derivative, drawing heavily upon tropes and themes established in the *The Hangover*, *Bridesmaids* and *Death at a Funeral* (where drugs, bizarre characters and mishaps threaten to ruin a wedding/funeral), as well as *Meet the Parents* (Jay Roach, 2000) (where a tough patriarch disapproves of, and monitors, his daughter's suitor). *A Few Best Men* recycles the basic plot formula of *The Hangover* – a group of guys acting badly almost derail a wedding. As such, there is a sense of déjà vu about the storyline and even the humour. While *Bridesmaids* also borrows from *The Hangover* by retelling this story from the perspective of bridesmaids, it also renews the formula. On the other hand, *A Few Best Men* essentially transposes the idea of a group of young men behaving badly in Las Vegas, to behaving badly at the wedding, and rather than almost derailing a wedding they actually succeed in doing so – a twist on the plotline that failed to impress the critics. While the movie is at times hilarious, the narrative and individual gags are so over the top that the comedy becomes absurd and ridiculous.

The movie is closely related to a strand of local comedy revolving around international protagonists, or 'outsiders', who struggle to acclimatize to Australian society/culture, which is typically characterized as outdoors, masculine and low-brow. *They're a Weird Mob* (Michael Powell, 1966), which was based on a popular comic novel about an Italian journalist who immigrates to Australia and struggles to come to grips with the Australian accent and cultural customs, is a primary example. *A Few Best Men*, written by a British screenwriter with input from Elliott, is told from an international perspective. Australian characters and the representation of 'Australianness' are based upon broad clichés and stereotypes – from 'ocker' yobbos and surf boards with shark bites in them to the notion that being Australian is all about booze and sunshine.

Moreover, the film is very much an attempt to produce a commercial movie targeting an international audience. As a result, the film is more concerned with being an outrageous comedy along the lines of *The Hangover*, than parodying or providing a satirical look at contemporary Australian culture. Overall, *A Few Best Men* is a movie that had potential but in the end is too clichéd and over the top to achieve the success of the films it mimics.

Mark David Ryan

References

Guilliatt, Richard (2012) 'Stephan Elliott is back, for better or for worse,' *The Australian*, 21 January, http://www.theaustralian.com.au/news/features/stephan-elliott-is-back-for-better-or-for-worse/story-e6frg8h6-1226245743811. Accessed 18 March 2013.

O'Neill, Phelim (2012) '*A Few Best Men*: review', *The Guardian*, 30 August, http://www.guardian.co.uk/film/2012/aug/30/a-few-best-men-review. Accessed 18 March 2013.

Schembri, Jim (2012) 'A Few Best Men', *Sydney Morning Herald*, 25 January, http://www.smh.com.au/entertainment/movies/a-few-best-men-20120125-1qhgw.html. Accessed 18 March 2013.

Wood, Sura (2011) 'A Few Best Men: Film Review', *Hollywood Reporter*, 17 October, http://www.hollywoodreporter.com/review/a-few-best-men-film-249306. Accessed 18 March 2013.

Kenny

Country of Origin:

Australia

Studio/Distributor:

Thunderbox Films

Director:

Clayton Jacobson

Producers:

Clayton Jacobson
Rohan Timlock

Screenwriters:

Clayton Jacobson
Shane Jacobson

Cinematographer:

Clayton Jacobson (credited as 'Camera A')

Composer:

Richard Pleasance

Synopsis

Kenny Smyth is a Melbourne plumber who works for the company Splashdown, installing and maintaining portable toilets at outdoor events such as music festivals and car rallies. Derided for his choice of employment by his father and brother, and despised by his ex-wife, Kenny remains philosophical about his profession and endearingly congenial to all. Sent by his company to a Portaloo convention in Nashville, Tennessee, it is here that Kenny's affable, down-to-earth attitude and honest work ethic enable him to secure an important business deal, establish cross-cultural friendships and ignite romantic interest. Upon returning home, Kenny cares for his ailing father and manages the most important occasion on Splashdown's calendar, the Melbourne Cup, during which his love for his young son, who he brings along to the event, is touchingly portrayed. Confronted with a final act of disrespect from a man who refuses to move his car to make space for Kenny to drive his parked sewage truck, Kenny the underdog finally fights back using the very tools of a trade which has earned him such condescension.

Critique

Kenny (Shane Jacobson), the eponymous hero of this Australian mockumentary, is an Aussie battler – a figure whose presence in

Editors:

Clayton Jacobson
Sean Lander

Duration:

97 minutes

Genres:

Comedy
Mockumentary

Cast:

Shane Jacobson
Eva Von Bibra
Ronald Jacobson
Ian Dryden
Chris Davis
Jesse Jacobson
Morihiko Hasebe

Format:

35mm

Year:

2006

Australian cinema, and especially in Australian comedy, has a long history dating back at least to the classic silent film *The Sentimental Bloke* (Raymond Longford, 1919). The unforgettable patriarch Darryl Kerrigan in *The Castle* (Rob Sitch, 1997) is perhaps the most prominent recent reference point. *Kenny* reconstitutes the battler for a twenty-first century audience, with Shane Jacobson triumphant in the title role as the exemplary Australian everyman whose decency, honesty and unshakably positive outlook represent the Australian spirit at its best. When Kenny arrives at the Cleaners and Pumpers Convention in Nashville, Tennessee – which he refers to as 'Poo HQ' – our wide-eyed protagonist seems at first to be out of his depth amidst the flashy, supersized US spectacle. But much like Australia's most iconic 'ocker' hero before him, Mick 'Crocodile' Dundee, Kenny's naivety and good will work in his favour as those he meets along the way cannot help but be drawn to his typically Australian self-deprecating humour and lack of pretension.

For a comedy premised on the travails of a Portaloo employee, *Kenny* mostly rises above cheap toilet humour to instead offer a far more subtle character study than might be expected. Filmed using a handheld camera, director Clayton Jacobson's mockumentary style allows for remarkable comedic tact in a film dominated by such crude subject matter, with the humour deriving largely from the deadpan presentation of grotesque situations. These are in turn cleverly juxtaposed with Kenny's philosophical insights, simple yet inspiring worldviews shared in direct addresses to the camera. 'I sometimes feel lucky I got this job,' he states at one point, 'and I work with a great bunch of blokes. That's more than anyone can ask for.'

We catch glimpses of this workingman's personal life in Melbourne's suburbia, and it is the overwhelming ordinariness of these scenes – picking up his son from his ex-wife's house and placating his disgruntled father about his choice of profession – which almost enables *Kenny* to be mistaken for a work of *cinéma-vérité*. Such a perception is further enhanced by the film having been shot entirely on location, including scenes at iconic Australian events such as the Melbourne Cup.

The film's committed investment in this singular character, however, comes at the expense of any significant narrative arc or development of the minor characters. And while it does as a result feel somewhat long, given a lack of any element of suspense and sometimes awkward dramatic structure, such qualms have not bothered audiences in Australia where *Kenny* has been a critical and commercial success, receiving a handful of industry awards including an Australian Film Institute (AFI) Award for Best Lead Actor.

Billed as 'a Jacobson Brothers film', the film was largely a family affair. It was written by and features a number of men from the Jacobson clan: the creative team of Clayton and Shane; their father Ronald who plays Kenny's father; and Shane's son Jesse who plays Kenny's son. Adding to the blurring of life and fiction, *Kenny* was in fact funded by the real-life Portaloo company featured in the film, Splashdown. Like its predecessor *The Castle*, being independently produced on a modest budget did not prevent *Kenny* from performing admirably at the Australian box office where it earned AU$7.7 million. Following a wave of 1990s films that satirized Anglo-Australian culture, *Kenny*'s success in 2006 confirms the resilience of the 'ocker' genre of Australian comedy and its continued resonance with local audiences.

Ilana Cohn

The Sapphires

Country of Origin:

Australia

Studio/Distributor:

Goalpost Pictures

Director:

Wayne Blair

Producers:

Rosemary Blight

Kylie Du Fresne

Screenwriters:

Tony Briggs

Keith Thompson

Director of Photography:

Warwick Thornton

Production Designer:

Melinda Doring

Synopsis

In the late 1960s, three Indigenous Australian sisters, Julie, Gail and Cynthia, enter a local talent contest in a small rural town but they are passed over for the prize due to racial prejudice. Their talent is noticed by drunken Irishman and former cruise ship entertainments officer, Dave, who offers to become their manager. After receiving consent from the girl's parents, they travel to Melbourne to ask their long-lost cousin Kay to complete the group. As a child, Kay was taken to a mission and raised as a white Australian. As a result she has tried to distance herself from her Aboriginal family and heritage. This generates tension between Kay and Gail, the oldest sister. Julie has a child she leaves at home during the tour. Cynthia was left at the altar and is determined to have a good time. Under Dave's guidance, the girls are reinvented as soul singers. They rehearse, change their image and learn to dance, before successfully auditioning before a US military panel to tour Vietnam. Their performances vary greatly: from their first shaky appearance in a small bar in Saigon, to intimate scenes inside a hospital singing to wounded soldiers, to packed performances for marines in army camps close to the front line. The tense relationship between Gail and their alcoholic manager Dave turns into romance just as the

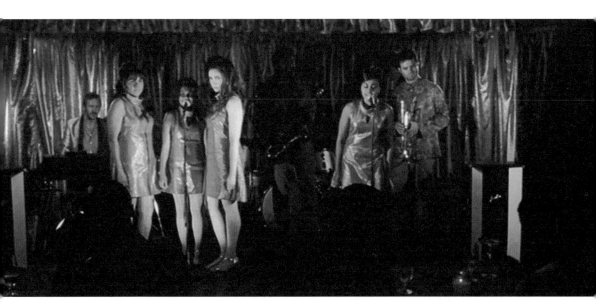

The Sapphires
(Wayne Blair, 2012)

Composer:

Cezary Skubiszewski

Editor:

Dany Cooper

Duration:

103 minutes

Genres:

Comedy
Musical

Cast:

Chris O'Dowd
Deborah Mailman
Jessica Mauboy
Shari Sebbens
Miranda Tapsell

Format:

35mm

Year:

2012

war catches up with them. After a full-scale attack on an army camp where they are performing, the group flees, but not all escape unscathed.

Critique

The Sapphires is an Indigenous Australian musical comedy. The movie could also be described as an international Indigenous film. By invoking the American struggle for racial equality in the late 1960s and through the use of famous African American music (such as 'I Heard It Through the Grapevine' [Norman Whitfield and Barrett Strong, 1966] and 'I Can't Help Myself' [Brian Holland, Lamont Dozier, Eddie Holland, 1965]), Wayne Blair has attempted to speak to an international audience. In so doing, Blair has created a universal story which does not silence or limit the presentation of specific Indigenous issues, such as the Stolen Generations, represented through the character of Kay. Similarly, setting the film during the Vietnam War (without representing it as a problematic period of American history) allows a reference point for western audiences. This is aided by the filming of many scenes on location in Vietnam. Nevertheless, at the time of writing, the movie had received only a limited release in the United States, although the movie has earned almost US$17 million at the box office in Australia, the United Kingdom and New Zealand.

One of the movie's strengths is its strategic casting. Chris O'Dowd is an Irish comedian who first came to prominence in the British television sitcom *The IT Crowd* (Retort, Channel 4, 2006–13) before taking roles in the hilarious British comedy *The Boat That Rocked* (Richard Curtis, 2009) and the US wedding comedy *Bridesmaids* (Paul Feig, 2011). His role as Dave, while still humorous, is heart-warming and complex as his character shows an appealing sympathy to the young Indigenous Australian girls. Like *Rabbit-Proof Fence* (Phillip Noyce, 2002) and its inclusion of English actor Kenneth Branagh, and the starring role played by Geoffrey Rush in *Bran Nue Dae* (Rachel Perkins, 2009), *The Sapphires* benefits from an international draw card such as O'Dowd. Deborah Mailman, well established in Australia as a leading actress in both film and television, won her second Australian Academy of Cinema and Television Arts (AACTA) Award (formerly the AFI Awards) for Best Actress for her role as Gail. She previously won the award in 1998 for her role in *Radiance* (Rachel Perkins, 1998). The presence of former *Australian Idol* (FremantleMedia Australia, Network Ten, 2003-09) contestant and emerging actor Jessica Mauboy (who also appeared in *Bran Nue Dae*) ensured that the film covers a wide range of both locally and internationally recognized talent.

Perhaps what sets *The Sapphires* apart from many other Indigenous films in Australia is the way that Blair prioritizes the glitz of the musical performances and a light-hearted, feel-good story, rather than making a serious socially conscious film that didactically examines sombre social/cultural/political issues. Blair uses humour and song to lighten what could be an intense film of racial struggle during the 1960s. He appears to have no real interest in sending a direct ideological or sociopolitical message to the audience – in contrast to Warwick Thornton's *Samson and Delilah* released in 2009 that examines the destructive world of substance abuse in remote Indigenous communities. (Thornton was also *The Sapphires*'s AFI/AACTA Award-winning Director of Cinematography.) Although social issues are addressed, as in Kay's story, they are handled softly. While these issues are clearly raised, they are merely a component of a story that focuses primarily on human relationships and personal challenges in a time of unrest. Again, by internationalizing the narrative and reinforcing the universal struggles of minorities regardless of ethnicity, *The Sapphires* becomes a local Australian story that successfully plays on a global stage.

Elizabeth Ellison

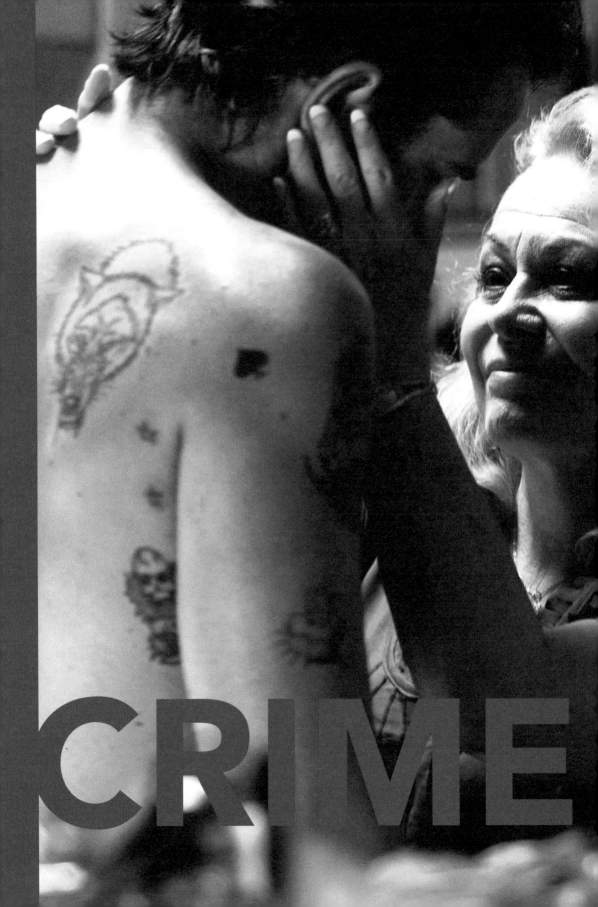

CRIME

Animal Kingdom
(David Michôd, 2010).
© Kobal Collection

Australian crime is an enduring and established genre that has recently enjoyed a surge in production and popularity. At a time when crime rates in Australia are falling there has been a steady increase in screen crime with audiences relishing criminal activity as a form of entertainment. Australian crime films have a robust national history with contemporary genre variations retaining a commitment to social-realist issues, true crime and naturalism with a domesticated focus and a powerful crossover with television crime drama. Australian crime cinema is defined by an ambivalent attitude towards depictions of evil where moral boundaries are hazy, police are compromised and audiences are asked to identify with criminals as anti-heroes perhaps recalling a trace of the bushranger mythology or the nation's celebrated anti-authoritarian streak. While the Australian crime genre is multifaceted and raises numerous issues for analysis, this essay focuses on four key issues central to crime narratives over the past decade: a fascination with 'true crime', an ambivalence about clear distinctions between good and evil, a high degree of crossover between film and television and a focus on ethnicity and crime.

The juxtaposition of good and evil that is central to crime narratives is blurred in the Australian genre variation. Representations of the police force as good, moral guardians are confined to television drama, while Australian crime cinema focuses predominantly on criminals, gangsters and vengeful victims. The rare instances when the police do appear in Australian cinema, they are invariably corrupt. The heroes of Australian crime dramas are ambitious young delinquents, prostitutes working their first trick, career gangsters, petty criminals and serial killers with firm family values. Depictions of evil are more slippery: corrupt cops, hardened killers and psychopaths make up the roll call but their malevolence is surreptitious. The moral compass is not clearly divided into sectors of good and evil. In a gambling den full of crooks, everyone plays the victim card. This ambivalence precipitates a search for authenticity.

Australian audiences have demonstrated an enduring fascination for the true-crime genre with its mix of naturalism, sensationalism and an explanatory social realism. There has been a stream of true-crime stories in Australian cinema since the mid-1970s including titles such as *Mad Dog Morgan* (Philippe Mora, 1976), *Money Movers* (Bruce Beresford, 1978), *Hoodwink* (Claude Whatham, 1981), *Heatwave* (Phillip Noyce, 1982), *Squizzy Taylor* (Kevin James Dobson, 1982), *The Boys* (Rowan Woods, 1998), *Chopper* (Andrew Dominik, 2000), *Bra Boys* (Sunny Abberton and Macario De Souza, 2007) and, more recently, *Animal Kingdom* (David Michôd, 2011) and *Snowtown* (Justin Kurzel, 2011). True crime has also featured regularly on television in such mini-series and series as *The Great Bookie Robbery* (Nine Network, 1986), *Blue Murder* (Southern Star, ABC [Australia], 1993) the *Underbelly* franchise (Screentime, Nine Network, 2008–), *Killing Time* (FremantleMedia, TV1, 2011) and *Bikie Wars: Brothers in Arms* (Screentime, Network Ten, 2012).

The best examples of Australian true-crime cinema (*The Boys*, *Chopper*, *Animal Kingdom* and *Snowtown*) creatively depict real events, invite ethical debate and contribute to the media history of the crimes on which they are based. For example, the daring real crime known as the 'Great Bookie Robbery' of 1976 spawned surprisingly different interpretations of the events. The robbery inspired a three-part miniseries (1986), a large section of *Underbelly: A Tale of Two Cities* (2009) and the heist at the heart of *The Hard Word* (Scott Roberts, 2002).

The tropes of the true-crime film blend the historical details of the bushranger films with the brutality and social realism of the prison film to create iconic Australian drama that honours the larrikin and an anti-authoritarian spirit while blaming a monstrous social environment. Rosalind Smith neatly summarizes the historical context of Australian true crime:

> The settlement of Australia as a penal colony, the violent and unresolved history of relations between settler and Indigenous cultures, and a tradition of national mythmaking surrounding criminal figures, also indicate the centrality of true crime and its narration to formations of Australian national identity. (Smith 2008: 17)

The focus of Australian true crime is on uncovering the ordinary in shocking and sensational, high profile, macabre and heavily mediated rapes, robberies and murders. Andrew Fraser, the underworld's former solicitor of choice before being imprisoned for cocaine importation, claims that understanding the public fascination for true crime is simple – 'it's like people watching a car accident – they can't help themselves. They are appalled by it, but at the same time they are fascinated by it' (Noble 2010). For audiences, part of the fascination is also negotiating what they know of an event, its presentation in the media and in various films and television shows. The Walsh Street murders and the Pettingill family entered into popular mythology; *Killing Time* and *Animal Kingdom* both examine the explosive family dynamics but with a different thematic focus. The banning or embargo on the TV screenings of *Killing Time*, *Blue Murder* and *Underbelly* because of ongoing court cases that could be compromised by the broadcasts add to the genre's social significance and popular impact.

True-crime films promise to explain criminal psychology, speculate as to the motivation of the killers and contextualize the events. They are implicitly understanding of the villains and seek to illuminate the context and process of the crime while eschewing narrative closure. The characters tend to be working class or socially marginal anti-heroes and their lifestyles are structured to create prurient audience interest. In the case of the two most recent and celebrated examples of true crime, *Snowtown* and *Animal Kingdom*, the action unfolds through the eyes of two passive young men, not yet villains, but implicated by their failure to extricate themselves from their adult criminal milieu. They oscillate between good and evil, failing to stake a clear position before being sucked down to the levels of their adult mentors. The protagonists of both films experience abuse and witness atrocities before becoming killers in their own right. Murder becomes a form of self-preservation. In these perverse coming-of-age narratives, these characters are presented compassionately, as befitting victims of circumstances.

The genre is most often fixated on heinous and inexplicable murders that are forensically explored through a detailed treatment of the criminals and the world they inhabit. The location of the events is invariably suburban with the crimes appearing more shocking as they occur unexpectedly amidst an otherwise mundane and dreary facade. *Snowtown*'s mass murderer, John Bunting (Daniel

Henshall), is all the more sinister because he appears to be a normal, family oriented man trying to support the community in an otherwise desperate suburban landscape. It is remarkable that killers in this genre are often presented as likeable. The first half of *Animal Kingdom* humanizes the everyday lives of the Cody crime family and in so doing creates audience empathy for characters and an ambivalent audience experience.

One of the reasons that true crime is so popular is that it asks important questions about truth, style and ethics. *Chopper* provokes the audience to judge notorious felon Chopper Read's reliability as a narrator. Making sense of the relationship between 'the real' and film style is essential in exploring the various approaches to the truth. *Animal Kingdom* studiously avoids the glamorous gangster style of *Goodfellas* (Martin Scorsese, 1990) and *Underbelly* while sharing something with the minimalist suburban decrepitude of *The Boys*, its psychotic, unpredictable energy, and avoidance of on-screen violence for as long as possible. The elegant cinematography of *Snowtown* aestheticizes the poverty and mundanity of suburban North Adelaide into a surrealistically de-saturated depiction of the banality of evil where horrendous crimes appear conventional in the absence of ethical authority.

Ethnic crime narratives offer a different view of suburban criminality. In films such as *Little Fish* (Rowan Woods, 2005), *The Jammed* (Dee McLachlan, 2007), *Two Fists One Heart* (Shawn Seet, 2008), *The Combination* (David Field, 2009), *Cedar Boys* (Serhat Caradee, 2009) and *Crawl* (Paul China, 2011), antagonistic ethnicities drive the narrative. While statistics do not point to higher incidences of crime among ethnic communities, ethnicity is significant in contemporary crime cinema in its activation of mainstream anxieties and denunciations of the failures of multiculturalism. Numerous ethnic criminals appear in a range of films that are not necessarily crime. There is the insane local crime lord Tony the Yugoslav to whom Dom owes money in *The Wog Boy* (Aleksi Vellis, 2000). Then there is Anton the Russian in Paul Cox's melodrama *Salvation* (2008); the Greek kidnappers in *Nirvana Street Murders* (Aleksi Vellis, 1990); Indigenous youth on the rampage in *Yolngu Boy* (Stephen Johnson, 2001); the ill-determined ethnic mercenaries in *Holidays on the River Yarra* (Leo Berkeley, 1991); and the Vietnamese petty criminals in *The Finished People* (Khoa Do, 2003). Ethnic crime narratives represent stereotypical views of minorities, but at the same time they shed light on social issues, the environmental difficulties and dislocation of second-generation youth tragically caught between two cultures.

Mainstream apprehension about ethnic crime is continuously neutralized by the 'wog boy' humour and gross-out parody style of *Fat Pizza* (Paul Fenech, 2003) and its inclusive performance of multicultural misbehaviour. Writer and director Fenech's approach, across a range of film and television projects, is to create delinquent comedies full of anti-authoritarian petty crooks and stereotyped wannabe mobsters. In the same way, the culturally diverse world of the Gold Coast portrayed by Chris Nyst in *Crooked Business* (2008) is full of clearly marked ethnic crims who are brought together in an energetic crime caper that connects a variety of underworld characters through a dodgy deal gone wrong. Russian Tony is tricked by (Lebanese) 'Stand Up Sam' who does a job for Bondi Bob by buying up Jewish – aka Four B Two – Lou Wiseman's stolen jewels. After Lou's Kiwi henchman starts looking for Sam, the briefcase containing the jewels is mixed up with another belonging to a Chinatown villain, which contains stimulants for racehorses. This is a hilarious representation of criminal multiculturalism where all crooks are ethnics and the gangs are culturally diverse. In contrast, what made the sophisticated multi-stranded narrative investigation of *Lantana* (Ray Lawrence,

2001) so effective was the implication that anyone who is not Anglo-Australian is implicitly stereotyped as a potential criminal. Similarly, in *Jindabyne* (Ray Lawrence, 2006) some of the townsfolk believe that racism motivated four friends to delay reporting the death of an Aboriginal woman. This becomes the real crime that divides the community, rather than the murder; the woman's killer goes unnoticed and unpunished.

Two films about Lebanese youth as aspirational criminals from Sydney's south-western suburbs emerged in the wake of racially motivated riots in Cronulla in 2005. *The Combination* and *Cedar Boys* independently examine the relationship between young Lebanese men, migrant-class poverty, the Anglo mainstream, the desire for blonde girlfriends and conflict with the established criminal milieu. Similar themes were explored in the SBS police procedural television series, *East West 101* (Knapman Wyld, SBS, 2007–11). The protagonists of *Cedar Boys* and *The Combination* are caught between two cultures. They are neither fully Australian nor traditionally Lebanese. They struggle with their identity and idealized performances of masculinity, and become caught up in a criminal culture from which they struggle to escape. Both films feature Lebanese youth seeking to come of age through drugs and violence while asserting a unique cultural identity. They too are victims of circumstances and their environment as they seek to negotiate a space between good and evil and their national identity.

In ethnic crime films, the character's ethnicity and relationship to an imaginary Anglo mainstream is central to the narrative. The ethnic criminal context determines the visual style, music, patois and performance style of the film. The characters in *Cedar Boys* and *The Combination* steal cars, deal drugs and are involved in violent assaults and actions that appear hostile to women and 'white' Australians. *Cedar Boys* and *The Combination* add to the cultural diversity of Australian crime cinema while at the same time resonating with the prevailing social context.

Greg Dolgopolov

References

Noble, Tom (2010) 'Why We Love True Crime', *The Weekly Review*, 27 May. http://www.theweeklyreview.com.au/article-display/Why-We-Love-True-Crime/2899. Accessed 21 January 2013.

Smith, Rosalind (2008) 'Dark Places: True Crime Writing in Australia', *Journal of the Association for the Study of Australian Literature*, 8, pp. 17–30.

Animal Kingdom

Country of Origin:

Australia

Studio/Distributor:

Porchlight Films

Director:

David Michôd

Producer:

Liz Watts

Screenwriter:

David Michôd

Cinematographer:

Adam Arkapaw

Production Designer:

Jo Ford

Composer:

Antony Partos

Editor:

Luke Doolan

Duration:

112 minutes

Genres:

Crime

Drama

Cast:

Guy Pearce

Joel Edgerton

Sullivan Stapleton

Jacki Weaver

Luke Ford

Ben Mendelsohn

James Frecheville

Laura Wheelwright

Format:

35mm

Year:

2011

Synopsis

After the overdose death of his mother, teenager Joshua 'J' Cody moves in with his grandmother 'Smurf' and three uncles – all exhibiting varying degrees of psychopathy – who drag him into a terrifying criminal underworld. The film traces the slow decline of the Cody family and their associates; a decline brought about by renegade police with a grudge against the family and by Melbourne's changing criminal structures. When one of the gang members is gunned down by police, the family decides to exact revenge. When J and his uncles are dragged in for questioning by the police, Detective Lechie realizes that J is the weak link in the family. He offers J support and understanding in exchange for information. J is caught between Detective Lechie, his vicious, panicking family, and a group of corrupt cops seeking to kill him. In order to survive, J has to outwit everyone and find his place in the animal kingdom

Critique

Animal Kingdom is a true-crime thriller loosely based on the Pettingill family and the 1988 Walsh Street killings in Melbourne. The crime and the eventual downfall of the family are seen through J's (James Frecheville) naive perspective. The film is strongly resonant with the Australian true-crime classic *The Boys* (Rowan Woods, 1998) in its menacing tone and quotidian depiction of dysfunctional family dynamics that provide the context for suburban violence. It is a dark and desperate film that does not celebrate the anti-hero, or the criminal lifestyle and eschews the gaudy glamour of the television series *Underbelly* (Screentime, Network Ten, 2008–). And yet it is a stylish, stark and naturalistically suburban depiction of a crime family deeply entrenched in Melbourne's underworld coming to the end of its reign. Cinematographer Adam Arkapaw (who also shot *Snowtown* directed by Justin Kurzel in 2011) creates a darkly stylish world of cluttered interiors and frantic suburban action. It is a sophisticated and innovative take on the gangster tale exploring family and power, betrayal and survival in an unspectacular suburban jungle of crazed crooks and crooked cops.

The Codys are notorious armed robbers, but this is not a classic gangster film featuring high octane hold ups (*Money Movers* [Bruce Beresford, 1978]; *The Hard Word* [Scott Roberts, 2002]) or slapstick bank jobs (*Two Hands* [Gregor Jordan, 1999]). Instead the narrative and conventions are suburbanized with a focus on the domestic lives of the Cody clan. The armed robbery pre-history is shown in the title sequence in a series of security footage stills. Once the Codys' revenge plan is enacted and the police commence their investigations, the majority of the film becomes an intense man-on-the-run, fugitive thriller.

Animal Kingdom is structured as a zoomorphic analogy comparing the Cody clan to the animal kingdom and specifically to a lion pride that is slowly losing its power and arrogance. While J is not entirely criminally naive, he is surrounded by frightening, unpredictable beastly characters in a world where, as the film's title suggests, the survival instinct dominates any social mores or legal codes. How does he survive or adapt? The concept of the animal kingdom is explored throughout the fabric of the film and is important to understanding the transmutation of the criminal species from an established order to one defined by diversity and survival of the fittest through better adaptation and natural selection. The film studiously avoids depicting animals, but regularly features off-screen dogs barking, growling and slobbering. The Cody family is likened first to a lion pride and then to cornered animals gnashing their teeth in a desperate bid to survive a police force that has turned rogue. J is caught like a rabbit between his savage family and the paternal Detective Lechie (Guy Pearce) who offers J protection and a biology lesson in natural selection: 'Things survive because they are strong. Everything reaches an understanding.' The title is also a red herring: it is not an animal kingdom in the sense of 'everything knowing its place in the scheme of things', but one where survival creates upheaval. After having survived life on the run, J understands where he belongs and it is not with the police. When he returns home and shoots Pope (Ben Mendelsohn) – the insane former leader of the pack – it is a form of adaptation; a heritable trait in selective breeding that ensures evolution and a continuation of the species.

After winning the Jury Prize at Sundance, *Animal Kingdom* enjoyed box office success domestically grossing AU$4.9 million and taking a further AU$2.5 million internationally. *Animal Kingdom* has become one of the most successful Australian crime films of recent years reinvigorating the genre with its innovative rhythm, naturalistically disturbing characters, brooding atmosphere and unexpected plot developments.

Greg Dolgopolov

Cedar Boys

Country of Origin:

Australia

Studio/Distributor:

Templar Entertainment

Director:

Serhat Caradee

Producers:

Matthew Dabner

Jeff Purser

Ranko Markovic

Screenwriter:

Serhat Caradee

Synopsis

Tarek is a young working-class Lebanese Australian man who dreams of a better life. He is a panel beater living with his non-English speaking father and housewife mother. His brother Jamal is in jail for an unspecified charge and cannot afford an appeal. Tarek's dream is to start a business of his own, save enough money to move from Sydney's south-west – where he is constantly monitored by his parents and is the regular butt of racist jokes from his co-workers – to the eastern suburbs, and finance his brother's appeal. His friends, Nabil and Sam, also dream of better lives. Nabil works in a family business cleaning apartment blocks. Sam is a club goer and junior drug dealer, making just enough money to rent his own apartment. Driving around the city one night, Tarek spots Amy, a blonde Anglo-Australian woman walking into a bar. Attracted to her difference – a seemingly affluent 'white' inner-city woman – Tarek becomes involved with Amy, only to realize that their differences are not

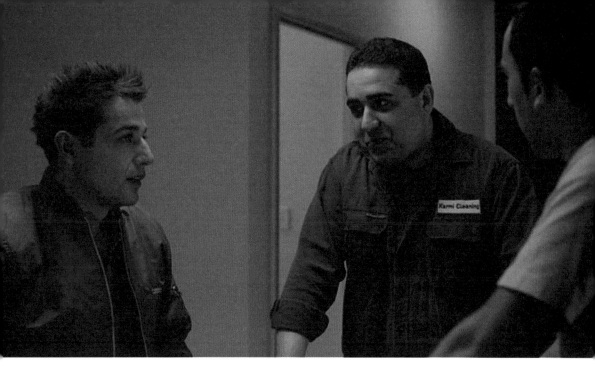

Cedar Boys
(Serhat Caradee, 2009)

Cinematographer:

Peter A. Holland

Production Designer:

Claire Granville

Composer:

Khaled Sabsabi

Editor:

Suresh Ayyar

Duration:

100 minutes

Genres:

Crime

Drama

Cast:

Les Chantery

Rachael Taylor

Bren Foster

Waddah Sari

Buddy Dannoun

Format:

35mm

Year:

2009

merely cultural. While working, Nabil suspects a drug drop at one of the apartments. Persuading Tarek to look out for him, Nabil searches the apartment and discovers a stash of drugs. The three young men are identified by the gangsters from whom they stole the drugs, with tragic consequences.

Critique

Cedar Boys is Serhat Caradee's feature film debut. Premiering at the Sydney Film Festival in 2009, the film won the Audience Award, and was nominated for other prestigious awards, including the Best Feature Film at the Inside Film Awards (popularly known as the IF Awards). Caradee was inspired by Martin Scorsese's *Mean Streets* (1973), with the desire to tell a story of 'outsiders wanting in'. With its fast-paced editing style, and Peter Holland's gritty handheld camerawork, *Cedar Boys* tells the story of those of 'Middle Eastern appearance' who struggle to move beyond ethnic stereotypes on the mean streets of Sydney. *Cedar Boys* is a crime film packed with nightclub scenes, fast cars, rap music, stacks of cash, hordes of drugs and sleazy bars, and a morality tale in which the trio's desire for success and recognition through crime fails to pay off. There is also a further element – ethnicity. The characters come from working-class immigrant families, and strive for recognition within society through unlawful acts. Their criminal acts are not purely due to inner conflict, however; rather, Caradee attempts to tell a tale where acts of crime arise from social, cultural and political circumstances and from the victimization of the characters as a result of their ethnic background.

Nevertheless, in terms of character and narrative development, rather than eliminating the ethnic stereotype that has been associated with crime over the last two decades, the film perpetuates it by projecting an apparently inevitable connection between crime and ethnicity. This is not to say that Caradee's narrative and dialogue do not attempt to challenge everyday ethnic struggles, especially in the relationship between Tarek (Les Chantery) and Amy (Rachael Taylor). The bar scene where Tarek meets Amy is cleverly packed with racial tension through Caradee's witty dialogue. Here the film-maker allows the issue being dealt with to surpass racial stereotype, mocking the prejudice and fixed misconceptions surrounding the geographical importance of Sydney's suburbia; and in particular the 'barbarian' south-west, where the majority of the population is vastly multicultural.

Yet *Cedar Boys*, and often the crime genre more generally, reduces ethnicity to crime, and crime to ethnicity. *Cedar Boys*'s director claims that the film breaks down the barriers of prejudice and typecasting through the complexity and vulnerability of the protagonists who fall into crime due to their sociocultural circumstances (Nicholson 2009). Nevertheless, Tarek's character – a vulnerable man who becomes a tragic hero in an attempt to get ahead and to escape these circumstances – is a historically familiar figure in crime films (see for example Robert Warshow's (1962) famous essay 'The Gangster as Tragic Hero'). Tarek and Nabil (Buddy Dannoun) are not portrayed as criminals, but they are destined to become so. Tarek's relationship with his parents is limited, and as such their culture is simplified. The film's handheld gritty feel allows the story to progress as a social-realist narrative, however this supposed reality does not account for the potentiality that Lebanese Australian individuals are neither villains nor victims. David Field's *The Combination*, released in the same year, follows a similar trajectory – suburban ethnic crime.

Overall, Caradee's effort in exploring Lebanese Australian culture and the issues individuals and the community face as an ethnic minority within Australian society is a unique endeavour that has rarely been undertaken in Australian cinema. But despite *Cedar Boys*'s ambition as a story, the film typically reinforces stereotypes associated with Lebanese Australian culture and insists on criminalizing ethnicity.

Batoul Amhaz

References

Nicholson, Anne Maria (2009) 'Film Aims to Break Down Stereotypes of Lebanese Youths', *ABC News* 23 July 2009.

Warshow, Robert (1962) 'The Gangster as Tragic Hero', in *The Immediate Experience: Movies, Comics, Theater, and Other Aspects of Popular Culture*, Cambridge: Harvard University Press, pp. 97–104.

The Combination

Country of Origin:

Australia

Studio/Distributor:

See Thru Films

Director:

David Field

Producer:

John Perrie

Screenwriter:

George Basha

Cinematographer:

Toby Miller

Production Designer:

Xanthe Highfield

Composer:

Labib Jammal

Editor:

Ken Sallows

Duration:

96 minutes

Genre:

Crime

Cast:

George Basha
Firass Dirani
Doris Younane
Rahel Abdulrahman
Claire Bowen
Michael Denkha

Format:

35mm

Year:

2009

Summary

In Sydney's west, Lebanese Australian John is released from prison and returns home to live with his younger brother Charlie and his mother Mary. He begins a relationship with Sydney, a young white woman, after rescuing her from sexual assault. Her parents openly disapprove of the relationship. Tensions soon arise between the brothers as Charlie's involvement in the local drug trade lures him deeper into the criminal underworld. When John discovers a cache of drugs in Charlie's bedroom he destroys it, leaving Charlie tens of thousands of dollars in debt to the dangerous drug lord, Ibo. Charlie is given a deadline to repay the money. John steps in, borrowing the money and negotiating a truce. Meanwhile, Sydney's parents offer her an ultimatum: leave John or move out of the family home. With tensions high, John struggles and ultimately fails to maintain peace on all fronts.

Critique

The Combination examines the subject of ethnicity through the lens of the crime drama. The movie effectively transposes the usual iconography, formulas and thematic concerns of the gangster film to the Lebanese Australian community and the ganglands of western Sydney. In so doing, the film-makers offer an alternative vision of a maligned ethnic minority within Australian society, one typically portrayed through the distortions of commercial television current-affairs programs focusing upon community anxieties about racial and gang warfare. Typical generic tropes common in cinematic crime are drawn upon to create a local, ethnic variation of the genre: the stock character of the gangster boss and his henchman; payback and exercises in cinematic violence; bungled drug deals; family bonds ruptured by disloyalty; and the sense of looming tragedy. However, these tropes may have been applied a little too efficiently. Although they dramatize the ugliness of racial conflict, the narrative's progression is somewhat inevitable and many of the characters are reduced to common caricatures (the ultimately cowardly gang boss, the tragic youth seduced by crime, and the idealistic Anglo love interest for the ethnic protagonist). The overall dramatic tone, a coalescence of realism and melodrama, is sometimes jarring, and the events that unfold are often improbable. But these crime conventions also allow the film-makers to make the film's more unfamiliar and nuanced racial and cultural themes more recognizable to audiences.

But perhaps most interestingly, *The Combination*'s portrayal of what is sometimes regarded as a separate world within Australian society is not based on the impression of an outsider, but is rather grounded in the personal experiences of screenwriter/actor George Basha as well as those of the young Lebanese Australian cast, many of whom are western Sydney residents and, with the exception of Firass Dirani, are not professional actors. The film also benefited from extensive informal community consultation regarding the representation of its political themes. For this reason, the film is more culturally significant than stylistically innovative, and the movie's ideas and aspirations are easier to engage with than the story itself. The humour, frankness and physical affection shared by the male characters sets *The Combination* apart from many other films in the predominantly masculine local crime genre. In their interactions with each other, and their Lebanese friends and family, the two brothers (particularly Charlie) partake in a distinctly emotional and non-patriotic form of mateship. This is a relatively novel contribution to the representation of masculinity in Australian cinema; one that builds upon a 'softer' and more diverse representation of masculinity developed since the 1990s.

The delicate treatment of the 2005 Cronulla riots, a key event in contemporary history, is a thematic undercurrent to gang warfare in the narrative. Different characters separately watch news reports of the riots and react internally and individually. The characters are united through their bewildering experiences of events that are beyond their control yet which have deep personal impacts. These current affairs are touched upon rather than laboured; playing out in the background of scenes (even as the subject becomes thematically dominant). As such, the film functions not merely as a 'reply' to specific race-related incidents, but as an effort by Lebanese Australians to tell their own 'self-representative' stories and as a distinctive contribution to Australian film culture by its Lebanese Australian screenwriter. Like *The Jammed* (Dee McLachlan, 2007) and *Jindabyne* (Ray Lawrence, 2006), *The Combination* uses the conventions of the crime film and the above narrative devices to explore marginalized communities. Through the interpersonal relationships of John, Charlie, Mary and 'whitebread' Sydney, *The Combination* shows how manifold external cultural and political concerns manifest in the identities of individuals and communities.

Lauren Carroll Harris

Snowtown

Country of Origin:

Australia

Studio/Distributor:

The Warp X Australia

Director:

Justin Kurzel

Producers:

Anna McLeish

Sarah Shaw

Screenwriters:

Shaun Grant

Justin Kurzel

Synopsis

Life is BMX bikes, ciggies and boredom in a junk-filled backyard for 16-year-old Jamie. He lives with his strung-out mother Elizabeth and younger brothers in an impoverished Adelaide suburb where the only fun is jousting with shopping trolleys. His mother's boyfriend is a pervert who takes naked photographs of Jamie and his brothers while his mother is playing the pokies. She lashes out with hopeless anger when she finds out. The police are unwilling to act, but a cheery neighbour, John Bunting, who despises paedophiles and homosexuals, helps organize a community response. With John's smiling support Jamie is able to take revenge on his abuser. As the neighbourhood campaign to clean up the suburb gathers momentum, John gradually becomes the father-figure that Jamie and his family so desperately need. John introduces Jamie to driving, guns and his hatred of child abusers and homosexuals. Jamie is seduced by John's philosophies and begins to follow his lead, eventually joining his small group of vigilantes. But as the

Cinematographer:

Adam Arkapaw

Production Designer:

Fiona Crombie

Composer:

Jed Kurzel

Editor:

Veronika Jenet

Duration:

119 minutes

Genres:

True crime
Psychological horror

Cast:

Lucas Pittaway
Daniel Henshall
David Walker
Bob Adriaens
Louise Harris
Frank Cwiertniak
Matthew Howard
Marcus Howard
Anthony Groves
Richard Green
Beau Gosling
Aaron Viergever

Format:

35mm

Year:

2011

gruesome extent of John's campaign is revealed, Jamie suddenly realizes his own entrapment. He is now caught up in the heinous actions of the vigilante gang and is drawn deeper and deeper into John's world of hatred, torture and murder.

Critique

Justin Kurzel's elegant, low-budget debut feature film won the Audience Award at the Adelaide International Film Festival and was awarded Special Mention by the President of the Critics' Week Jury at Cannes in 2011. *Snowtown* was nominated for ten Australian Academy of Cinema and Television Arts (formerly the Australian Film Institute) Awards in 2012, winning six including Best Direction. The film was well-received critically and earned more than AU$1 million at the local box office.

Snowtown is a true-crime film that traces the origins and context of the infamous Bodies-in-Barrels murders that took place in South Australia between 1992 and 1999. The murder and torture spree is considered to be Australia's worst serial killing with eleven grisly deaths. A brilliant study of the dangerous implications of boredom and the harsh realities of social disadvantage, the true horror of *Snowtown* is the seeming normality of the violence and casual perversions. The horror stems from the bleakness of suburban life in a welfare-dependent housing estate. Drab monotony and the tedium of hopelessness (thematic terrain also explored in Rolf de Heer's *Bad Boy Bubby* [1993] and *The King is Dead!* [2012]) mark the lives of the underclass of Salisbury North. Shot on location in the same suburbs where the murders occurred and employing a cast of locals, *Snowtown* is a stylish, social-realist tale of a young man and his manipulative father figure who is a serial killer. The film examines the social and community context that gave rise to the killing spree through the vulnerable eyes of Jamie Vlassakis.

John Bunting, as portrayed by Daniel Henshall, is not a typically evil character. He appears as an affable saviour to this disadvantaged community who are seeking to protect their children from violence and abuse. He is focused, intelligent, resourceful, a charismatic speaker and a good cook who sees value in a family sitting down together for dinner and eating healthy food. Ironically, this good natured patriarch is also a brutal sadist who despises homosexuals and those he considers 'perverts'. He tortures and murders his victims, concealing their disappearances by forcing them to leave telephone messages saying that they have left town, before disposing of their bodies in barrels filled with acid. The film presents a complex portrait of a dangerously charming man who justifies murder through a skewed sense of child protection. By the end of the film, however, it is clear that Bunting and his henchman Wagner (Aaron Viergever) are looking for any excuse to kill. While there may have initially been a warped sense of purpose behind the killings, as the narrative unfolds, the torture and mutilation is increasingly driven by a sadistic lust for power and domination.

Snowtown is a serious, methodical serial killer film that surprisingly avoids easy moral condemnations. It examines all eleven murders in detail from the perspective of Bunting's young protégé (Lucas

Pittaway). Himself a victim of abuse, the real Jamie Vlassakis would become the Crown's key witness at the trial.

The socialist-realist cinematic tradition that *Snowtown* engages with suggests that the perpetrators of the killings are as much victims as the people they callously torture, and all are victims of their environment and inherited social disadvantage. However, director Kurzel tempers this assessment with a highly stylish approach that aestheticizes the bleak landscape and finds moments of great beauty punctuating scenes of violence and dread. Adam Arkapaw's cinematography mixes the brutality and dreariness of the suburbs with moments of dreamlike, arty exposition and lush gentle landscapes.

While it is not a horror film, despite the horrors of the events, there are detailed portrayals of the techniques employed by Bunting and his accomplices. The scene in which Jamie's half-brother, Troy (Anthony Groves), is tortured is extraordinary in its length and brutality, and in the lack of fetishization of the pain and gore. Jamie is finally transformed from an observer to a murderer, albeit to end Troy's suffering. The intimate close-up of Bunting, an expression of ferocious concentration on his face as he administers pain in controlled bursts, provides a fascinating insight into the workings of a sadist that sees torture as scientific inquiry.

Snowtown is an extraordinarily difficult film on many levels. Many of the victim's families are still alive, and at the time of writing court suppression orders were still in place. Actors were drawn from the community where the murders occurred and some commentators have condemned the use of taxpayer's money to fund a film that glorifies the murders. It is a powerful and ethically complex film that highlights the ambiguity of evil in the naturalistic depiction of Australia's worst serial killer.

Greg Dolgopolov

Two Hands

Country of Origin:

Australia

Studio/Distributor:

CML Films

Meridian Films

Director:

Gregor Jordan

Producer:

Marian Macgowan

Screenwriter:

Gregor Jordan

Director of Photography:

Malcolm McCulloch

Synopsis

Eighteen-year-old Jimmy is a strip club spruiker and aspiring criminal living and working in Sydney's Kings Cross. On the same day that he lands his first job as a courier for crime boss Pando, he meets Alex, the girl of his dreams. Jimmy's good fortune quickly turns bad, however, when street kids steal the $10,000 he is meant to deliver for Pando while he takes an ill-advised swim at Bondi Beach. To make matters worse, the car Jimmy borrows from Acko – Pando's right-hand man – to make the delivery is also stolen. Desperate for a quick score to pay them back, Jimmy manages to line up a job on a bank robbery. But before the robbery takes place he is apprehended by Pando and his gang. With supernatural help, Jimmy escapes, but he must still repay his debts.

Critique

Two Hands was written and directed by Gregor Jordan, whose short film *Swinger* won the Tropicana Short Film Festival in 1995.

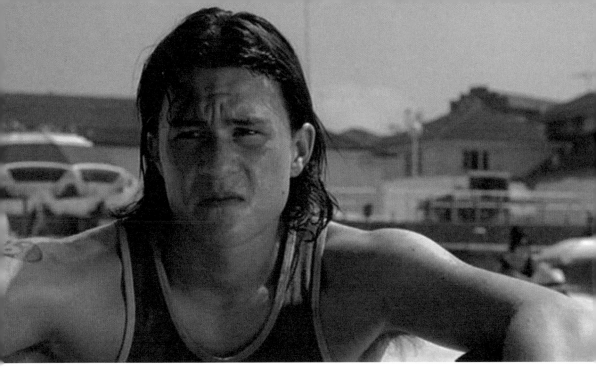

Two Hands
(Gregor Jordan, 1999)

Production Designer:

Steven Jones-Evans

Composer:

Cezary Skubiszewski

Editor:

Lee Smith

Duration:

103 minutes

Genre:

Crime

Cast:

Heath Ledger
Bryan Brown
Rose Byrne
Susie Porter
David Field

Format:

35mm

Year:

1999

Jordan then went on to win the Jury Prize at Cannes later the same year. He followed up his success with the development of *Two Hands*, which Jordan describes as 'a black comedy gangster film with a supernatural subplot' (Urban n.d.). The writer/director won two Australian Film Institute (AFI) Awards for the film: one for Best Direction, the second for Best Screenplay.

Two Hands features a stellar cast that includes a young Heath Ledger in the role of the not-so-bright Jimmy, the renowned Australian actor Bryan Brown as Kings Cross crime boss Pando, and a 19-year-old Rose Byrne as the country girl with a heart of gold, Alex. Ledger would go on from *Two Hands* to begin a meteoric rise in Hollywood (although he briefly returned to Australia to star in Jordan's *Ned Kelly* in 2003). In 2005, he was nominated for an Academy Award for Best Actor for his role in *Brokeback Mountain* (Ang Lee, 2005), and in 2009 he was posthumously nominated and subsequently won the Academy Award for Best Supporting Actor for his role as the Joker in *The Dark Knight* (Christopher Nolan, 2008). Ledger and his fellow cast members create a surprisingly believable set of characters for the larger-than-life story world of *Two Hands*.

Inspired primarily by gangster films such as *The Godfather* (Francis Ford Coppola, 1972) and *Goodfellas* (Martin Scorsese, 1990), *Two Hands* also owes debts to Shakespeare and George A Romero. The film opens with direct-to-camera narration by a ghost who is digging his way out of hell with what is later revealed to be the intention of helping his younger brother, Jimmy, to wise up. Jordan reveals that the character was inspired by the Greek chorus of *Henry V* and visually patterned after the zombies of Romero's *Night of the Living Dead* released in 1968 (Schwartz 1999: 5). Having the film open with narration by a character from beyond the grave gives *Two Hands* a unique magic-realist dimension that is sadly underdeveloped in the film. It is also interesting to note that the non-linear narrative device employed at the outset of the film is similar to that used in *Fight Club* (David Fincher, 1999), released in the same year as *Two Hands*. *Two Hands* opens with Jimmy facing his seemingly imminent death at the hands of Pando and his men, which is then followed by a flashback that returns viewers to the beginning of the action to explain how Jimmy had arrived at this fate.

The dark comedic tone of *Two Hands* is one of the film's highlights. Indeed, there are several scenes in the film that are genuinely funny. For instance, the bank robbery that goes wrong, or the Tarantino-esque final shoot-out featuring the second instance of a gun jamming that creates a laugh-out-loud moment in a highly tense and fatal scene. In addition, there is the motif of the family-man/criminal, shown planning bank robberies or even murders in the presence of his children: Pando plots his revenge on Jimmy while doing origami with his preschool-aged son. In another scene, after the heist with Jimmy, one of the bank robber's children accidently fires a shotgun while money from the robbery is being counted. The juxtaposition of the domestic and 'professional' lives of the criminals creates an interesting and humorous counterpoint to the violence and darker themes of the film. It is also an example of the film's prescience, considering the HBO television series *The Sopranos* (David Chase, HBO, 1999–2007), which is built around a similar concept, was in its first season when *Two Hands* was released. In fact, this domestic/criminal juxtaposition, along with the anachronic plotting and magic-realist elements, points to the fact that *Two Hands* was well attuned to the *fin de siècle* zeitgeist in which it emerged.

Matthew Campora

References

Urban, Andrew L (n.d.) 'Two Hands On Location', *Urban Cinefile*, http://www.urbancinefile.com.au/home/view. asp?a=1302&s=features. Accessed 3 April 2013.

Gillard, Garry (2007) *Ten Types of Australian Film*, Perth: Murdoch University.

Schwartz, Larry (1999) 'Handy Business', *Sunday Age*, 25 July, p.5.

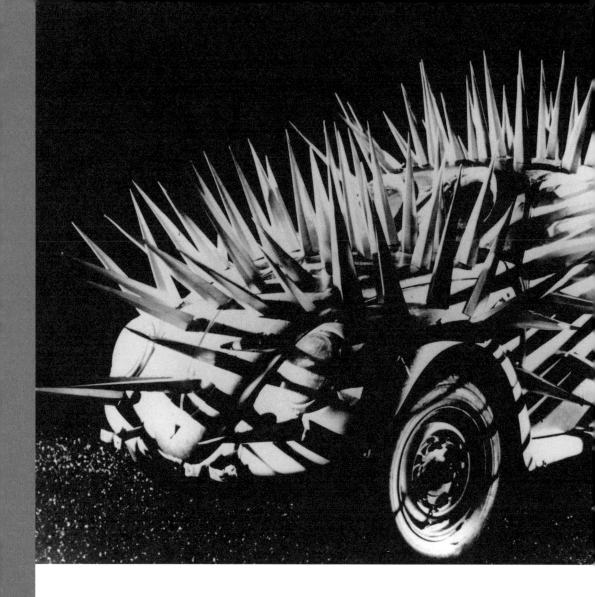

AUSTRALIAN
GOTHIC

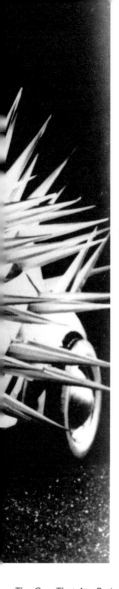

The Cars That Ate Paris
(Peter Weir, 1974).
© Kobal Collection

*Mos depth /
longest
mode in
Aussie cinema*

The aesthetic, thematic and textual nexus which constitutes the Australian Gothic can claim to represent the most persistent, fertile, articulate and therefore significant trend within Australian cinema over the past forty or more years. Yet at the same time it must also be conceded that a critical consensus on or indeed a working definition of what constitutes the Gothic as a recognizable style, narrative consistency or tonal predisposition within Australian film-making remains contestable and elusive. Like late classical *film noir*, the viewer knows it when s/he sees it, but other viewers see it in something else, somewhere else. Just as the violence, visual style, wit and cynicism of noir can be seen to grow from, through and amidst the impetuous gangster films of America in the 1930s, the paranoia and pessimism of post-classical and Cold War 1950s Hollywood, and all the in-between shades of crime, detective and psychological 'melodrama' made in the 1940s, so Australian Gothic infiltrates many genres (or 'types' to acknowledge Garry Gillard's highly pragmatic categorizations) of the national cinema (Gillard 2007). As a result, though Gothic itself cannot always be easily defined, its universal occurrence has come to define Australian film-making.

How then is this category with multiple definitions and identifications to be discussed? Assertions of textual, textural and thematic consistency characterizing the malleable canon of *film noir* run into similar difficulties, and can therefore prove useful guides. How does the summary definition of that category, as metropolitan, down-beat, ideologically-vexed and expressionistically-styled B-picture cope with the Caribbean settings of *Lady from Shanghai* (Orson Welles, 1947), the A-list stars of *Double Indemnity* (Billy Wilder, 1944) or the arch, screwball-comedic dialogue of *The Big Sleep* (Howard Hawks, 1946)? In essence, by acknowledging a diverse contemporary production context on the one hand, and a retrospective, critically-imposed unity on the other. The Gothic requires a similar open-mindedness and attention to detail to be positioned and appreciated as a significant element in the narratives, motifs and tendencies of a considerable cross-section of Australian cinema. This does not mean circumscribing a delimited and exclusive canon, or conversely expanding a category to inclusive meaninglessness, but rather engaging in constructive critical thinking

Definition

about the frequent, coherent inclusion of uncanny and unnerving content, in Australian films both inside and outside the accepted boundaries of horror cinema as an international commodity. It is necessary therefore to consider the Gothic as a conglomeration of tonal, thematic and stylistic elements, which both articulate aspects of nationally relevant narratives for home audiences and distinguish the brand of Australian horror overseas.

Although the Gothic carries associations of horror, not all horror films (Australian or otherwise) deserve the label of 'Gothic'. Equally, the Gothic inhabits and inflects films, often only in brief and in detail, which conventional criticism places readily in other categories. That viewers thus form and ascribe the filmic category is not an inappropriate evaluative act but a recognition of the films' cumulative cultural significance in the consciousness of the target audience. Australian Gothic explores significant cultural interactions with several key imagistic and ideological concerns: troubled relationships with the land and landscape; problematic evaluations of the past; and individual conflicts with the pressures of authority and conformity. These structuring principles permeate Australian films which might otherwise be placed in myriad generic categories (horror, thriller, science fiction, crime drama), and which are consequently stretched and enriched by the uneasy, uncanny and unpalatable elements with which the Gothic endows them.

The Gothic emerges with the resumption of feature production, with some of the first productions of the 1970s laying down the landmarks around which later films are orientated. *Walkabout* (Nicolas Roeg, 1971) and *Wake in Fright* (Ted Kotcheff, 1971), despite their non-Australian directors, initiate the othering of the landscape and the anxiety-inducement of the remote, outback town which come to characterize so many subsequent films. The small town as inverted idyll, as trap and site of secret perversion becomes a staple of the Gothic, concretized in examples such as *The Cars That Ate Paris* (Peter Weir, 1974) and extended to quasi-westerns like *Shame* (Steve Jodrell, 1988) and science fiction films such as *Incident at Raven's Gate* (Rolf de Heer, 1989). Outsiders straying into the rural interior encounter only hostility, secrecy and traumatic experience, forcing a revaluation of their identity, and that of the country itself. The continent's interior, both in the acculturated form of the rural, isolated town and the unadulterated natural form of the vast uninhabited wilderness, at once hides, facilitates and inspires deviant behaviour, or confronts characters with adversaries in the flora and fauna which defy human logic, technology and strength. These traits and givens in the Gothic's organization and articulation of tainted relationships with the land persist into recent examples such as *Rogue* (Greg McLean, 2007) and *Black Water* (Andrew Traucki and David Nerlich, 2007), just as *Wolf Creek* (Greg McLean, 2005) recalled but updated the rural–urban divide of *Wake in Fright* and *Shame*. Discernible in these examples is a key to the Gothic's narrative patterning, in the hero's gathering awareness of the secret malevolence of paternalistic authority. In turn this realization entails the defamiliarization of the world and the values which that authority upholds. Part of the problematization of heroic status and action that these films emphasize is a recognition of the inability to act justly, or more often simply an inability to act at all, within the prejudicial social reality which this debased form of authority maintains.

If the countryside and the country town are discovered to be false idylls and fallen paradises, the portrayals of Australian cities and suburbs import the Gothic and its disconcerting realizations to urban citizens and situations. In Gothic portrayals, it is the capacity of the outback and its flora and fauna to confound logic and categorization (in *Walkabout*); of the rural landscape to secrete or indeed foster perversion and transgression (in *Cars* and *Shame*) and of the modern urban environment to obfuscate individual or institutional iniquity, social inequality and even national shame, in examples such as *The Last Wave* (Peter Weir, 1977), *Heatwave* (Phillip Noyce, 1982) and *Georgia* (Ben Lewin, 1988). Like *Wolf Creek*'s channelling of the reverberations of notorious crimes, both Noyce's and Lewin's films probe past lives and mysteries in semi-fictional scenarios. *The Last Wave* in particular represents the potential of the Gothic to wed generic materials to contemporary, national issues and universal art-cinema dilemmas. On one level a science fiction film (with its intimations of imminent apocalypse), it is also an exploration of individual, existential breakdown (depicting a Sydney lawyer's transformative encounter with Aboriginal defendants in a murder case). The landscape maintains its Gothic significance in this film, despite its metropolitan setting, because of the fictional, metaphorical location of Aboriginal tribal sites literally beneath the modern Australian city. Bringing the cultural-historical repressed into the heart of modern urban Australia, and making its resurgence indivisible from the spiritual, emotional and professional crisis of the protagonist, are this film's most eloquent manifestations of the Gothic's fascination with the convergence of notions of the past, valuations of the land and understandings of the self. Suburbia's compromises and covert activities have received treatment again more recently in *Beautiful* (Dean O'Flaherty, 2009), an Australian response to the depiction of a family's or community's undercurrents in *American Beauty* (Sam Mendes, 1999) and *Donnie Darko* (Richard Kelly, 2001).

Forty years on, the Gothic still permeates, complicates and articulates the themes of Australia's cinema and the work of its film-makers, even in Hollywood, as in *The Truman Show* (Peter Weir, 1998) or *Hearts in Atlantis* (Scott Hicks, 2001). The Gothic version of horror in Australian cinema maintains a distinctive, recognizable flavour, which is all the more welcome as an evolving, expressive continuity when, in comparison, contemporary American horror has only the acid-reflux of recapitulative remakes of seminal films of the 1970s. When newer Gothic films invoke their forbears, it is generally for recognition of their updating and extension of familiar patterns and plots in the light of persisting or renewed relevance (for example, *Wolf Creek* and *Jindabyne* [Ray Lawrence, 2006] reuse and reappraise the conceptions of rural towns and outback masculinity found first in films of the revival). The continued presence of Gothic traits in Australian films in the second decade of the twenty-first century underlines their uninterrupted importance to cultural expression and debate, post-Mabo, post-multiculturalism and post-reconciliation, and on for as long as the same searching questions need to be asked of Australian identities.

Jonathan Rayner

Reference

Gillard, Garry (2007) *Ten Types of Australian Film*, Perth: Murdoch University.

Bad Boy Bubby

Country of Origin:

Australia

Studio/Distributor:

Bubby Productions
Fandango
South Australian Film Corp.
AFFC

Director:

Rolf de Heer

Producers:

Rolf de Heer
Giorgio Draskovic
Domenico Procacci

Screenwriter:

Rolf de Heer

Director of Photography:

Ian Jones

Production Designer:

Mark Abbott

Composer:

Graham Tardif

Editor:

Suresh Ayyar

Duration:

114 minutes

Genres:

Comedy
Drama

Cast:

Nicholas Hope
Claire Benito
Ralph Cotterill
Carmel Johnson

Format:

35mm

Year:

1993

Synopsis

Bubby is a 30-year-old infant, who has been hidden from the world in a filthy urban refuge by his ageing mother. She holds him in an abusive and incestuous thrall with violent punishments and tales of the lethal 'poison' of the world outside. After unwittingly murdering her and the degenerate priest who may be his father, Bubby emerges into the world as an impressionable innocent. His random encounters with an atheistic scientist, the Salvation Army and a rock band reveal the full range of human potential for violence, generosity, egotism, altruism, zealotry and love. He gains popular cultural celebrity for the words he spouts alongside the rock band's music, which amalgamate the observations, catchphrases and slogans he has overheard on his travels. He appears to meet the same woman, Angel, repeatedly during his odyssey. After a fateful encounter with her judgmental, religious parents, Bubby starts a family with Angel.

Critique

As an allegory of processes of colonization, immigration and multicultural integration, and a rewriting of the story of Kasper Hauser, *Bad Boy Bubby* epitomizes the fundamental and comprehensive defamiliarization of the social structure and individual's subjection within it, of which the Gothic perspective is capable. The feckless male's entrapment within an adult world complicated by rules, relationships and cultural difference had previously received a blackly comedic Gothic treatment in *Death in Brunswick* (John Ruane, 1990). Where *Shame* (Steve Jodrell, 1988) recruits Gothic materials to accompany realist gender politics within a framework of western and thriller motifs, Ruane's film mixes them with broad humour and occasionally gross spectacle, while ironically accommodating Australian cinema's contemporary agenda for positive multicultural representation. Even amidst its comedy and redemptive cross-cultural romance, Ruane's film depicts an older, conservative Anglo-Australian generation continuing to blight the potential of a younger and more tolerant generation. Cast adrift in a world he has been taught contains only poison, Bubby responds to every encounter as either a temporary blessing or immediate danger: he is the blank canvas on which every selfish prejudice, charitable gift and societal expectation is imprinted. He is equally unable to understand why a wealthy middle-aged woman might want his company, or why a working-class man should want to cut down a tree. Yet his freedom and ultimate self-realization are dependent, like those of Ruane's hero, on the forcible removal of a malignant parental presence. Having been exhorted to 'think God out of existence', Bubby achieves a messianic status, more indicative of his followers' superficiality and desperation than his potential as a prophet. While his impressionability and mimicry of everyone he meets may be excusable, his audiences copy his words and mirror his dress in an empty, commodified display of every vain search for meaning. Like Ray Lawrence's *Bliss* (1985), de Heer's film

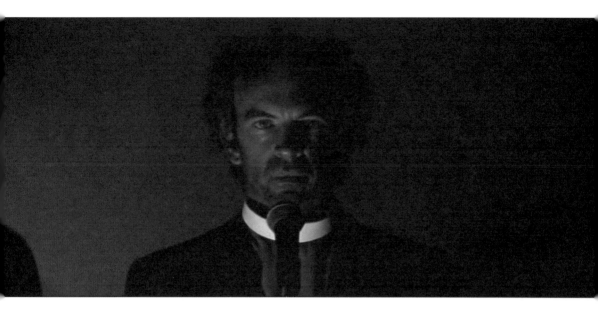

Bad Boy Bubby
(Rolf de Heer, 1993)

appears on the surface to be a one-off, an ambitious digression in the style and scope of Australian cinema. Yet they are not only kin beneath the skin, in their active confrontation of and challenges to their audiences, they are also illustrative of the pervasiveness of the Gothic scrutiny of societal structures. In bridging popular genres and eroding distinctions between them, the Gothic can also assume, as *Bliss* and *Bubby* demonstrate, the aspiration and capacity of art cinema.

Jonathan Rayner

Bliss

Country of Origin:
Australia
Studio/Distributor:
Window III Productions
Director:
Ray Lawrence
Producer:
Anthony Buckley

Synopsis

Harry Joy is an apparently contented family man, with a wife and children and a job in advertising. In reality his wife is having an affair, and his daughter is addicted to the drugs his son peddles. When he suffers a near-fatal heart attack, Harry has a terrifying vision of his own damnation, and of the hellishness of human existence even before death and final judgement. After recovering in hospital, he embarks upon a series of tests to reveal the truth of his family's existence, and becomes convinced he must change his lifestyle. He becomes infatuated with a young woman who leads a pure and natural life away from the consumerism and self-destructiveness of the city. Although Harry wishes to leave his former life behind

Screenwriters:

Ray Lawrence
Peter Carey, adapted from the
novel *Bliss*, by Peter Carey
(1981)

Cinematographer:

Paul Murphy

Art Director:

Owen Paterson

Composer:

Peter Best

Editor:

Wayne LeClos

Duration:

112 minutes

Genres:

Gothic comedy
Drama

Cast:

Barry Otto
Lynette Curran
Helen Jones
Gia Carides
Miles Buchanan

Format:

35mm

Year:

1985

to embrace a more natural lifestyle, his wife and family cannot,
and Harry loses everything. Retreating into the forest and growing
flowers, he takes years to woo back the women he loves.

Critique

An adaptation from Peter Carey's novel, Ray Lawrence's first feature
defies description in its mixing of satiric and horrific genres, its
subjective and objective narration, its self-reflexivity, awkward
black comedy and final gauche environmentalism. Although *Bliss's*
deliberate stylistic oddity underwrites its art-cinema credentials as
much as its overtly spiritual and ecological concerns, its Gothicism,
at its most pronounced in the earlier parts of the film, portrays the
protagonist's burgeoning consciousness of his parlous metaphysical
state and elucidates these very thematic concerns. Harry's
experiments to establish either his sudden madness in the real world
or his sanity in a newly-recognized hell condense the same vertiginous
fears which afflict the protagonists of *The Cars That Ate Paris* (Peter
Weir, 1974), *Summerfield* (Ken Hannam, 1977), *Shame* (Steve Jodrell,
1988) and other examples of the Gothic, when the world's veil slips
and the true nature of a debased and debasing existence is revealed.
The psychological trauma of Harry's revelation stands in contrast to
the banality of the faults and disillusionments which it uncovers: his
son is not an aspiring doctor but a mercenary drug dealer, and his
daughter a drug addict; his wife is unfaithful in a workmanlike fashion
with his business partner. Yet these disclosures are made apparent in
bizarrely self-conscious scenes: the son appearing in a Nazi arm band;
the adulterous couple having sex in a restaurant; the wife's guilt being
exposed by a repulsive manifestation of live fish. The subversion of
suburban normalcy which the film essays in its first half is therefore
on a par with *Cars's* dark parody of modern economics, which shows
the town's doctor wielding a power-drill bearing the red cross, and
a hillside of wrecked cars arranged like a graveyard. Although *Bliss*
may appear quite unlike any contemporary or subsequent Australian
film in its stylistic and tonal variation, and particularly in the way in
which it recovers from Harry's personal and familial apocalypse to
offer peace and transcendence, it is comparable with the surreal
exploration of America's underside which is undertaken in the near-
contemporary *Blue Velvet* (David Lynch, 1985). In comparison with
Lynch's later films, which have maintained the stylistic oddity, generic
hybridity and confrontation with audience expectation exhibited by
Blue Velvet, Lawrence's other features (*Lantana* [2001] and *Jindabyne*
[2006]) might appear to fit more comfortably within the contexts of
international art cinema and realism, but closer scrutiny reveals even
these highly respected films' tendency towards *Bliss's* Gothic themes
and nightmarish inflections. *Lantana's* ensemble examination of adult
relationships is grounded, like *Picnic at Hanging Rock* (Peter Weir,
1975), in a disappearance which defies explanation, and *Jindabyne*,
like *Bliss*, turns on the disorientating revelation of unbearable truths
for individuals, families and communities.

Jonathan Rayner

Celia

Country of Origin:

Australia

Studio/Distributor:

Seon Film Productions

Director:

Ann Turner

Producers:

Gordon Glenn

Timothy White

Screenwriter:

Ann Turner

Cinematographer:

Geoffrey Simpson

Production Designer:

Peta Lawson

Composer:

Chris Neal

Editor:

Ken Sallows

Duration:

102 minutes

Genres:

Gothic fantasy

Horror

Cast:

Rebecca Smart

Nicholas Eadie

Victoria Longley

Mary-Anne Fahey

William Zappa

Alexander Hutchinson

Format:

35mm

Year:

1988

Synopsis

Melbourne, the 1950s: Celia Carmichael lives with her parents and her paternal grandmother. She is deeply affected by the fairy-tale story of evil creatures called the 'Hobyahs'. Her Cold War childhood is overtaken by a series of arbitrary, concatenating and transformative events. Her grandmother dies; the Tanners, a young couple with left-wing beliefs, move in next door; and the ownership of pet rabbits is outlawed because of an agricultural crisis caused by wild rabbits. Simultaneously Celia witnesses a series of increasingly disturbing events: her father destroys his mother's books and papers because of the embarrassment her Communist sympathies caused him in childhood; Celia's pet rabbit is tortured by her cousin, and then forcibly taken away from her (by her uncle, a policeman) along with all domestic rabbits in line with government policy; Celia's father is sexually attracted to the new female neighbour and tries to blackmail her when he discovers her political beliefs and causes her husband to lose his job. Dynamized by these injustices, Celia starts to act. With her mother's help and despite her father's opposition, Celia campaigns for the release of the pet rabbits, writing directly to the premier of Victoria, Henry Bolte. When her rabbit dies in the local zoo, she vows vengeance on her uncle.

Critique

As a Gothic evocation of Australia's Cold War history, *Celia* taps the same vein of institutionalized injustice which the near contemporary *Ground Zero* (Michael Pattinson and Bruce Myles, 1987) explores in plot-driven conspiracy-thriller fashion. Where Pattinson's film treats an old family mystery as the stimulus for a retrospective and revelatory investigation of a shameful chapter of Australia's past, Turner's offers a fictional narrative at once historical and symbolic, a mid-twentieth century version of the allegorical Gothic to match *Picnic at Hanging Rock*'s (Peter Weir, 1975) nineteenth-century period-piece horror. On the surface, Celia's characterization may appear to fit with countless horror depictions of preternaturally perceptive children, only half understanding the vicissitudes of adult motives and actions, but answering them with a ruthless natural justice. The ancient fairy tale of *The Hobyahs* (collected in Jacobs 1894) with which she becomes obsessed (carrying its warnings of nightmarish creatures threatening domestic security and adults failing to heed portents of doom) stands as both a parallel to the naivety and paranoia of Cold War prejudices, and as an uncanny warning to the adult-like child that your enemies might well share your home. Celia's gang war with a bullying cousin replicates in the childhood realm the strong-arming and blackmail her father levels at Alice and Evan Tanner, and his own wife, but both reflect in miniature on the Cold War prejudices and conservative crackdown for which the rabbit purging itself is the most pertinent metaphor. The little girl's whimsical treatment of her rabbit's incarceration at the local zoo as politically motivated imprisonment ('Please release my rabbit – she's innocent') simply underlines how Celia herself, and in fact (in an echo of *Shame* [Steve Jodrell, 1988]) all the female characters in Turner's film are political prisoners, victims of oppression and in some cases activists and avengers. The compact between mother and daughter to circumvent politicized masculine control may appear as an anachronistic outpacing of the Cold War setting, but it establishes Celia as the representative of the next generation (after her grandmother in the 1930s and her mother in the 1950s) ready to confront chauvinism and political conservatism in the 1960s and 1970s. The film's Gothic elements then, in place in an uncomfortably scrutinized past, speak to both the historical and allegorized injustices, and the real and fictive losses of innocence.

Jonathan Rayner

References

Jacobs, Joseph (eds) (1894) *More English Fairy Tales*, London: D.Nutt.

The Piano

Country of Origin:

Australia/New Zealand/France

Studio/Distributor:

CiBy 2000
Jan Chapman Productions

Director:

Jane Campion

Producer:

Jan Chapman

Screenwriter:

Jane Campion

Cinematographer:

Stuart Dryburgh

Production Designer:

Andrew McAlpine

Composer:

Michael Nyman

Editor:

Veronika Jenet

Duration:

121 minutes

Genres:

Period romance
Melodrama

Synopsis

In the 1850s, Ada, a Scotswoman who has chosen to be mute since the age of six, arrives with her young daughter, Flora in Aotearoa (New Zealand) as a mail-order bride for landowner Stewart. She brings her primary means of expression, her piano, but Stewart refuses to haul it across the untamed bush back to his home. Stewart's Pakeha (European New Zealanders) estate manager, Baines arranges for the piano to be brought to his home in a trade with Stewart for more land. Baines then makes a 'bargain' of his own; Ada can have the piano back if she visits him, one visit for each of the piano's black keys. Stewart, who has not yet consummated his marriage with Ada, spies her having sex with Baines and becomes increasingly jealous of their intimacy. Ada gives Flora a piano key with a note to give to Baines, but she instead gives it to Stewart. Infuriated, Stewart brutally chops off one of Ada's fingers, and forces Flora to give it to Baines as a warning of what he will do if they meet again. It is decided that Ada, Flora, Baines and the piano will return to Scotland, but Ada has other plans.

Critique

Jane Campion made *The Piano* as a way to come to grips with being a part of colonial culture, as well as to explore female eroticism:

> I belong to a colonial culture and I had to invent my own fiction. I wanted to speak of the relationship between men and women, of the complex character of love and of eroticism, but also of the repression of sexuality. (Quoted in Wexman 1999: 105)

Notwithstanding the overt emphasis on sexuality, the film adopts more of a feminine gaze and at times a Victorian sensibility. Sexuality exudes even when little skin is shown, such as the scene

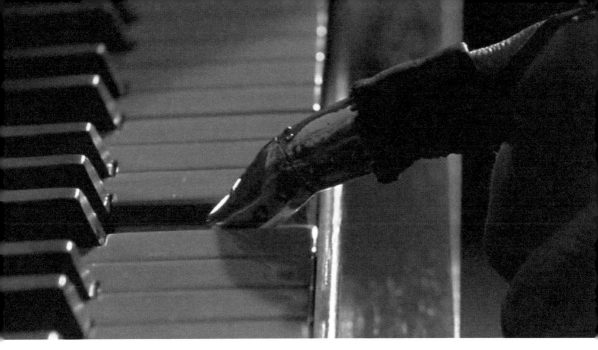

The Piano
(Jane Campion, 1993)

Cast:

Holly Hunter
Harvey Keitel
Sam Neill
Anna Paquin

Format:

35 mm

Year:

1993

when Baines (Harvey Keitel) peers at the tiny hole in Ada's (Holly Hunter) stocking, his first small glimpse of her bare skin.

Campion likened the film to a nineteenth-century novel, and credits Emily Brontë and Emily Dickinson as her primary literary inspirations. The film seems to combine elements of two of Campion's earlier films, the poetry of *Sweetie* (1989) and the narrative of *An Angel at My Table* (1990). Inspired by Roman Polanski's short film *Two Men and a Wardrobe* (1958), Campion also wanted to make a film centred around a large object (Wexman 1999: 114). Besides the attention to a female protagonist dealing with some sort of mental illness or trauma (what caused Ada's decision to become mute?), another recurring Campion motif is that of outdoor female urination (found in *Peel*, *Sweetie* and most memorably in *Holy Smoke* [1999]). Here it is not to emphasize the humiliation of her protagonists, but rather Aunt Morag's hypocrisy of criticizing Ada's piano playing as being improper because it is not 'plain and true', all the while her servants try to cover up her embarrassing alfresco behaviour with blankets shielding her, afterwards covering her urine with dirt like a cat.

In her first film, Anna Paquin (Flora) won several awards, including the 1994 Academy Award for Best Actress in a Supporting Role. The film's stars were arguably at their creative peaks; Hunter (who is an accomplished pianist) also won an Academy Award (for Best Actress in a Leading Role), starred in *The Firm* (Sydney Pollack, 1993) and won an Emmy for a made-for-TV film, *The Positively*

True Adventures of the Alleged Texas Cheerleader-Murdering Mom (Michael Ritchie, 1993). Sam Neill (Stewart) achieved stardom in *Jurassic Park* (Steven Spielberg, 1993), and Keitel had made *Bad Lieutenant* (Abel Ferrara, 1992), *Sister Act* (Emile Ardolino, 1992) and *Reservoir Dogs* (Quentin Tarantino, 1992) the previous year. (Keitel would return to work with Campion later in the decade, producing a memorable performance in *Holy Smoke*.) *The Piano* won the Palme d'Or at Cannes, making Campion the first female director to win the award. Miramax picked up the film for US distribution, where it was a success among critics and audiences. Besides Paquin's and Hunter's Oscars, Campion won the Academy Award for Screenplay Written Directly for the Screen. It was also nominated for five others, including Best Picture.

The Piano's reception revealed a diversity of interpretations of the film. Many noted its complex psychology. Ada's severed finger functions as a castration (a displacement of Stewart's castration at the hands of Ada and Baines?), but the phallus is restored with the silver finger and Ada is intact again, able to play piano. Some viewers were curious about Flora's spying and betrayal of her mother, especially since there are no scenes really showing Stewart becoming closer to her. But Flora apparently sees the impotent Stewart as much less of a threat to her relationship with her mother than the passionate Baines. For that matter, where does Stewart's violent turn come from? He has not forced on Ada her 'marital duties', and just as the relationship between Ada and Baines heats up, her relationship with Stewart becomes more amiable.

Although *The Piano* received almost universal acclaim, some critics did fault the ways in which Campion 'others' the Maori, as she would later troublingly 'other' India in *Holy Smoke*'s depiction of New Delhi, where all the Indians appear to be either beggars or bogus gurus who dupe unsuspecting westerners. In *The Piano* the sexually obsessed Maori confuse a Bluebeard shadowplay with reality, and mostly act as comic relief. As Maori critic Leonie Pihama states, 'We are left with the notions that Maori women cook and talk continually about sex and that Maori men carry pianos around in the bush, are irrational, and are unable to control their "native warlike instincts"' (Pihama 2000: 130). Controversy over accusations of plagiarism also arose, since there are several similarities between Campion's tale and Jane Mander's 1920 novel *The Story of a New Zealand River*, or as one scholar puts it, 'The case is not one of overt plagiarism in that Campion's characters do not literally speak Mander's lines, but the shape of their personalities, their situations, and their attitudes are identifiably similar' (Hoeveler 1998: 113). Although claims of plagiarism are certainly exaggerated, a rival production filming an adaptation of Mander's novel at the same time as *The Piano* was halted due to these similarities. Despite these criticisms, *The Piano* remains one of the essential Australian/New Zealand films, one that censures sexism, racism and capitalism.

Zachary Ingle

References

Hoeveler, Diane Long (1998) 'Silence, Sex, and Feminism: An Examination of *The Piano*'s Unacknowledged Sources', *Literature/Film Quarterly*, 26: 2, pp. 109–16.

Pihama, Leonie (2000) 'Ebony and Ivory: Constructions of Maori in *The Piano*', in Harriet Margolis (ed.), *Jane Campion's 'The Piano'*, Cambridge: Cambridge University Press, pp. 114–34.

Wexman, Virgina Wright (ed.) (1999) *Jane Campion: Interviews*, Jackson: University Press of Mississippi.

Shame

Country of Origin:

Australia

Studio/Distributor:

United American & Australian Film Productions
Barron Films

Director:

Steve Jodrell

Producers:

Paul D Barron
Damien Parer

Screenwriters:

Beverley Blankenship
Michael Brindley

Cinematographer:

Joseph Pickering

Production Designer:

Phil Peters

Composer:

Mario Millo

Editor:

Kerry Regan

Duration:

94 minutes

Genres:

Thriller
Drama

Cast:

Deborra-Lee Furness
Tony Barry
Bill McCluskey

Synopsis

Asta, a female biker, crashes her motorcycle on a country road and is forced to stay in a rural town while it is repaired at a local garage. The immediate, instinctive sexism she encounters from all the male inhabitants (except the garage owner Tim) leads her to investigate the town's culture of violent, chauvinistic behaviour. She discovers that the town's male youth habitually rape and sexually assault the local girls. The victims (among them the garage owner's daughter, Lizzie) are intimidated into silence. When it becomes obvious that the local police are not only aware but in collusion with the gang, Asta, a barrister from the city, embarks upon her own crusade to bring all the guilty parties to justice.

Critique

In *Northanger Abbey* (1817), Jane Austen's affectionate parody of the eighteenth-century literary Gothic, the heroine Catherine Moreland goes looking for the evidence of the uncanny and supernatural enervation in a country house. She finds only the prosaic evils of socio-economic injustice and gender inequality: in other words, the real horrors of her society which contemporary fiction screens or sublimates. In *Shame*, the heroine is not a naive innocent, venturing from the sophisticated town to a less complex but more ruthless rural setting, but a capable professional, flabbergasted rather than surprised by the vicious prejudice she finds, and infuriated rather than dismayed by the compromises and conspiracies which maintain it. The rural town of *The Cars That Ate Paris* (Peter Weir, 1974) and the imperatives of masculinity from *Wake in Fright* (Ted Kotcheff, 1971) attain a pointed, contemporary, politicized realism in Jodrell's film.

The film's impact is strengthened by the series of unexpected turns and incongruities with which the conspiracy, conflict and quest for justice are established. The gender of Asta the biker is revealed only when she removes her crash helmet (to be met with an immediate wolf-whistle); the secretiveness of the garage owner belies shame at his own powerlessness rather than guilt for his own transgression; it falls to Asta to become the daughter's avenger, but when the climactic tragedy overwhelms her, it becomes a communally accepted duty to enact justice. Masculinity, constantly

Allison Taylor
Simone Buchanan

Format:

35mm

Year:

1988

ironized and compromised within the Gothic, in *Shame* is judged in a social-realist observational mode, with an additional western aura which adds to rather than detracts from its impact. Similarly *Cars'* subversion of the western's definitions of heroism works through the incongruity of both American cinematic conventions appearing in Australian settings, and of the discernible echoes of the Spaghetti western's own complex relationship with the same source materials. The undermining and redefinition of stereotypes of Australian masculinity, itself a Gothic project through examples such as *Mad Max* (George Miller, 1979) is enhanced in its significance through the (ab)use of this generic framework. *Shame*, outstripping its precedent *Bad Day at Black Rock* (John Sturges, 1954) redoubles the updating and subversion of the western in its setting, timing and characterization, proving that even the most modern and mundane, idyllic and unexpected settings can harbour deviance and monstrousness. Crucially, however, *Shame* like *Cars* shows that the horrors the Gothic probes are not simply those of the groups that perpetrate, but also those of the individuals, communities and authorities which accept, deny or condone them.

Jonathan Rayner

Summerfield

Country of Origin:

Australia

Studio/Distributor:

Clare Beach Films

Director:

Ken Hannam

Producer:

Patricia Lovell

Screenwriter:

Cliff Green

Cinematographer:

Mike Molloy

Production Designer:

Graham 'Grace' Walker

Composer:

Bruce Smeaton

Editor:

Sara Bennett

Duration:

95 minutes

Genres:

Gothic

Synopsis

Teacher Simon Robinson arrives in a small country town to take over at the local school, following the unexplained disappearance of the previous incumbent of the post. He meets Jenny Abbott, who lives on a secluded farm with her brother David and her daughter Sally. Invited to visit the Abbotts' island estate, Simon drives the wrong way over a bridge to a high fence and locked gate. Retracing his steps, he accidently runs over Sally, breaking her leg. While he visits Sally at home to maintain her schooling, Simon becomes increasingly drawn to Jenny. Deciding to investigate what happened to his predecessor, Simon discovers photos of the former teacher with the Abbotts. Simon spends an evening with David and Jenny, but is forced to walk back to the house when his car does not start. Approaching the house, he discovers the Abbotts' secret and solves the mystery of his predecessor's disappearance.

Critique

'Nothing will prepare you for the end' claimed the advertisements for *Summerfield*. In fact, every facet of the film announces and affirms the inevitability of the film's conclusion, castigating the audience and the film's protagonist for the audacity of assuming alternatives for or agency over its narrative. Its mystery is not a mystery, and the enigma which the teacher excavates is a barely concealed secret. On release and in subsequent criticism, *Summerfield* has been viewed as an unsuccessful investigative thriller, and hence a 'bad' Australian film, because of this very transparency. One might as well reprove Simon (Nick Tate) for investigating a non-mystery to dire effect as

Thriller

Cast:

Nick Tate
John Waters
Elizabeth Alexander
Michelle Jarman

Format:

35mm

Year:

1977

criticize Oedipus for asking questions whose answers will prove fatal. The paradigm must be played out. The hero's actions are tied into a pattern and precipitate an outcome that only he (then again, perhaps *not even* he) cannot see. *Summerfield* was initiated and completed as a project by many of those associated with *Picnic at Hanging Rock* (Peter Weir, 1975): producer Patricia Lovell, screenwriter Cliff Green and composer Bruce Smeaton all worked on both productions (though the intended director Peter Weir was subsequently replaced by Ken Hannam).

The narrative evasion and obfuscation of *Picnic* provides a fertile comparison for the indirect consummation of *Summerfield*. The Gothicism of the earlier film resides in its assumption of art cinema's open-endedness, as the only fitting structural answer to its aestheticized and allusive exploration of sexuality, longing and landscape. It is impossible to really know of, through, or in a 'dream'. The Gothic in *Summerfield* arises from an ignorance or blindness undone by too little agency, and overcome by too much knowledge. While it appears to maladroitly short-circuit its thriller wiring, actually the film deliberately and (in an echo of *The Cars That Ate Paris* [Peter Weir, 1974]) subversively undermines the hero figure in his generically designated role. What results is only chaos, the exacerbation of a transgressive taboo. The unwise and impotent hero's investigation of the Summerfield estate reveals a consistent Gothic thematic element: incest, also a feature of *Cassandra* (Colin Eggleston, 1986), *Bad Boy Bubby* (Rolf de Heer, 1993) and *The Loved Ones* (Sean Byrne, 2009). The seclusion of the island farm, symbolizing the continent and its colonizers (the Abbott family can trace its line back to nineteenth-century seafarers) combines heritage with exclusivity, the past with a wrongdoing which continues to taint the present. In this respect, the enigmatic past the hero tries vainly to fathom is displaced in the film's discussion by the past of the country estate, and the estate which stands for the country. A mystery of paternity becomes subsumed in a secret of inherent transgression, the punishment of which consumes all affected individuals and generations.

Jonathan Rayner

The Cars That Ate Paris

Country of Origin:

Australia

Studio/Distributor:

Australian Film Development Corporation
Royce Smeal Productions
Salt Pan Films

Synopsis

In the midst of a nationwide economic crisis, Arthur Waldo and his brother George take to the roads in rural New South Wales. Coaxed off the main highway by signs promising food, lodging and gasoline, they approach the isolated town of Paris, but are suddenly involved in a car crash. Arthur is traumatized by the event and incapable of driving, and thus unable to leave town. He convalesces in the mayor's house, and gradually realizes that Paris's population subsists on the spoils of car accidents deliberately staged on the rural roads. He also discovers the local doctor has a collection of other crash victims who have been reduced to mindless 'veggies' in his debased 'experiments'. Tensions between the town's youth,

Director:

Peter Weir

Producers:

Hal McElroy
Jim McElroy

Screenwriters:

Peter Weir
Keith Gow
Piers Davies

Cinematographer:

John McLean

Art Director:

David Copping

Composer:

Bruce Smeaton

Editor:

Wayne LeClos

Duration:

91 minutes

Genres:

Horror
Comedy

Cast:

Terry Camilleri
John Meillon
Kevin Miles
Bruce Spence
Rick Scully

Format:

35mm

Year:

1974

who appear to incarnate the town's ambiguous relationship with the automobile, and the older generation, who shy away from the violent realities of the town's existence, come to a head on the night of the Paris Pioneers' Ball.

Critique

Peter Weir's first feature fleshes out the promise of his short film *Homesdale* (1972) while also synthesizing (perhaps to debatable degrees of success) aspects of British and American horror, black comedy and astringent social criticism. *Homesdale* itself represented a memorable early foray into the Gothic's thematic concerns, portraying the machinations of a manipulative authority supervising the 'treatment' of several secretive and malleable inmates at a secluded asylum. Its experimental-film funding and black-and-white cinematography underpinned an approach and aesthetic combining a Kubrickian criticism of authority with the paranoid black comedy of Polanski. With a colour palette more reminiscent of Hammer horror and an instinctive suspicion of the rural community comparable with the aura of *Straw Dogs* (Sam Peckinpah, 1971), *The Wicker Man* (Robin Hardy, 1973) and *The Texas Chainsaw Massacre* (Tobe Hooper, 1974), *Cars* essays simultaneously a universally applicable allegory of modern society and consumerism, and a nationally-specific parable of Australia's *amour fou* for the automobile.

Mad Max (George Miller, 1979) and its sequels may delineate a similar story of societal collapse and traumatic individual transformation on the roads across an Australian blankness with more gleeful destruction, kinetic editing and masculine angst, but Weir's film, in its evasiveness of tone, its Spaghetti western and George A Romero parodies and its probing of the true horrors of conformity, offers more complex concepts and many more filmic connections to ponder. The superficial resemblance of the outback hamlet to a rural idyll masks its stronger kinship with the frontier town, resembling but ridiculing the pattern of the western, where the law and lucrative lawlessness are viewed with similar, cynical pragmatism. In the conspicuous, musically accompanied montage sequences (which detail the division of the spoils of a crash and their subsequent conversion into a barter currency by the town's inhabitants), Weir's film becomes a self-conscious sociopolitical allegory to rival *Weekend* (Jean-Luc Godard, 1967).

Cars's western motifs – in its costuming and music as much as its liminal location and attendant masculine dilemmas of (in) action – belie the film's essentially comic and parodic stance towards the conventions of cinema and society which it cites and satirizes. Arthur (Terry Camilleri) the outsider may be forced into an incongruous heroic role, but he cannot save himself or indeed the town from *itself*. His impotence and ostracism (as the traffic warden unable to drive) underline his failure to meet the expectations of either an American (cowboy) or an Australian (car driver) definition of masculinity in action. His climactic resumption of driving is essentially another type of compliance, to the town's habitual car-based violence, rather than an independent, redemptive or revenging act. *Cars* opens with a pre-credit sequence showing, in mock-commercial form, a complacent young consumerist couple driving to their deaths in the idyllic Australian countryside, and ends with Paris's consumers let loose into the night-time rural landscape. In-between it absorbs and parodies a host of cinematic conventions, offers a scathing criticism of society on the road to moral and material breakdown, and in its amalgamation of hybrid styles and cross-bred concepts, goes some way towards demarcating the Gothic's agendas and themes. Virtually ignored on release, in retrospect it has gained recognition for its role in defining the Gothic and grounding its director in the uncanny territory which distinguished his films in the 1970s.

Jonathan Rayner

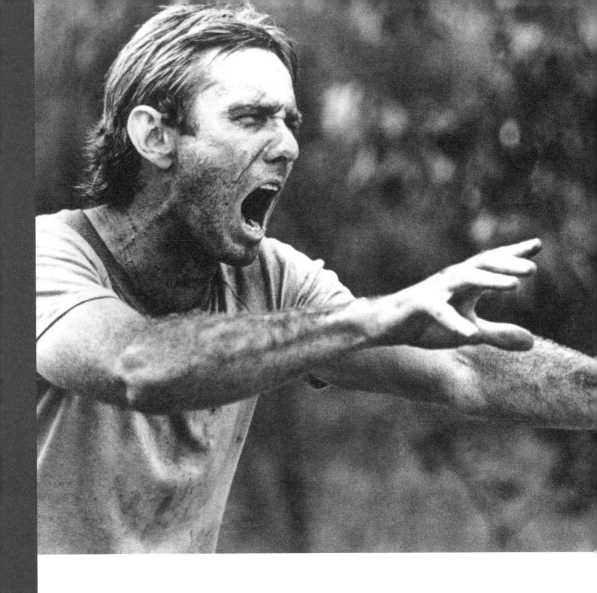

HORROR

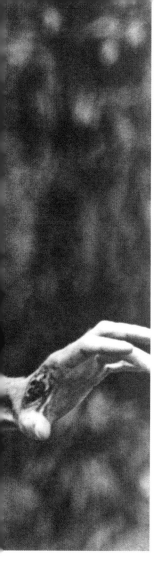

Long Weekend (Colin Eggleston, 1978). © Kobal Collection

The monstrous landscape and the revenge of nature are recurring motifs in Australian cinema. In the horror genre, the idea of the monstrous landscape emerges from, and builds upon, an established tradition in Australian cinema in which landscape functions not just as a setting for action, but also as a character in its own right. Rather than a picturesque wilderness or countryside, or a serene natural world untainted by civilization – representations common in landscape cinema celebrating positive aspects of the Australian outback – the monstrous landscape is a dangerous, malevolent and threatening force. Drawing upon themes also common in Australian Gothic narratives such as entrapment in a hostile environment, isolation and fear of the unknown (Turcotte 1988; see also Jonathan Rayner's essay in this volume), the monstrous landscape acts according to its own logic indecipherable to non-Indigenous Australians and is represented in terms of its alien-ness and inhuman horror.

A key movie which popularized the idea of the monstrous landscape in terms of horror-specific themes – particularly in terms of anxieties towards the landscape and the negative forces it exudes – is the eerie classic *Picnic at Hanging Rock* (Peter Weir) released in 1975. The movie revolves around the disappearance of a group of schoolgirls and their teacher during a picnic at the eponymous rock on St Valentine's Day in 1900. An arthouse movie shot like a horror film, the narrative suggests that an ancient supernatural force emanating from Hanging Rock abducts and consumes the girls. Throughout the narrative, tension arises from the alien-ness of the natural environment, and the eerie portrayal of the rock as a force of nature. Primordial faces are etched into monolithic rocks weathered by thousands of years, bird flights are disturbed, watches stop. In a classic scene – the last time the girls are seen – they walk dreamlike as though in a trance into a cavity in the rock and disappear. Only one is ever found.

Two contemporary films that borrow from, and build upon, these themes include the iconic slasher *Wolf Creek* (Greg McLean, 2005) and the eerie mockumentary *Lake Mungo* (Joel Anderson, 2008). As *Wolf Creek*'s director Greg McLean famously stated in the movie's 'making of' documentary, landscape can be regarded as the fifth main character in the narrative. While Mick Taylor is the primary villain, the three protagonists are also at the mercy of an ethereal landscape. Rain falls oddly and unexpectedly in the desert, watches mysteriously stop, and the outback seems to oppose the central characters at every turn. Ravines appear from nowhere during Liz and Kristy's dash for freedom. Ben escapes Mick's lair only to find himself trapped in the isolated emptiness and at the mercy of rugged terrain that threatens his life. And at the end of the movie, Mick Taylor fades into the twilight as though part of the desert – a 'monster' sent to cleanse it of intruders. In *Lake Mungo*, landscape is represented as a supernatural force in a more literal sense. The story is about the mysterious drowning of 16-year-old Alice Palmer and the haunting of her family by what appears to be her ghost. While on a high school excursion to Lake Mungo – a dry lake bed and an ancient Indigenous Australian burial site – Alice is confronted by an eerie supernatural spectre of her corpse (as though an apparition generated by the lake) revealing her fate – albeit one she cannot escape from – which sets in motion a series of events that lead to her death. Alice's ghost haunts her family in their suburban home to reveal her darkest secrets, including an affair with a neighbour.

In addition to a supernatural force, the monstrous landscape is also reified in the form of killer animals. As such, a dominant theme closely associated with the monstrous landscape, and often in conjunction with it, is the revenge of nature. In contemporary society, the harmonious co-existence of humanity and nature is under pressure, from the sharp rise in the extinction of endangered species to the relentless human encroachment on natural habitat. In the horror narrative, nature fights back. Non-Indigenous Australians, typically from the city with little understanding of the outback and its ways, are attacked by monstrous animals, or become victims of the revenge of nature.

Black Water (Andrew Traucki and David Nerlich, 2007) explicitly addresses the clash between the expansion of civilization and the sustainability of the animal world. Over the top of grainy footage of an ominous mangrove estuary, the movie is introduced by the text, 'the Salt Water Crocodile population in Northern Australia is expanding, so is the human population'. In *Black Water*, crocodiles are tourist attractions, and their natural habitat, once free of humans, is now a tourist playground. Crocodiles are also hunted or farmed for their skins with 'four feet being the optimum size for the handbag market'. But with the crocodile population growing, a rogue crocodile has returned to the placid waterway to reap revenge on humans. Killer crocodile movies *Rogue* (Greg McLean, 2007) and *Dark Age* (Arch Nicholson, 1987) contain similar themes in relation to the clash of nature/civilization and modern/primitive worlds. However, in these films, such issues are closely tied to Indigenous themes. In *Rogue*, a monster crocodile is the guardian of a sacred Indigenous waterway and attacks trespasses (poachers and tourists); and in *Dark Age*, attempts by park rangers to destroy a killer crocodile are complicated by Indigenous beliefs that the reptile is a Dreamtime spirit (Simpson 2010).

In the 'Ozploitation' classic, *Long Weekend* (Colin Eggleston, 1978; Jamie Blanks, 2008), protagonists are pitted, quite literally, against nature in the form of an entire ecosystem. In what has become a rediscovered cult-classic in recent years, the movies follow an urban couple who travel to a remote beach to repair their failing marriage. Unconsciously polluting and destroying the landscape and wildlife (crushing ant colonies and sea hawks' eggs, and shooting wildlife among many other attacks against nature), an entire ecosystem – snakes, sea hawks, dugongs, spiders, ants, possums and dogs – attacks the protagonists as revenge for their destruction of nature.

Animals in Australian horror films have an ability to adapt and hybridize in order to survive in a changing ecosystem. From killer crocodiles and marsupial werewolves to gargantuan boars and Tasmanian tigers, 'creatures' in Australian horror are feral animals that have adapted to harsh and changing natural environments only to become 'bigger, hungrier and angrier' (Simpson 2010: 43). Ultimately, these animals 'wreak revenge on humans who may have done them [or their natural habitat] injustice' (Simpson 2010: 43). The creature-feature *Razorback* (Russell Mulcahy, 1984) for example, contains themes around the dangerous implications of ravaging the land for commercial gains (in this case opal mining and kangaroo-shooting) and animal cruelty. Deep in the desolate outback, the landscape has spawned a monstrous freak of nature, a giant man-eating boar the size of a rhinoceros which terrorizes the town and its inhabitants. In *Howling III: The Marsupials* (Philippe Mora, 1987), a narrative more about hybridization for survival than the revenge of nature, a rare species of marsupial werewolf exists in the outback – spawned from the amalgam of the widely believed extinct Tasmanian tiger (in reality hunted by farmers into extinction in the early twentieth century) and the werewolf.

Two recent creature-features venture away from the outback and explore the dangers of the ocean and the implications of climate change. *The Reef* (Andrew Traucki, 2010), Australia's first shark horror, is a cautionary tale that preys on the timeless fear of the unknown and the great white shark. The movie suggests that humans are merely prey for sharks in their natural habitat and although humans may be able to traverse through or over the ocean they are unable to tame it. The 3D shark movie, and surprise international box office hit, *Bait* (Kimble Rendall, 2012), is a story about survivors of a tsunami who are trapped in a shopping centre and stalked by great white sharks. The movie draws on contemporary anxieties about the potentially devastating implications of climate change; and in addition to the destructive power of tsunamis, *Bait* alludes to the changing feeding patterns of sharks which are bringing more of the creatures closer to the coastline – and by implication popular swimming spots – due to dwindling fish stocks and global warming (a theme also implicit in *The Reef*).

The representation of the monstrous landscape has been and remains a powerful theme in Australian horror cinema. Although the peculiarities of the outback (the unique flora and fauna and the ancient geography) have become more familiar, and even banal, for Australians in the twenty-first century – particularly in comparison to early settlers who found the Australian bush alien and exotic – the harsh extremes and often ethereal nature of the landscape, clashes with dangerous animals and natural disasters remain prominent in the popular imagination. Large red-dust storms fuelled by drought engulfed cities along the east coast in 2009 (see Ramachandran 2009), shark and crocodile attacks occur every year, and floods that swamp metropolitan cities (the Brisbane floods in 2011), bush fires (the Black Saturday fires in 2009 claiming 173 lives) and cyclones are reminders of the power of nature and the extremes of the Australian landscape. Consequently, as climate change brings new challenges for the Australian population and threats from the landscape evolve, so too will the monsters and the representation of monstrous landscape in Australian horror movies.

Mark David Ryan

References

Ramachandran, Arjun (2009) 'Sydney turns red: Dust storm blankets city', *Sydney Morning Herald*, 23 September, http://www.smh.com.au/environment/weather/sydney-turns-red-dust-storm-blankets-city-20090923-g0so.html. Accessed 3 April 2013.

Simpson, Catherine (2010) 'Australian Eco-Horror and Gaia's Revenge: Animals, Eco-Nationalism and the New Nature', *Studies in Australasian Cinema*, 4: 1, pp. 43–54.

Turcotte, G, (1998) 'Australian Gothic', in Mulvey Roberts (ed.), *The Handbook to Gothic Literature*, Basingstoke: Macmillan.

Bait

Country of Origin:

Australia/Singapore

Studios/Distributor:

Bait Productions
Pictures in Paradise
Story Bridge Films

Director:

Kimble Rendall

Producers:

Peter Barber
Todd Fellman
Gary Hamilton

Screenwriters:

Shayne Armstrong
Duncan Kennedy
John Kim
Shane Krause
Justin Monjo
Russell Mulcahy

Director of Photography:

Ross Emery

Production Designer:

Nicholas McCallum

Composers:

Joe Ng
Alex Oh

Editor:

Rodrigo Balart

Duration:

91 minutes

Genre:

Horror

Cast:

Richard Brancatisano
Xavier Samuel
Sharni Vinson
Julian McMahon
Dan Wyllie
Alice Parkinson
Phoebe Tonkin
Lincoln Lewis
Cariba Heine
Adrian Pang
Martin Sacks

Synopsis

Josh works as a lifeguard on the Gold Coast in Queensland, a holiday destination popular for its beaches. Guilt-ridden over a fellow lifeguard's death, Josh's relationship with his girlfriend Tina deteriorates, and she moves to Singapore. A year later, Josh is working in a local supermarket stacking shelves when he bumps into Tina. She is back in town with – it is suggested – her new boyfriend Steven. They are in Australia to visit Steven's father Jessup who manages the supermarket. A few aisles away, Jaimie, a teen delinquent struggling to cope with the death of her mother, is caught shoplifting. Her father Todd, a local police officer, arrives to arrest her. Two masked men, Doyle and Kirby, hold up the supermarket. During the robbery, a giant tsunami swamps the Gold Coast. The survivors are trapped in the flooded supermarket and an underground car park. Great white sharks, washed in with the wave, now lurk in the murky waters preying on victims. Trapped on top of supermarket shelves, or in submerged cars on the lower level, the survivors must find a way out.

Critique

The shark horror, or 'sharksploitation' subgenre, has produced some terrible movies. The genre, by its very nature, is limited to stories about giant or marauding packs of sharks stalking, terrorizing and devouring hapless victims. Movies that attempt to tell a serious story risk being unfair compared with, or falling a long way short of, Steven Spielberg's landmark classic *Jaws* (1975). On the other hand, film-makers who take the route of exploitation trade upon high body counts, gore, absurdity and ridiculous or implausible plots. *Shark in Venice* (Danny Lerner, 2008), *Mega Shark vs Giant Octopus* (Jack Perez, 2009), *Mega Shark vs Crocosaurus* (Christopher Ray, 2010) and *Sand Sharks* (Mark Atkins, 2011) are a handful of awful examples. To the director's credit, *Bait* is a movie aware of the genre's limitations and attempts to entertain without taking itself too seriously.

Bait was originally penned and was to be directed by Russell Mulcahy, the Australian director of cult classics *Razorback* (1984), *Highlander* (1986) and *Highlander II: The Quickening* (1991). It was reported that Mulcahy pulled out of the project to direct episodes of the television series *Teen Wolf* (Southern Star Productions/ Hanna-Barbera Australia/Atlantic/Kushner Locke, CBS, 1986-88) (Bernstein 2011). He was replaced by former Hoodoo Gurus guitarist and one-time feature film director Kimble Rendall. Rendall's first feature film as director was the teen slasher movie *Cut* (2000), which was a dismal failure at the box office and was universally savaged by critics. Over the next decade, Rendall slowly won back favour with producers as a second-unit director on the local blockbusters *Knowing* (Alex Proyas, 2009) and *Killer Elite* (Gary McKendry, 2011), and Hollywood action movies filmed in Australia including *Ghost Rider* (Mark Steven Johnson, 2007) and *I-Robot* (Alex Proyas, 2004).

Yuwu Qi

Format:

D-Cinema, 3-D

Year:

2012

Despite a novel premise for a shark horror, and a huge production budget, *Bait*'s script was underdeveloped. In all, six screenwriters are credited with writing or redeveloping the script, something that is almost unheard of in Australian cinema. Australia's first 3D horror movie, *Bait* was produced on an estimated budget of AU$30 million – making it the highest-budget Australian horror movie of all-time – and involved the creation of two major sets: a 'fully-working supermarket and a multi-storey car park' (Swift 2012). An official Australian/ Singapore co-production, the movie was filmed at the Village Roadshow Studios on the Gold Coast where the narrative is set. Most of its budget was secured from Australian and Singaporean investors, with approximately AU$5 million from Chinese investors. The film was edited and graded in Singapore. Rather than using live sharks (like the lower-budget Australian shark thriller *The Reef* [Andrew Traucki, 2010]), *Bait*'s sharks were constructed from animatronics and CGI.

Bait was a surprise box office hit. While struggling to scrape AU$1 million at the Australian box office despite a strong marketing campaign, and earning less than US$150,000 in Singapore, the movie did achieve respectable box office earnings in other international markets. The film earned almost US$2 million in Italy, US$1.3 million in Malaysia and US$2.5 million in Russia. The movie's most successful market, by a significant margin, was China. Taking over AU$7 million on its opening weekend across 2,000 screens (*Screen Daily*, 15 November 2012), *Bait* earned almost US$25 million in its first three weeks at the Chinese box office. At the time of writing, *Bait* had become the most successful Australian movie ever released in China, outperforming the high-budget Australian titles *Happy Feet Two* (George Miller, 2011), which earned AU$6 million at the Chinese box office, *Killer Elite* (Gary McKendry, 2011), which earned AU$5 million, and even the unofficial UK/Australian co-production and Academy Award winner *The King's Speech* (Tom Hooper, 2010), which earned AU$1 million. *Bait*'s success in China was in part a result of the producers' efforts to tailor the movie for Chinese audiences. As a condition of Chinese investment, new scenes (with a focus on the movie's Asian characters) were required and an extra '15 minutes of new material' was recorded (3 minutes of this footage was added to the Chinese version of the film) (Quin 2012). Moreover, characters with broad Australian accents were re-dubbed with 'mid-Atlantic'/ US accents after producers deemed them too difficult for Chinese audiences to understand (Quin 2012).

Bait is bad, but entertaining. Despite a relatively strong cast of young emerging actors (Samuel, Vinson, Tonkin and Lewis) and seasoned Australian television veterans (McMahon and Sacks), the acting is over the top. As a reviewer for the *Sydney Morning Herald* put it, 'everybody here has been issued with a licence to over-act, the aim being to push audiences to that orgasmic point where they want to shriek, laugh and jeer at the same time' (Hall 2012). Some elements are forced and overwrought: actors deliver overblown performances and bizarre dialogue over a dramatic violin score, and then a CGI shark chomps a character in half. When combined with characters slipping between poor American and Australian accents, the movie is little more than 'old-fashioned B-movie silliness' (Adams

2012). But laughing at the absurdity and wondering what will happen next is precisely part of the appeal of this subgenre for audiences. The couple Kyle (Lincoln Lewis) and Heather (Cariba Heine) spend most of the movie trapped in a submerged car arguing. Standing on top of the car's roof waiting to swim across the water to safety, Kyle throws Heather's dog to the shark to try and save himself, but is instead devoured while the dog survives. Steven jumps into the water to turn off the power in a ridiculous diving suit, reminiscent of a Ned Kelly suit of armour, made from shopping trolley mesh; while in the final action sequence, Josh hangs upside down from a ceiling like an action hero to stun a shark bursting from the water with a Taser gun.

In the end, humorous scenes like these and the movie's self-conscious tongue-in-cheek style result in a fun, B-grade popcorn movie. To date, the movie also has the honour of being the most successful Australian creature-feature of all time at the box office.

Mark David Ryan

References

Adams, Mark (2012), 'Bait 3D', *ScreenDaily.com*, http://www. screendaily.com/reviews/the-latest/bait-3d/5045811.article. Accessed 24 February 2013.

Bernstein, Abbie (2011), '"Teen Wolf"—Seriously', Fangoria.com, 3 June, http://www.fangoria.com/index.php?option=com_content&view=article&id=4681. Accessed 27 February 2013.

Hall, Sandra (2012), 'Underwater, over-acted, but lots of bite in Bait 3D', *Sydney Morning Herald*, 20 September, http://www.smh.com.au/action/printArticle?id=3646365. Accessed 24 February 2013.

Quin, Karl (2012), 'Sinking our Teeth into China', *Sydney Morning Herald*, 30 October, http://www.smh.com.au/entertainment/movies/sinking-our-teeth-into-china-20121024-285n9.html. Accessed 26 February 2013.

Swift, Brendan (2012), 'Director Kimble Rendall talks Bait 3D', *IF Magazine.com.au* (online), http://if.com.au/2012/09/20/article/Director-Kimble-Rendall-talks-Bait-3D/JITBTEUZMS.html. Accessed 26 February 2013.

Body Melt

Country of Origin:

Australia

Studio/Distributor:

Australian Film Commission
Bodymelt Pty Ltd
Dumb Films
Film Victoria

Director:

Philip Brophy

Synopsis

The suburban estate of Homeville has become the focus of dangerous and unlicensed scientific experimentation. The residents of Pebbles Court are the unwitting guinea pigs for lifestyle enhancements and dietary supplements from Vimuville, a company operating from an abandoned chemical works. The company's products have affected one former scientist at the facility, whose offspring are mutants with murderous tendencies. All the free drugs supplied to the suburbanites are highly addictive and bring horrific, fatal side-effects. Body parts expand, mutate, explode or implode, with the victims forming a complete cross-section of the community in terms of gender, age and ethnicity. A police investigation into the

Producers:

Rod Bishop
Daniel Scharf

Screenwriters:

Rod Bishop
Philip Brophy, based on four
unpublished short stories by
Philip Brophy

Director of Photography:

Ray Argall

Production Designer:

Maria Kozic

Composer:

Philip Brophy

Editor:

Bill Murphy

Duration:

81 minutes

Genres:

Horror
Comedy

Cast:

Gerard Kennedy
Andrew Daddo
Ian Smith

Format:

35mm

Year:

1994

frequent gory deaths eventually locates the site and identifies the discredited scientists responsible for the disaster, just as one family visits the 'health spa' created within the former chemical plant. Several family members and the plant's employees themselves succumb to the effects of the drugs before order is restored.

Critique

'The first stage is glandular; the second is hallucinogenic …': self-conscious body culture is explored as a target for satire in Brophy's sole, memorable feature film. The outlandishness and trauma of the transformation and destruction of the human body which the film details underlines the forms of physical and psychological dependency which body consciousness imposes on a vulnerable, gullible population. Subjected to televised images of ideal physiques and lifestyles, attempting to fit impossible gendered expectations, obsessively seeking fleeting physical pleasure, and conforming to the demands of the elitist sporting culture and beach environment, the modern Australian proves a willing accomplice in their own subjugation. The film's relentless and escalating victimization of naive suburbanites evokes little sympathy, suggesting (in a way comparable to the brutal social critiques displayed in David Cronenberg's films) that *Body Melt* does not express or expect sympathy for them. It is not that their susceptibility to products promising improvements to the body, and therefore to lifestyle, reflects their guilt or merits punishment, but simply that any product patronage and consumption carries risk in a capitalist moral vacuum. The middle-class's belief in endless and accelerating self-improvement is ripe for mockery, for the very reasons that popular depictions of its existence seldom admit threats of the enormity and abject status which *Body Melt* inflicts with such aplomb. The film's masterstroke is the appearance of Ian Smith (known world-wide as Harold Bishop, from the cast of the long-running Australian soap opera *Neighbours* [Grundy Television, Seven Network 1985-86; Network Ten 1986-]) in the role of the degenerate and unrepentant scientist. That 'Harold' is capable of such villainy, and that Pebbles Court, a polite, representative suburban cul-de-sac twinned with *Neighbours*'s Ramsay Street, could be his target and afflicted with genuine, overwhelming tragedy, attacks several sacred popular cultural certainties. The film's laughably graphic spectacles of bodily disintegration, framed in familiar, safe surroundings register as a cultural assault as excessive and gory as Peter Jackson's contemporary Kiwi Gothic. Although poised between Canadian and New Zealand body horrors, Brophy's film is actually more accurately attuned than either in national and cultural terms.

Jonathan Rayner

Long Weekend

Country of Origin:

Australia

Studio/Distributor:

Dugong Films
Film Victoria
Australian Film Commission

Director:

Colin Eggleston

Producers:

Colin Eggleston
Richard Brennan

Screenwriter:

Everett De Roche

Cinematographer:

Vincent Monton

Production Designer:

Larry Eastwood

Composer:

Michael Carlos

Editor:

Brian Kavanagh

Duration:

92 minutes

Genre:

Horror

Cast:

John Hargreaves
Briony Behets

Format:

35mm

Year:

1978

Synopsis

Peter and Marcia, a young, childless couple, embark on a weekend camping trip. The infidelities of both partners lie behind their constant bickering. The short holiday exposes rather than heals their animosity. On the way, their discarded cigarettes start bush fires, and they run over a kangaroo on the highway. Peter and Marcia heedlessly attack the wildlife encroaching on their campsite; they chop down trees, spray insecticide, shoot ducklings and take eggs from the nest of a bird of prey. Peter kills a dugong which Marcia has mistaken for a shark in the surf, and subsequently they are disturbed by moaning cries that may come from an abandoned calf. Their machines and appliances start to break down, and fresh food unaccountably starts to rot. They discover another campsite which seems to be abandoned, apparently overwhelmed by growing vegetation, and a van submerged on the beach nearby. Slowly the natural world begins to take revenge.

Critique

Long Weekend's premise literalizes the meeting point between urban and rural Australia, Indigenous and non-Indigenous perceptions and valuations of the landscape, and natural and acculturated notions of justice. As a forceful and inescapable allegory for the acquisition and exploitation of the Australian continent, the film picks up where *Walkabout* (Nicolas Roeg, 1971) leaves off, replacing an inscrutable and impassive environment, indifferent to the presence and problems of urban white Australians, with an actively malign landscape, bent on sloughing off the heedlessly destructive intruders. Where Hitchcock's *The Birds* (1963) leaves unstated the single or accumulated acts which provoke nature to violence, *Long Weekend* confronts and condemns the specific and repeated inflictions upon the fertile body of the landscape of which the colonizing culture stands accused. The impetus and economy of the film's screenplay (written by Everett de Roche, also responsible for a later depiction of nature's vengeance in *Razorback* [Russell Mulcahy, 1984]) delays the demise of the utterly unsympathetic characters only for the purpose of exacerbating the suffering they experience, to counterbalance their senseless and mechanical destruction of the environment.

Criticism of the film has often decried its over-determination of the couple's guilt and injured nature's justified revenge. In eschewing the arbitrariness of Hitchcock's enigmatic forbear, *Long Weekend* can appear brutally mechanical in its narrative logic and hectoringly obvious in its ecological message. At the time, De Roche's other credits in Australian horror – *Patrick* (Richard Franklin, 1978), *Harlequin* (Simon Wincer, 1980) and *Road Games* (Richard Franklin, 1981) – were commercially-oriented and internationally-targeted productions, which downplayed their national specificity with the over-dubbing of accents and casting of American stars. By comparison, *Long Weekend* emphasizes its national relevance at every stage, from the couple's jeep equipped with roo-bars (which do indeed fulfil their purpose) and their negligence in starting a bush fire with a discarded cigarette, to their instinctively ingrained movement towards the beach for recreation. However, from the film's first image the beach has been invested with as much menace as the bush: a crab on a rocky shore, about to be washed away by the waves, stands as the perfect metaphor for the fleeting and fragile colonial presence on the continent, halted at the coastline and permanently insecure in its territorial claim. It is from the beach that the husband glimpses a threatening shadow in the surf, and on the shoreline that he discovers evidence of other campers swallowed up by the sand and landscape. And a suitably Australian ending is determined, when the crazed husband is mown down on the highway by a landtrain, carrying sheep to the slaughterhouse. Notably, the relevance if not the reputation of *Long Weekend* has led to a recent remake – *Nature's Grave* (Jamie Blanks, 2008), also written by De Roche – starring the American actor Jim Caviezel and Australian Claudia Karvan as the troubled husband and wife. If the film's message has always been obvious, equally obviously it has never gone away.

Jonathan Rayner

The Loved Ones (aka The Loved Ones: Pretty in Blood)

Country of Origin:

Australia

Studio/Distributor:

Ambience Entertainment
Omnilab Media

Director:

Sean Byrne

Producers:

Mark Lazarus
Michael Boughen

Screenwriter:

Sean Byrne

Director of Photography:

Simon Chapman

Production Designer:

Robert Webb

Composer:

Ollie Olsen

Synopsis

Brent is recovering from a road accident in which his father was killed. Lola asks him to their high school prom, but he turns her down, as he plans to attend with his girlfriend Holly. Lola kidnaps Brent, subjecting him to prolonged physical torture in her home, which has been decked out as an alternative prom dance setting by her father. Father and daughter silence Brent and attempt a makeshift lobotomy, before throwing him into a cellar filled with their previous victims, who have become mindless cannibals. Brent fights back, and manages to escape, but Lola pursues him, now intent on harming Holly too.

Critique

The Loved Ones bears a passing resemblance to the visceral torture narratives seen in recent American horror (for example, the series of *Saw* [*Saw* (James Wan, 2004); *Saw II* (Darren Lynn Bousman, 2005); *Saw III* (Darren Lynn Bousman, 2006); *Saw IV* (Darren Lynn Bousman, 2007); *Saw V* (David Hackl, 2008); *Saw VI* (Kevin Greutert, 2009)] and *Hostel* films [*Hostel* (Eli Roth, 2005); *Hostel: Part II* (Eli Roth, 2007); *Hostel: Part III* (Scott Spiegel, 2011)]). But remarking on the similarity of the graphically violent acts creates a largely inappropriate comparison. Byrne's film is not a slavish copy of an American franchise or phenomenon, but a self-consciously referential and typically Australian example of the Gothic.

Both the broad outline and the fine detail of *The Loved Ones* evoke comparison with Peter Weir's *The Cars That Ate Paris* (1974): the hero traumatized by a car crash; the deviant family's collection of lobotomized 'veggies'; the retributive, climactic road violence, indulged with relish in the film's closing minutes, in both an assertion

Editor:

Andy Canny

Duration:

84 minutes

Genre:

Horror

Cast:

Xavier Samuel
Robin McLeavy
Victoria Thaine
John Brumpton
Suzi Dougherty

Format:

35mm

Year:

2009

and complication of heroism. At the same time, there are inclusions of other Gothic consistencies – the suggestions of incest between Lola (Robin McLeavy) and her father (John Brumpton) – and odd appropriations of horror Americana – the deranged alternative prom and Lola's vengeful self-righteousness produce vague echoes of *Carrie* (Brian de Palma, 1976) – which demand deeper scrutiny. Such facets make the film appear more like a deliberate addendum to 1970s Australian Gothic than a cannily commercial parallel to the contemporary trends of international horror. The odd timelessness of the prom costumes perhaps places the film connotatively in that decade, or function to suggest that the importation of the American institution itself is to blame for the precipitation of violence.

If *Body Melt* (Philip Brophy, 1994) taps the rampant insecurities inspired by pressures towards physical conformity, then *The Loved Ones*, while insisting on the family as the site of character strength and inherited weakness, also asserts the teenager's vulnerability to perceptions and expectations of emotional expression. (Suzi Dougherty, who plays Brent's mother Carla, made her film debut in a supporting role in *Body Melt*.) We do not necessarily choose who or how we love. The production is markedly circumscribed (most of the action takes place within the bounds of Lola's family home) and this conscious limitation, allied to the camera's impassive, static observation of the most violent acts, facilitates the film's slow and inexorable progress. Although Byrne's film does not display the tonal variability of *Cars*, it shares the earlier film's black comedy to leaven the violent spectacle. Under different circumstances, maybe *Muriel's Wedding* (PJ Hogan, 1994) could have ended like this.

The Loved Ones premiered at the 2009 Toronto International Film Festival, where the film won the Midnight Madness Cadillac People's Choice Award. The following year, the film won the Best International Feature Award at the 2010 Lund International Fantastic Film Festival in Sweden. Sean Byrne received an Australian Academy of Cinema and Television Arts Award nomination for Best Original Screenplay in 2012.

Jonathan Rayner

Primal

Country of Origin:

Australia

Studio/Distributor:

Primal Films
AV Pictures
Known Associates
Talisman Films

Director:

Josh Reed

Synopsis

In a brief prologue set thousands of years in the past, an Indigenous man is attacked and killed by an unseen creature. In the present day, a group of students travel by car into the outback. Dace is intent on studying Indigenous rock paintings in remote caves as part of an academic project. Anja appears to be recovering from an undisclosed personal trauma and suffers episodes of claustrophobia which make it impossible for her to enter the caves. The others are along for a weekend of camping, drinking and sex. On arrival, two of the party encounter a mutated rabbit, which tries to attack them. Later, Mel goes skinny-dipping in the lake next to the caves and emerges covered in leeches. She rapidly becomes ill, and degenerates into a

Producers:

Nigel Christensen

John Cordukes

Rob Gibson

Josh Reed

Screenwriters:

Nigel Christensen

Josh Reed

Director of Photography:

John Biggins

Production Designer:

Gypsy Taylor

Composer:

Rob Gibson

Editor:

Josh Reed

Duration:

80 minutes

Genre:

Horror

Cast:

Zoe Tuckwell-Smith

Krew Boylan

Lindsay Farris

Wil Traval

Rebekah Foord

Format:

Digital

Year:

2010

carnivorous and cannibalistic animal. The group attempts to escape through the caves, not realizing the dangers that lurk within.

Critique

'Where are we?' 'How specific do you want me to be?' 'Try … Australia?'

The obvious formulaic bases of *Primal*, in films of carnivorous zombie invasions and high teenage body-count slasher horror, should not distract from the definitively, defiantly Australian slant to its rendering of an uncanny horror landscape. *Rogue* (2007), Greg McLean's bigger budget follow-up to *Wolf Creek* (2005), took as Australian a topic as possible (a killer crocodile) but failed to capitalize on the potential of uninhabited Northern Territory landscapes and predictable *Jaws*-like set pieces. *Black Water* (Andrew Traucki and David Nerlich, 2007) achieved a tauter and unrelentingly downbeat effect in realist-inflected horror with the same subject matter, without succumbing to modish, recapitulative 'found-footage' stylization or outsize CGI crocodiles. By contrast, *Primal* deploys equally familiar narrative elements located within the same picturesque, sublime and quintessentially Australian outback environment, and provides concise, conventionalized, blackly comedic horror on a substantially lower budget.

The clichéd aspects of the lost, imperiled teenage expedition, with the physical, animalistic deterioration of one member of the party provoking a moral, behavioural decline in the rest, do not impede the film's undaunted logic and pace, or devalue the underlying cultural specificity of its horror landscape. In a comparable Indigenization of horror, *Dying Breed* (Jody Dwyer, 2008) connects the fatal impact of colonialism on Tasmania (the extinction of unique species and peoples) with the inherent degeneracy of the imported human society (from criminality into cannibalism via inbreeding). Adding historical detail to a formula epitomized by *Wrong Turn* (Rob Schmidt, 2003), it portrays a student group's searching for evidence of the survival of the Tasmanian tiger and instead discovering a crazed community descended from the nineteenth-century penal colony. By contrast, *Primal* embeds its horror in an environment which is inherently violent, alien and alchemical, in its effects on groups and individuals. It does not take revenge so much as, after the model of *Long Weekend* (Colin Eggleston, 1978), simply harvest and prey upon a human presence it predates by millennia. In *Primal* a natural pre-history not only triumphs over contemporary human society but also apparently trumps Indigenous cultural history: none of the complex arguments over Australian land rights has acknowledged any pre-human occupiers, the kind of unimaginable Lovecraftian presence which the film's climax reveals. The apparent simplicity of this coup – reasserting the unfathomability of the landscape by explicitly divorcing its difference from associations of Indigeneity – should not distract from its revealing audacity: how many more, and older, inhabitants must white Australia confront?

Jonathan Rayner

Razorback

Country of Origin:

Australia

Studio/Distributor:

McElroy & McElroy
UAA Films
Western Film Productions

Director:

Russell Mulcahy

Producer:

Hal McElroy

Screenwriter:

Everett De Roche, adapted
from the novel *Razorback* by
Peter Brennan (1981).

Synopsis

On a desolate windswept property, a giant wild boar – the
eponymous razorback – crashes through the wall of a homestead
and steals off with Jake's grandson. Jake is tried by a 'kangaroo
court' for the child's disappearance but is released due to a lack
of evidence. Jake becomes obsessed with tracking and killing the
animal to prove his innocence. Several years later, an American
broadcast journalist, Beth Winters, arrives in town to film a
controversial story on kangaroo hunting and animal cruelty. She
raises the ire of the townsfolk most of whom work for the local
Pet Pak abattoir (which specializes in kangaroo meat). When Beth
disappears, her husband, Carl Winters arrives from New York to
investigate. Tracking down a lead, posing as a kangaroo shooter,
Winters becomes lost in the desert and during a long journey back
to civilization he catches his first glimpse of the razorback. Carl
learns of the boar's role in his wife's disappearance, and prepares
for a final showdown.

Razorback (Russell Mulcahy, 1984). Sourced from
the AFI Research Collection with permission from
Hal McElroy (McElroy All Media) and Jim McElroy
(McElroy and McElroy)

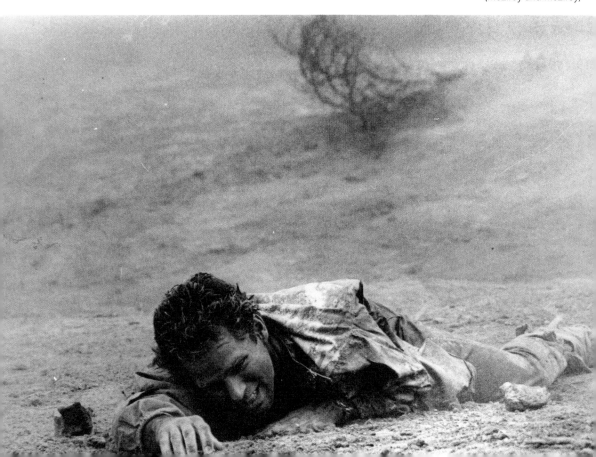

Cinematographer:

Dean Semler

Production Designer:

Bryce Walmsley

Composer:

Iva Davies

Editor:

William M. Anderson

Duration:

95 minutes

Genre:

Horror

Cast:

Gregory Harrison
Arkie Whiteley
Bill Kerr
Chris Haywood
David Argue
Judy Morris
John Howard
John Ewart

Format:

35mm

Year:

1984

Critique

Razorback, a creature feature about a giant boar terrorizing a remote outback community, is one of the most iconic Australian horror movies of all time. Yet upon the movie's release, *Razorback* was viewed as an oddity and was a box office flop. With a premise revolving around a man-eating pig the size of a rhinoceros, eccentric characters and references to Lindy Chamberlain and her persecution – with a boar replacing the baby-snatching dingo – the movie was received as a horror comedy even though it was originally marketed as a serious genre picture. Nevertheless, even though aspects of the movie have not stood the test of time (the boar, for example, looks like a scruffy marionette), the movie's style and premise are timeless and it has become a cult classic.

The film was adapted from a novel with the same title by Australian journalist Peter Brennan, and produced by Hal McElroy, co-producer of the classic Peter Weir films *Picnic at Hanging Rock* (1975) and *The Last Wave* (1977). Having been sent the manuscript, McElroy recalled finding it a thrilling read and immediately thought it was 'an out there idea' with potential for a movie (McElroy 2012). McElroy hired Everett De Roche, an 'Ozploitation' specialist to pen the screenplay, and Russell Mulcahy to direct. Mulcahy had established his credentials as a talented director of music videos including The Buggles's 'Video Killed the Radio Star' (1981) – the very first video played on the MTV channel in the United States in 1981 – The Vapors's 'Turning Japanese' (1980) and Duran Duran's 'Planet Earth' (1981) among many others. According to De Roche, the original story was difficult to adapt to screen. Perhaps because of this, as the above synopsis suggests, the movie's narrative is not a conventional creature feature, and is comprised of several interwoven sub-plots.

Much has been written about *Razorback*'s visual style and for good reason. It has been described as a 'video-clip horror' (Barlow 1995: 151), and Mulcahy's signature style is evident in the use of smoke machines and flares among other techniques familiar from his music videos. Perhaps because of this, the movie has a surreal quality. Sometimes labelled as style over substance, *Razorback* is indeed visually stunning. Mulcahy and cinematographer Dean Semler masterfully capture the beautiful, ethereal colours of the outback. Semler deservedly won the 1984 Australian Film Institute (AFI) Award for Best Achievement in Cinematography for *Razorback* along with the Australian Cinematographers' Society's highest award, the Cinematographer of the Year, for his body of work. In moody dusk scenes, eerie elongated shadows creep across the red desert in the bruised auburn twilight. Windmills beat through ghostly light. The *mise-en-scène* is reminiscent of the post-apocalyptic wasteland of *Mad Max 2* (George Miller, 1981), which was also shot by Semler. Rusted car hulks hang from twisted trees. Dwellings are ramshackle shanties made from scrap, or abandoned mine shafts, and the town itself is a degenerate collection of roughly hewn buildings. In a hallucination sequence after Winters (Gregory Harrison) becomes stranded in the desert, the audience is introduced to a visual netherworld.

Ghostly skeletons sway in the wind against a backdrop of endless desolation. Towering shards of salt jut from the desert floor like frozen lightning bolts and flares of colour burst on the horizon like min-min lights.

Like countless Australian genre films, *Razorback* paints a bleak picture of the outback and its inhabitants. The landscape is barren and desolate, the township is a cesspool of drunkards and degenerates. Only a handful of individuals manage to retain their civility in the oppressive isolation and maddening heat. The highways are sites of death and boredom-fuelled road rage overrun by yahoos and rapists. The Baker brothers (David Argue and Chris Haywood) are character types typical in 'Ozploitation' movies. Employees of the Pet Pak abattoir, they are crazed hooligans with a taste for mayhem, rape and slaughter. The razorback and other vermin have stripped the land bare of vegetation and fouled the waterholes. The landscape could be viewed as a monstrous entity, one more frightening and deadly than the monster itself. The landscape is portrayed as a wasteland that destroys all who enter it – with the unbearable heat, shimmering mirages, harsh and deadly terrain, and the killer animals waiting to consume those – especially city folk – who stumble into the wilderness.

Almost thirty years after its release, *Razorback* is a movie that has grown in stature over time. It is a standout title in the vaults of 'Ozploitation' and Australian horror cinema and one that deserves to be celebrated for many years to come.

Mark David Ryan

References

Barlow, Helen (1995), 'Razorback', in Scott Murray (ed.), *Australian Film 1978–1994: A Survey of Theatrical Features,* Oxford University Press: Melbourne, p. 151.

McElroy, Hal (2012). Interview with author (Mark David Ryan), 12 November.

The Tunnel

Country of Origin:

Australia

Studio/Distributor:

Distracted Media

Director:

Carlo Ledesma

Producers:

Enzo Tedeschi
Julian Harvey

Synopsis

A news team, led by the ambitious journalist Natasha, investigate a catacomb of subterranean tunnels beneath Sydney's metropolitan railway system. Originally built for a new railway network, an official government plan to convert the tunnels into an underground water reservoir to cope with a crippling drought threatening the city has been suspiciously abandoned. Unable to secure official permission to enter the tunnels, Natasha breaks in with cameraman Steve, sound recordist Tangles and producer Pete. They venture deep underground. While filming, Tangles begins hearing interference through his headphones. Fearing for their lives, and with their torch and camera batteries running low, the news team flee for the surface. Not all of them make it out alive.

Screenwriters:

Enzo Tedeschi
Julian Harvey

Cinematographer:

Steve Davis

Production Designer:

Kate Newton

Composer:

Paul Dawkins
Katie Newton

Editors:

Enzo Tedeschi
Julian Harvey

Duration:

90 minutes

Genres:

Horror
Thriller

Cast:

Bel Deliá
Andy Rodoreda
Steve Davis
Luke Arnold

Format:

35mm

Year:

2011

Critique

The Tunnel is a found-footage movie in the vein of ultra-low budget horror films such as *The Blair Witch Project* (Daniel Myrick and Eduardo Sánchez, 1999), and more recently the *Paranormal Activity* franchise (Oren Peli, 2007; Tod Williams, 2010; Henry Joost and Ariel Schulman, 2011; Henry Joost and Ariel Schulman, 2012) and the low-budget Australian film *Lake Mungo* (Joel Anderson, 2008). The film was financed through crowd-sourcing and released for free via peer-to-peer downloading sites to recoup returns through DVD sales via their website, ancillary markets and donations from viewers. And yet while much has been written about *The Tunnel*'s innovative online financing, distribution and marketing models (see for example Bodey 2010 and Bartlett 2011), like many horror films, *The Tunnel* remains largely a cult phenomenon with very little critical attention paid to the text itself.

As a horror movie, *The Tunnel* trades upon suspense and suggestion over explicit violence and gore. By avoiding well-worn conventions typical of trite 1980s slasher movies – absurd weapons, extreme camera angles, countless limbs chopped off and discordant orchestral strings – the film-makers have produced a slow-burn movie, more of a psychological thriller in tone than a shock horror. Indeed, *The Tunnel* is the type of horror movie that favours quiet terror above grotesque brutality, and constructed realism above overt symbolism. This understated style extends to *The Tunnel*'s narrative structure. As the synopsis suggests, the spine of the plotline is the team's wandering in empty tunnels and the pursuit. The mockumentary format is not a radical innovation, but it does bring a degree of novelty to the premise: interviews with the surviving members of the news crew are interspersed with flashbacks of their experiences underground and moments of melancholy reflection. The flashbacks are presented through 'real' footage captured by the camera crew while in the tunnels and time-stamped CityRail CCTV tape. This style results in a gritty, 'low-fi' aesthetic typical of contemporary found-footage films.

Though the audience catch glimpses of the creature's pale skeletal form and piercing eyes, its actual nature and identity are never revealed. Demon, ghost or some other form of monster, it is implied that the beast is supernatural rather than human. This approach opens up realms of horrifying possibilities, all of which are left to the spectator's imagination. As *The Tunnel* declines to paint an explicit picture of the mutant killer, the setting itself becomes prominent as an active force in the narrative, capable of inflicting trauma and crushing hope.

The idea of a monstrous landscape that threatens the lives of characters is typical in Australian horror. But in *The Tunnel*, this idea is transplanted from the desolate outback, to a vast concrete wilderness beneath the city. 'I didn't realize how vast they were,' says Natasha (Bel Deliá) referring to the tunnels. 'There's virtually a whole other city beneath us.' In the movie, the notion of a city beneath a city is an unnerving concept due to its proximity to everyday life. The underground tunnels are uncharted, claustrophobic and isolated, although they are at times only metres away from the bustle of inner-city train stations. The struggle for survival in an isolated, yet urban, scape is evident in a scene in which Natasha struggles to open a manhole in a ceiling leading directly onto a busy road – cars zoom overhead, oblivious to her screams.

The tunnels are not imagined, but actually based on several different locations in and around Sydney's city centre. Though the monster is inhuman, the tunnels are a killing trap for people, designed by people. The use of man-made, confined subterranean spaces sets *The Tunnel* apart from the typical Aussie horror flick – where protagonists are threatened in wide, open spaces generally set in the outback – and renews the conventions of Australian landscape horror.

Lauren Carroll Harris

Reference

Bartlett, Myke (2011) 'The Pirates and the Tunnel', *Metro*, 167, p.114.

Bodey, Michael (2010) 'Filmmakers Build Funds, Frame by Frame', *The Australian*, 5 July, p.7.

ROAD MOVIE

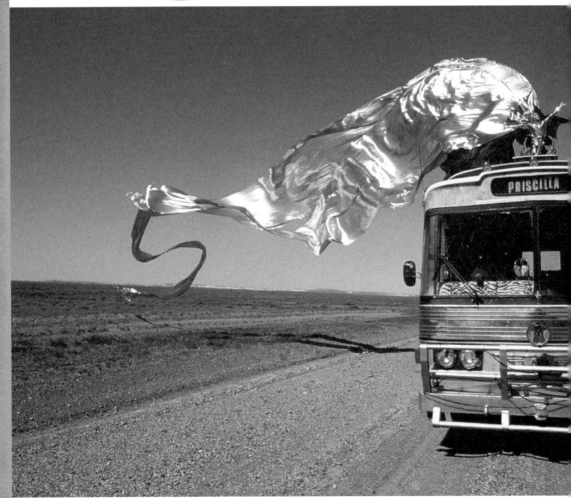

The Adventures of Priscilla, Queen of the Desert
(Stephen Elliott, 1994). © Kobal Collection

[T]he road movie is [...] like the musical or the western, a Hollywood genre that catches peculiarly American dreams, tensions and anxieties, even when imported by the motion picture industries of other countries.

(Cohan and Hark 1997: 2)

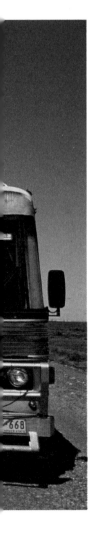

Undoubtedly Australia, like the United States, provides a natural fit for the road movie with its vast geography offering suitable spatial and temporal terrain for nomadic protagonists to traverse. In the road movie, Australia is often represented by a set of stylistic norms in cinematography, also common in the US road movie, such as the extensive deployment of wide-angle and fish-eye lenses, panorama scope and long-shots of landscapes with human figures diminished and isolated, high-angle aerial and crane-mounted travelling shots, exaggerated depth and ubiquitous shots of the road stretching to a limitless horizon. Both nations are also settler societies that were significantly transformed by the technological intervention of the motor car, with the pre-motorized western and the Australian equivalent, the bushranger/drover film, argued to be forerunners to the road movie (Venkatasawmy, Simpson and Visosevic 2001: 77).

In spite of these apparent similarities, Australian film-makers have made concerted attempts to differentiate the local road movie by accommodating specific national contexts, themes and tendencies resulting in an indigenous expression of the genre. This is perhaps not surprising given Australian cinema's ongoing nationalist project of self-definition, which has been attached, in varying degrees, to government funding objectives since the 1970s.

The documentary *The Back of Beyond* (John Heyer, 1954), tracking the journey of outback mailman, Tom Kruse, has been argued to be the first Australian road movie (Venkatasawmy, Simpson and Visosevic 2001: 79). However, as Jonathan Rayner (2000: 149) notes, it was not until the mid-1970s that Australian film began to explore the motifs of the car and the road more earnestly in films such as *The Cars That Ate Paris* (Peter Weir, 1974) and *Backroads* (Phillip Noyce, 1977). While this development may have partly been influenced by the post-*Easy Rider* (Dennis Hopper, 1969) growth of the American road movie, it also coincided with the revival of Australian cinema during the early 1970s. It can also be aligned to the consolidation of a youth car culture in Australia in the late 1960s and 1970s, in which cars were valued both as status symbols and for entertainment, which was forged partly as the result of young people's access to higher levels of independent disposable income. In fact, Australian road movies cultivate a particular attachment to the mythic value of car culture, a point enthusiastically endorsed by Quentin Tarantino in the documentary, *Not Quite Hollywood: The Wild Untold Story of Ozploitation!* (Mark Hartley, 2008). Tarantino remarks that 'nobody shoots a car the way Aussies do. They manage to shoot with this fetishistic lens that just makes you want to jerk-off'. This point has also been made, albeit not in such explicit terms, by Australian directors, George Miller (*Mad Max* [1979]; *Mad Max 2* [1981]; *Mad Max: Beyond Thunderdome* [1985]) and Jasmine Yuen-Carracun (*Cactus* [2008]), and by film critic Adrian Martin (Venkatasawmy, Simpson, and Visosevic 2001: 80), among others.

American road movies often feature a nihilistic rebel-outlaw mentality to a greater extent than their Australian counterparts, with a few exceptions, such as the Tarantinoesque *Kiss or Kill* (Bill Bennett, 1997). This may be in part because America fetishizes gun culture to a greater degree via its constitutional legitimization. Australian 'outlaw' or thriller road movies, such as the Mad Max cycle, *Stone* (Sandy Harbutt, 1974), *The Cars That Ate Paris* and *Road Games* (Richard Franklin, 1981), by contrast have depicted the road as a contested space whereby vehicles rather than guns are predominantly deployed as weapons. As George Miller observes in *Not Quite Hollywood*, 'in Australia we have autocide rather than homicide'.

This emphasis on car culture helps ensure the road movie's attachment to the trope of masculinity; the road is hardly a traditionally feminized domestic space (Cohan and Hark 1997: 3). This is also reinforced by the road movie's direct descendance from the highly masculinized genre of the drover/bushranger film, and the western. However, Australia does have a social and cinematic tradition of privileging and problematizing masculinity, and the road movie undoubtedly allows for the ongoing expression of these concerns. Certainly this is evident in the road movies reviewed for this collection, which in varying ways 'use the road as a space where masculinity is free to change' (Butterss 2000: 227).

The American road movie is bound up in notions of freedom, forging 'a travel narrative out of a particular conjunction of plot and setting that sets the liberation of the road against the oppression of hegemonic norms'; and as such, 'road movies project American western mythology onto the landscape traversed and bound by the nation's highways' (Cohan and Hark 1997: 1). The extent that these values of liberty and individualism have been transposed onto the Australian road movie is questionable. The foundation of the American frontier myth is enshrined in the expansionist notion of 'manifest destiny' in relation to land acquisition, which led to the American west being 'civilized' by large-scale development, such as the railroad. In contrast, while the car undoubtedly enacted a form of mastery and progress in pioneer Australia, colonial Australia was forged out of the (erroneous) doctrine of Terra Nullius, 'a land belonging to no one'. While both doctrines confer a similar sense of entitlement in relation to the displacement of Indigenous inhabitants and land settlement, Terra Nullius also embodied notions of geographical emptiness, and of a land that, for the most part, has refused widespread and dense settlement other than along the coastline.

This perhaps explains why Australian road movies tend to explore off-road potential to a greater degree than their American counterparts. As Stephan Elliot, the writer/director of *The Adventures of Priscilla, Queen of the Desert* (1994) notes, 'the key to all road trips is don't stay on the main roads' (Knight 2009: 8). Thus, while the road can initially be configured as a symbol of freedom and escape in Australian road movies, it often transpires that it serves as a constraining, civilizing force; a barrier to the possible monstrosities, barbarism or bigotry that may lie in wait for the person who strays off the road into the isolated, uncharted terrain of the Australian bush or outback. In *Priscilla*, a quirky detour off the main road allows for an encounter with a series of off-beat, but mostly homophobic, inhabitants of Australia's sparsely populated interior. In *Wolf Creek* (Greg McLean, 2005), it allows for the murderous encounter with the monstrous inversion of Crocodile Dundee, Mick Taylor. This has also been expanded on in an Australian context to include films that involve off-road journeys by foot, often featuring the character archetype of the Indigenous Australian tracker, such as *Walkabout* (Nicholas Roeg, 1971), *The Tracker* (Rolf de Heer, 2002) and *Rabbit-Proof Fence* (Phillip Noyce, 2002) (see Probyn 2005).

Both American and Australian road movies are generally infused with a pronounced degree of generic hybridity, whether it is horror, noir, crime, thriller or comedy. However, in contrast to American film, Australian cinema has a tendency to mobilize social realism as a key aesthetic mode. This often takes the form of a low-key egalitarian ordinariness, exemplified by a social typology of 'Australianness', represented by 'dagginness, quirkiness, ugliness or excess of some kind' (Venkatasawmy, Simpson and Visosevic 2001: 82). The Australian road movie is no exception to this, providing a stylistic variation on the more glamorous American road movie, which is often 'too cool to address seriously socio-political issues' (Atkinson 1994: 16). For example, in the 1970s a range of 'suburban' road movies, such as *FJ Holden* (Michael Thornhill, 1977) and *Summer City* (Christopher Fraser, 1977), offered brutally honest portrayals of suburban youth culture, alcoholism, teen sex and misogyny. In these instances, while the car is configured as a symbol of freedom and mobility, the protagonists ironically remain trapped within the banality of the suburban sprawl.

In the past few decades these sociopolitical issues have been largely 'structured through the themes and/or characters associated with white Australia's relationship to either Indigeneity or "ethnic" immigrancy', whereby 'the logic of the genre's setting has combined with its narrative logic to produce a "non-white" landscape traversed by refugees from hegemonic white society' (Harris 2006: 99–100). This has been explored in a number of key Australian road movies, including *Beneath Clouds* (Ivan Sen, 2002), and a series of 'road movies by foot' such as *Rabbit-Proof Fence* and *Lucky Miles* (Michael James Rowland, 2007). More social-realist works such as *Mad Bastards* (Brendan Fletcher, 2010) and *Samson and Delilah* (Warwick Thornton, 2009), while not fitting squarely within the genre, have incorporated the road and the journey as key motifs in their explorations of Indigenous Australian identity. However, the social dimension of the Australian road movie is often mediated by a national project of self-exhibition that uses cinema to promote Australia as a tourist destination. Road movies such as *Last Ride* (Glendyn Ivin, 2009), *Charlie & Boots* (Dean Murphy, 2009) and paradoxically *Wolf Creek*, afford the opportunity to foreground distinctive qualities of the remote Australian landscape for both international and national audiences, thus producing an interesting set of tensions between the aesthetic pleasures offered by Australia's spectacular natural wonders offset by the raw ugliness and/or ordinariness of its inhabitants.

Deborah J Thomas

References

Atkinson, Michael (1994) 'Crossing the Frontiers', *Sight and Sound*, 4: 1, pp. 14–17.

Butterss, Philip (2000) 'Australian Masculinity on the Road', *Media International Australia Incorporating Culture and Policy*, 95, pp. 227–36.

Cohan, Steven and Hark, Ina Rae (1997) *The Road Movie Book*, London and New York: Routledge.

Harris, Hilary (2006) 'Desert Training for Whites: Australian Road Movies', *Journal of Australian Studies*, 29. 86, pp. 99–110.

Knight, Anneli (2009) 'Get this Show on the Road', *Sydney Morning Herald*, 1 May, p. 8.

Probyn, Fiona (2005) 'An Ethics of Following and the No Road Film: Trackers, Followers and Fanatics', *Australian Humanities Review*, http://www.australianhumanitiesreview.org/archive/Issue-December-2005/Probyn.html. Accessed 29 September 2013.

Rayner, Jonathan (2000) *Contemporary Australian Cinema: An Introduction*, Manchester: Manchester University Press.

Venkatasawmy, Rama, Simpson, Catherine and Visosevic, Tanja (2001), 'From Sand to Bitumen, From Bushrangers to Bogans: Mapping the Australian Road Movie', *Journal of Australian Studies*, 25: 70, pp. 75–84.

The Adventures of Priscilla, Queen of the Desert

Country of Origin:

Australia

Studio/Distributor:

Specific Films
Latent Image Productions

Director:

Stephan Elliott

Producers:

Michael Hamlyn
Al Clark

Screenwriter:

Stephan Elliott

Director of Photography:

Brian J Breheny

Production Designer:

Owen Paterson

Composer:

Guy Gross

Editor:

Sue Blainey

Duration:

103 minutes

Genres:

Road movie
Musical
Comedy

Cast:

Hugo Weaving
Guy Pearce
Terence Stamp
Bill Hunter
Sarah Chadwick
Julia Cortez
Mark Holmes
June Marie Bennett

Format:

35mm

Synopsis

Two drag queens, Mitzi aka Tick and the flamboyant Felicia aka Adam and an acerbic transsexual, Bernadette, travel from Sydney to Alice Springs in a lavender-coloured tour bus called Priscilla. Marion, Tick's ex-wife, has offered them a cabaret gig at the Alice Springs casino she runs. All three protagonists seize on the opportunity to take a break from the dissatisfaction of their city lives, and to give Tick a chance to reunite with his son who he has not seen since his separation. On the way they encounter various colourful locals, as well as the dark side of the Australian outback and less accepting attitudes of rural Australia. When Priscilla breaks down in the middle of the desert they set up camp and later meet a group of welcoming Indigenous people for whom they perform. Eventually they are towed to a small outback town where the bus is repaired by a helpful mechanic, Bob, who joins them on their journey. They arrive in Alice Springs where Tick is reunited with his son, and the group fulfils Adam's long-held dream of climbing Kings Canyon in drag. All of the travellers must decide whether to stay or return to Sydney.

Critique

Priscilla is arguably the most iconic Australian road movie of all time. At the time of its release, the film was praised for making a contribution to Australian cinema beyond the seemingly ubiquitous costume dramas of the 1970s and stereotypical, hetero-normative configurations of 'Australianess' embodied in the likes of *Crocodile Dundee* (Peter Faiman, 1986). Instead, *Priscilla* situates itself within a cycle of Australian kitsch or camp, which feature 'the retrospective idolisation of 1970s Glamour' (Rayner 2000: 21). Certainly much of the narrative drive and comedic pleasure of this film is enabled by the incongruous juxtaposition apparent in the flamboyant excess of urbanized drag culture with the vastness and parochialism of the Australian outback. Summed up in one of the film's most memorable lines, 'cock in a frock on a rock', it is this quality that lends a 'joy ride' element to Priscilla, 'which literally dresses up the road movie in drag' (Venkatasawmy, Simpson and Visosevic 2001: 82).

As Katie Ellis (2006) has documented, there was also a focus in 1990s Australian cinema on marginal and identity politics. To this end *Pricilla* deploys the road movie's generic hospitality 'to the marginalised and alienated' (Cohan and Hark 1997: 12), by mapping the political geography of outback Australia around themes of sexuality, gender, race and other cultural agendas. As with much of Australian cinema, masculinity is to the fore, but in a way that challenges the hegemony of highly normative constructions of Australian 'ocker' masculinity. *Priscilla* makes good use of Australia's off-road potential as a means of exploring this displacement and difference via its exposé of rural bigotry and homophobia, which culminates most powerfully in the anti-gay graffiti sprayed on Priscilla. The film purposefully advocates models

Year:

1994

of tolerance in its depiction of Bob (Bill Hunter) and Bernadette's (Terence Stamp) enduring relationship, and the consolidation of familial bonds as Tick (Hugo Weaving) assumes the mantle of father to his son, Benjamin (Mark Holmes), within the paradigm of queer difference.

Priscilla, however, is a bundle of contradictions. Seemingly transgressive and progressive with its positive focus on queerness and transexuality, and its open-minded portrait of an 'ocker' male, the film is also profoundly regressive in its marginalization of femininity and race. The grotesque representation of Bob's Filipino wife, Cynthia (Julia Cortez), who consistently embarrasses herself (and us) with her drunken lewdness, and the ability to shoot ping pong balls out of her vagina, provides a highly problematic racial stereotype, one which configures the Asian 'mail-order bride' as 'castrating, foreign, manipulative and perversely sexualised' who does not, and never will, belong in Australia (Robertson 1997: 279). Similarly, Bernadette's tirade on a rather butch white woman, Shirley (June Marie Bennett), in the Broken Hill pub, who admittedly is crudely homophobic, appears excessively misogynistic. The representation of the Indigenous people that the three chief protagonists encounter on their travels has also been criticized for portraying an 'egregious' racial stereotype (Robertson 1997: 280) which is schematic at best.

Cohan and Hark argue that the 'road movie provides a ready space for exploration of the tensions and crises of the historical moment during which it is produced' (1997: 2). While this is undoubtedly true of *Priscilla*, it is a sobering thought that the social tensions the film exposes still have profound ongoing relevance in Australia two decades later. While drag and gay culture is tolerated as a spectacle of difference bound-up in values of performance and entertainment, achieving recognition and rights in Australia is still problematic, with debates over the legitimatization of gay marriage and surrogacy rumbling on at the time of writing.

Somewhat paradoxically, the film also taps into other contemporary national agendas on racism and sexism. The parochial racism depicted in *Priscilla* is still alive and well in Australia as evident in Joe Hildebrand's recent television series, *Dumb, Drunk and Racist* (Cordell Jigsaw, ABC [Australia], 2012). Similarly Prime Minister Julia Gillard's high profile parliamentary attack in October 2012 on the misogyny of opposition leader, Tony Abbott, highlighted the inherent sexism that continues to manifest itself in the Australian social fabric.

Regardless of these troubling aspects of the film, *Priscilla* has become firmly embedded in the Australian cultural imagination. There have been subsequent successful Broadway and West End musical adaptations of the film, while one of Australia's commercial television networks recently ran a talent quest to find a drag performer for the Broadway production in the Australian television reality show, *I Will Survive* (FremantleMedia Australia, Network Ten, 2012).

Deborah J Thomas

References

Cohan, Steven and Hark, Ina Rae (1997) *The Road Movie Book*,
London and New York: Routledge.

Ellis, Katie (2006) 'Rehabilitating 1990s Australian National Cinema',
Senses of Cinema, 39, http://sensesofcinema.com/2006/39/
rehab_australian_cinema_1990s/. Accessed 5 November 2012.

Rayner, Jonathan (2000) *Contemporary Australian Cinema: An
Introduction*, Manchester: Manchester University Press.

Robertson, Pamela (1997) 'Home and Away: Friends of Dorothy on the
Road in Oz', in Steven Cohan and Ina Rae Hark (eds), *The Road
Movie Book*, London and New York: Routledge, pp. 271–86.

Venkatasawmy, Rama, Simpson, Catherine and Visosevic, Tanja
(2001), 'From Sand to Bitumen, From Bushrangers to Bogans:
Mapping the Australian Road Movie, *Journal of Australian
Studies*, 25: 70, pp. 75–84.

Charlie & Boots

Country of Origin:

Australia

Studio/Distributor:

Instinct Entertainment

Director:

Dean Murphy

Producers:

David Redman
Shana Levine
Dean Murphy

Screenwriters:

Stewart Faichney
Dean Murphy

Cinematographer:

Roger Lanser

Production Designer:

Ralph Moser

Composer:

Dale Cornelius

Editor:

Peter Carrodus

Duration:

100 minutes

Genres:

Road movie
Comedy

Synopsis

After the death of his mother, Boots McFarland assists his estranged
father Charlie on his dairy farm in Warrnambool, Victoria. In order
to help Charlie recover from his chronic grief and depression, Boots
persuades his father to join him on a long discussed road trip to go
fishing at Cape York Peninsula, the northernmost tip of Australia.
Together they set off in a classic Holden Kingswood up the east coast.
Along the way they have a series of misadventures and encounters
with a host of colourful local characters, including a teenage female
hitchhiker near the country-music capital of Australia, Tamworth, and a
female trucker who takes a particular shine to Charlie. Initially, Charlie
seems unable to overcome his reclusive melancholia but then begins
to relax. After Boots reveals another tragedy, both characters start to
come to terms with their grief.

Critique

Charlie & Boots is moulded along the generic lines of the 'buddy'
road movie, but, at the same time, is overtly marked as a national
project of self-exhibition. Its tourist travelogue presentation of the
east coast of Australia, comprising a series of episodic vignettes,
showcases a land populated by eccentric rural characters. The
film also makes the most of Australian icons, including the classic
Holden Kingswood car, and various 'big' kitsch landmarks, such
as the 'Giant Koala' and Tamworth's statue of an oversized golden
guitar.

A gentle, low-key comedy, punctuated by dramatic moments,
Charlie & Boots resolutely avoids the 'coolness' that can
characterize American road movies. Instead, it proposes a more
genial, egalitarian space that explores the distinctive regionalism
of Australia and its inhabitants, within a storyline revolving around
the father-and-son relationship. Aimed at a broad audience, the film
was released to coincide with Father's Day in 2009, and succeeded

Cast:

Paul Hogan
Shane Jacobson
Morgan Griffin
Roy Billing
Peggy Thompson
Anne Phelan
Baxter James Thomson

Format:

35mm

Year:

2009

in achieving the best opening weekend for any Australian film that year (ABC News 2009). This was probably in large measure due to its resurrection of popular iconic Australian actor, Paul Hogan (aka Crocodile Dundee) and, to lesser extent, the popularity of Shane Jacobson after his performance as the eponymous lead character in the successful 'mockumentary' comedy, *Kenny* (Clayton Jacobson, 2006). There is even an in-joke at the end of the credits, referring to Hogan's previous occupation as a rigger on the Sydney Harbour Bridge; as the duo drive across the bridge, Boots remarks, 'amazing piece of engineering', to which Charlie replies, 'Yeah! But imagine painting the bastard!'

Like countless Australian films, masculinity is to the fore as the two protagonists hesitantly consolidate filial bonds abetted by two of the defining features of the road movie genre itself: the shared intimacy of the 'confined space' of the car (Cohan and Hark 1997: 8) and the time taken in the journey itself. *Charlie & Boots*'s lighter comic moments are offset by a palpable sense of grief. While the film is somewhat clichéd in its portrayal of the death of Grace (Peggy Thompson) at the beginning of the film, it avoids undue heavy handedness in the almost incidental revelation of the death by drowning of Ben (Baxter James Thomson), Boots's son, part way through the film. Also, to an extent, Paul Hogan as an actor lacks the emotional range necessary for this portrayal of grief and tension. As a result, his performance is, at times, rather flat and stilted in spite of the fact that Charlie's clumsy, inarticulate attempts to communicate his grief cohere with his character type. Overall, however, the film manages to impart a genuine and touching sense of emerging tenderness and connection wrought between these two somewhat rough-hewn Aussie blokes in the face of loss.

Their journey exemplifies how 'the road has always functioned in movies as an alternative space where isolation from the mainstream permits various transformative experiences' (Cohan and Hark 1997: 5). As usually happens in this genre, 'life on the road ends and a new form of home is established' (Butterss 2000: 233). Charlie and Boots can travel no further than the uppermost point of Australia, which also signals a decisive end to conflict. The differences between the two protagonists are reconciled so that in a sense the two protagonists arrive, in somewhat cyclical fashion, 'home' to a less conflicted, more accommodating space.

Deborah J Thomas

Reference

ABC News (2009) 'Charlie & Boots Storm Aussie Box Office', http://www.abc.net.au/news/2009-09-08/charlie-and-boots-storms-aussie-box-office/1421022. Accessed 17 January 2013.

Butterss, Philip (2000) 'Australian Masculinity on the Road', *Media International Australia*, 95, pp. 227–36.

Cohan, Steven and Hark, Ina Rae (1997) *The Road Movie Book*, London and New York: Routledge.

Last Ride

Country of Origin:

Australia

Studio/Distributor:

Talk Films

Director:

Glendyn Ivin

Producers:

Nicholas Cole
Antonia Barnard

Screenwriter:

Mac Gudgeon, adapted from
the novel *Last Ride* by Denise
Young (2004)

Cinematographer:

Greig Fraser

Production Designer:

Jo Ford

Composer:

Paul Charlier

Editor:

Jack Hutchings

Synopsis

Ex convict, Kev and his 10-year-old son, Chook, embark on a desperate journey across the South Australian outback on the run from the police. A series of flashbacks of the boy's fragmented memories reveals that Kev has committed a violent assault on his friend Max. Kev and Chook make their way by bus, foot, hitchhiking and in stolen cars. They survive by pilfering food along the way, sometimes eating rabbits they have shot. Most nights they sleep under the stars and Kev tells Chook stories. Kev is a damaged and conflicted man who, in spite of his love for his son, is at times unable to restrain his violence. This culminates as the two arrive at Lake Gairdner, a vast, empty salt lake.

Critique

The coupling of father and son in *Last Ride* provides a variation on the well-established road movie trope of the 'outlaw couple on the run'. Glendyn Ivin's feature debut (after winning the Palme d'Or for Best Short Film at Cannes in 2003) adopts a treatment of mood, tone, pacing, character and setting reminiscent of other contemporary Australian films, such as *Cactus* (Jasmine Yuen-Carracun, 2008) and *Samson and Delilah* (Warwick Thornton, 2009). While Kev (Hugo Weaving) and Chook's (Tom Russell) journey appears doomed from the outset, the film is devoid of the nihilistic glamour and sustained action often apparent in American 'outlaw' road movies. Instead it adopts a more socially honest examination of its themes, with the laconic pacing and spasmodic dialogue,

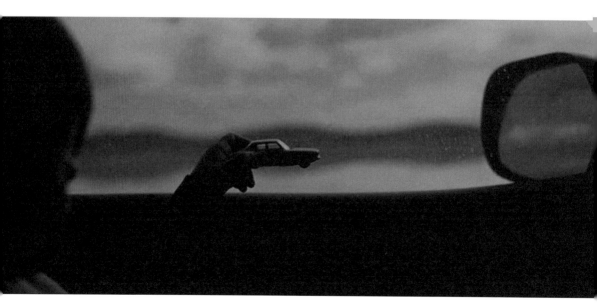

Last Ride
(Glendyn Ivin, 2009)

Duration:

100 minutes

Genres:

Road movie
Drama
Coming of age

Cast:

Hugo Weaving
Tom Russell
Anita Hegh
John Brumpton

Format:

35mm

Year:

2009

punctuated by violence, providing a disturbing and hard-hitting portrait of a desperate man and his child on the run.

Kev is undoubtedly an intensely hard-bitten ex-con who, in many respects, is patently ill-equipped to provide the material stability and nurturing that a 10-year-old child needs. In contrast, the more sensitive and compassionate Chook assumes the moral centre of the film; much of the action is filtered through his subjectivity as the film reflects on a child trying to reconcile his life on the run, and his father's erratic, sometimes violent behaviour and warped morality, with displays of extreme tenderness and protectiveness. In spite of the film's relatively slow pace there is a palpable sense of suspense and anticipation built up around the unpredictable edginess and fragility of Kev's behaviour, which constantly threatens to erupt and impinge on Chook's safety. In one particular scene, Kev brutally and repeatedly holds his son under water in an effort to teach him how to swim. In another scene, the film interrogates masculine identity as Kev beats Chook when he discovers that his son, in childlike fashion, has applied make-up and lipstick to his face. However, the 5000 km journey not only affords the opportunity for a slow reveal of the events that led father and son to be fugitives, but also the pedagogy of Kev's abusive behaviour. It transpires that Kev endured abuse from his own father as well as abuse during his time served in prison ('All sorts of shit goes on in prison, mate. I was young … easy prey').

The film's director expressed in a television interview on ABC's *At the Movies* (1 July 2009) that he intended to make a 'brutiful' film. This is manifest in the way in which the social realism of *Last Ride* is offset by the beautiful but distant and alienated landscape of the South Australian outback, which not only provides a parallel to the marginalization of its central protagonists, but also their beauty/ cruelty relationship. This is presented as a project of self-exhibition with sweeping panoramic shots of various landmarks, such as the Flinders Ranges and culminating with the vast flat salt lake, Lake Gairdner, which provides the stunning backdrop to the film's final poignant moments. There is also an interesting momentary reference in the film to Australia's often forgotten multicultural history when Chook and Kev take shelter in a defunct Afghan Heritage Museum. The film was praised for the subtle and evocative depth of its lead performances, and generally attracted a positive critical response both nationally and internationally with noted American critic Roger Ebert giving it four out of four stars (Ebert 2012).

Deborah J Thomas

Reference

Ebert, Roger (2012) '*Last Ride*' [review], *Chicago Sun-Times*, 27 June, http://rogerebert.suntimes.com/apps/pbcs.dll/ article?AID=/20120627/REVIEWS/120629977. Accessed 27 January 2013.

Rabbit-Proof Fence

Country of Origin:

Australia

Director:

Phillip Noyce

Producers:

Phillip Noyce
Christine Olsen
John Winter

Screenwriter:

Christine Olsen, based on the book *Follow the Rabbit-Proof Fence* by Doris Pilkington (Nugi Garimara) (1996)

Cinematographer:

Christopher Doyle

Production Designer:

Roger Ford

Composer:

Peter Gabriel

Editors:

Veronika Jenet
John Scott

Duration:

94 minutes

Genres:

Adventure
Road movie

Cast:

Kenneth Branagh
Everlyn Sampi
Tianna Sansbury
Laura Monaghan
David Gulpilil

Format:

35mm

Year:

2002

Synopsis

1931, Jigalong, Western Australia. Three Indigenous children, 14-year-old Molly, her younger half-sister Daisy and their younger cousin Gracie, are captured by authorities and taken under the terms of the 1905 Aborigines Act to the Moore River Native Settlement, hundreds of kilometres away from their home. Determined to return home, Molly plans their escape from the settlement after a storm, as the rain will wash away their footprints. The girls rely on the charity of strangers for food on their trek northward. All the while they are pursued by the authorities, led by Chief Protector of Aborigines, AO Neville.

Critique

This is a tale of the 'Stolen Generation' – in reality around 100,000 Indigenous children from around Australia who were removed from their homes without parental consent and without a court order, and placed in far distant settlements, fostered or adopted by non-Indigenous families between the turn of the twentieth century and the early 1970s. The 'rabbit-proof fence' of the title was in fact three fences, constructed in Western Australia (WA) between 1901 and 1907 in a vain attempt to prevent rabbits reaching the farmlands of western WA. In the film, the children walk along the No. 3 and No. 2 Fences before finally joining up with the No. 1 Fence that leads them all the way back home.

Kenneth Branagh plays A.O. Neville (called 'Devil' by the Moore River children), the legal guardian of every Indigenous person in Western Australia. Neville believes his heart is in the right place, even when what he advocates could be labelled genocide. He wants to enforce the state's 1905 Aborigines Act, under which 'mixed-blood' children were not only placed under his guardianship, but could also be removed from their families. Neville wanted all 'half-castes' (i.e. children of mixed Indigenous and non-Indigenous descent) 'absorb[ed] into the white race' until the 'Aboriginal is bred out', as he rationalizes it in the film. (The Act remained on the statute books until it was repealed by the Native Welfare Act 1963, under which responsibility for 'native minors' passed from the Commissioner to the Department of Native Welfare. This Act, and the policy of removal, was finally repealed by the Aboriginal Affairs Planning Authority Act 1972.) This telling of Australia's racist history sets it apart from notable films such as *Jedda* (Charles Chauvel, 1955), *Walkabout* (Nicolas Roeg, 1971) and *The Last Wave* (Peter Weir, 1977), which also explored Indigenous issues, but did not so overtly explore the history of Australia's mistreatment of its Indigenous population.

Noyce had earlier examined racism and Indigenous issues in *Backroads* (1977), but had not made a film in Australia since *Dead Calm* (1989). By 2002 – a notable year for the director, with the release of his critically acclaimed adaptation of Graham Greene's novel *The Quiet American* – he had established himself as one of the more notable directors of the Hollywood thriller. Discussing the motivation for his return, Noyce said 'I no longer knew what it was like to feel Australian, but then along came this story' (Pendreigh 2002).

Primarily known for his work with Wong Kar-Wai, Christopher Doyle's cinematography captures the Western Australia landscape as few others have, to the point where it becomes a character in the narrative. Doyle and Noyce also employ a subjective camera at times to capture the children's point of view. Peter Gabriel created a fitting soundscape with his Golden Globe-winning score that incorporates Indigenous sounds. Everlyn Sampi's performance as Molly stands out, even if life imitated art – Sampi rebelled against the demands of film-making and tried to run away (Pendreigh 2002). David Gulpilil, known for his major roles in *Walkabout*, *Mad Dog Morgan* (Philippe Mora, 1976), *The Last Wave* and *Crocodile Dundee* (Peter Faiman, 1986), plays Moodoo the tracker, and received significant award attention the same year for his leading role in Rolf de Heer's film, *The Tracker* (2002).

Rabbit-Proof Fence contains several notable sequences, including the heart-wrenching scene where Molly and Daisy (Tianna Sansbury) are taken away from their mother. The film begins with Molly's voice-over in the language of her people, Martuwangka, but the viewer is not entirely sure of the film's veracity until the final minutes, when we see the real Molly and Daisy, now octogenarians. This powerful moment evokes one last tear, as Molly admits to never having seen Gracie (Laura Monaghan) again after their parting. Yet it is the cinematography that keeps this film, albeit one based on a heartfelt true story, from becoming a pedestrian, inspirational movie-of-the-week. It captures their arduous, mammoth undertaking with shots of battered feet in ragged, dusty shoes treading slowly over the rocky, arid landscape. The book describes the children taking horses and a boat for small portions of the journey, but the film's artistic licence omits this. The film won several awards, including Best Film at the 2002 Australian Film Institute Awards. *Rabbit-Proof Fence* received almost universal critical acclaim from North American critics, but was shut out at the Academy Awards, despite the marketing efforts of distributor Miramax films.

Zachary Ingle

Reference

Pendreigh, Brian (2002) 'Leaping the Fence of Australia's Past', *Film Inside Out*, http://www.iofilm.co.uk/feats/interviews/r/rabbit_proof_fence_2002.shtml. Accessed 1 May 2013.

Walkabout

Country of Origin:
Australia/UK
Studio/Distributor:
Max L.Raab-Si Litvinoff Films

Synopsis

A teenage girl and her younger brother are taken into the outback by their father for a picnic; and, in a premeditated attack, he attempts to kill them. The children manage to escape and confronted by his actions, the father burns the family car and commits suicide. Lost in the unforgiving heat of the desert, the children embark on a journey with some food and water from the picnic, a transistor radio

Director:

Nicolas Roeg

Producer:

Si Litvinoff

Screenwriter:

Edward Bond, adapted from the novel *Walkabout* by James Vance Marshall (1959)

Cinematographer:

Nicolas Roeg

Production Designer:

Brian Eatwell

Composer:

John Barry

Editors:

Antony Gibbs
Alan Patillo

Duration:

100 minutes

Genres:

Drama
'No road' movie

Cast:

Jenny Agutter
Luc Roeg
David Gulpilil
John Meillon

Format:

35mm

Year:

1971

and the school uniforms they wore on the day. Their resources dwindling, the siblings cross paths with a young Indigenous man on a 'Walkabout' – a rite of passage for young Indigenous men who undergo a journey to live apart from their families for a period of time. The young man guides the siblings through the rough terrain, providing them with food and water and sharing his intimate knowledge of the landscape and nature. The young Indigenous man and his fellow travellers form a bond, but cultural misunderstanding leads to tragedy.

Critique

Walkabout is a carefully constructed representation of an encounter between two contrasting cultures that, despite their differences, also have fundamental similarities. The opening scenes of *Walkabout* are critical in setting up these binaries. In a dramatic montage of city life in Sydney, the director Nicolas Roeg effectively depicts the notion of a 'civilized world': bustling city streets, suited men entering office buildings, women wearing colourful dresses and traffic lights controlling the flow of cars. Inasmuch as these beautifully filmed shots depict a modern capitalist society, Roeg neatly juxtaposes these visuals with the humming sound of a didgeridoo and images of the outback. The opening scenes imply that beneath the surface of white Australian society lie the complex histories of Australian colonialism.

Apart from introducing the binary opposites of culture and nature, the opening scenes introduce the movie's main characters: the father (John Meillon) is shown at work in a large sterile office building; his teenaged daughter (Jenny Agutter) is at school receiving voice training; while the young boy (Luc Roeg) is running around in the yard of a boy's school. All the gender roles are neatly delineated and the nuclear family is completed with a shot of the mother, who, unaware of the tragedy that will unfold, prepares the family picnic.

Far removed from the inner city and the family's upper-middle-class lives, the plot takes a dark twist when the children are taken for a drive into the bush. The father's emotional distance from his children is signified by a number of shots in which he is depicted looking at his children, as if to analyse their behaviour, yet appears unable to comprehend who they are. As indicated by harmonious music and sweeping tracking shots, the film initially represents the children's escape from their father into the bush as a journey of new opportunities. However, the impending dangers of the harsh desert are suggested by a close-up shot of ants feasting wildly on picnic scraps. The journey is punctuated by a number of potential threats: wild animals, unforgiving terrain, and, above all, the scorching heat of the sun. In spite of this, the girl clings to the world that she has left behind as she tells her brother to look after his blazer: 'we don't want people to think that we are a couple of tramps'. The boy aptly retorts, 'What people?'

Following their fortuitous encounter with the Indigenous man (David Gulpilil), the girl's insistence on keeping up a good appearance softens. In a famous scene in which they look for water, the girl briefly touches the man's bare chest. This scene establishes a sexual tension fused with race relations as a powerful reoccurring motif throughout the film. Additionally, the representation of the girl – who was sixteen at the time of filming – is highly voyeuristic. In one scene she is depicted skinny-dipping in a creek. The height and the distance of the camera turn her body into a cinematic spectacle amidst the luscious nature of the Australian outback. Yet the scene is filmed as if this spectacle is purely for the benefit of the viewer and not the Indigenous man. In other words, while the relationship between the girl and the man remains sexually innocent, it is the viewer who is encouraged to visually 'consume' her body for spectatorial pleasure.

Perhaps because the film was made by a non-Australian director and largely a non-Australian cast and crew, *Walkabout* represents an extremely unusual case in which nudity is featured in Australian cinema. After the relaxation of censorship laws, so-called 'ocker' comedies and Australian commercial television only featured nudity from the early to mid-1970s onwards. Roeg's iconoclastic approach is reaffirmed by a strong penchant for fantasy and surrealistic satire. Possibly in a reference to Federico Fellini, *Walkabout* includes a stunningly bizarre scene which includes mainly Italian meteorologists lusting after the only woman in their team. In another scene, a brash gold-shirted Australian man reveals himself as the gang master of a group of Indigenous children producing kitschy 'Aboriginal' art objects. The clash and the parallels between the two cultures is emphasized in a dramatic montage: images of the young Indigenous man slaughtering wild animals are interlaced with a shot of a Sydney butcher putting meat through a grinder. Roeg twists and bends the language of cinema to create a multifaceted depiction of two cultural binaries constantly at play with each other.

Towards the end of the film, the children's first contact with western society is with a grumpy manager of an abandoned mine who is apparently stuck in perpetual limbo as he awaits orders from his superiors. The contrast between the Indigenous man's kindness and the rudeness of the mine manager could not be greater. *Walkabout* ultimately can be read as a powerful homage to Australia's Indigenous population, the country's complex colonial past, and the beauty of the outback.

Marco Bohr

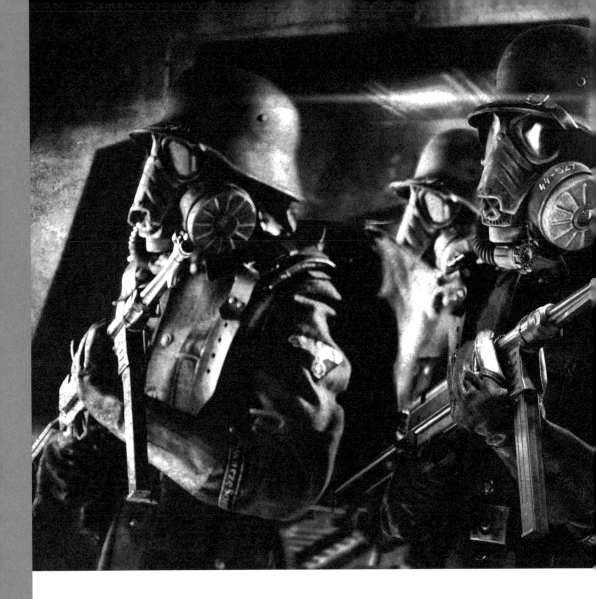

SCIENCE FICTION

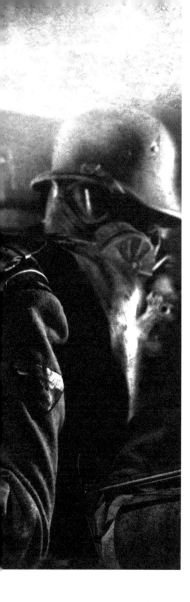

Iron Sky
(Timo Vuorensola, 2012).
© Kobal Collection

Few science fiction films have been made in Australia by Australians for Australian audiences, with most of the handful of locally-produced films made since the mid-1990s. Yet there has always been a solid Australian audience for non-Australian science fiction films and a strong international niche audience for the genre. While Australia has provided below-the-line crews and heads of departments (cinematographers, production designers, and so on) for many non-Australian science fiction films produced domestically, few Australian film directors have specialized in the genre. This is somewhat surprising considering that Alex Proyas achieved a degree of international success for his Gothic science fiction film *Dark City* (1998), and George Miller achieved international fame following the worldwide success of *Mad Max 2* (1981). Although the science fiction element of *Mad Max 2* is tenuous – and even more so in the case of the original *Mad Max* (George Miller, 1979) – Miller is credited with creating a new (sub)genre which incorporates science fiction elements and has been widely imitated internationally: the dystopian, post-apocalyptic movie. Nevertheless, Australia has only produced a small number of science fiction movies. In addition to the above films, key titles include: *Mad Max Beyond Thunderdome* (George Miller, 1985), *Shirley Thompson versus the Aliens* (Jim Sharman, 1972), *The Time Guardian* (Brian Hannant, 1987), *The Chain Reaction* (Ian Barry, 1980) and, more recently, *Knowing* (Alex Proyas, 2009), *Daybreakers* (Michael and Peter Spierig, 2009) and *Iron Sky* (Timo Vuorensola, 2012).

A problem when discussing Australian science fiction movies is that a corpus of films that constitute what could be regarded as a local tradition is poorly understood. At the core of this issue is the nexus between international and local production. As local high-end science fiction movies are often produced within a globalized industry structure – *Dark City* is a primary example (see Helms 1998) – and international runaway productions are often filmed at local studio facilities and draw upon Australian technical crews, supporting casts (sometimes leads) and department heads, the demarcation between local and international production can be blurred. *The Matrix* (Andy and Lana Wachowski, 1999), for example – although officially classified by government screen agencies as an international production – was filmed locally, received local investment, and contained input from key Australian creatives (Australian producer, Andrew Mason, was a significant player involved in the film, and the cast includes Hugo Weaving, among others). The issue of what delineates an Australian and an international production has been further complicated since the inception of the Producer Offset in 2007. An incentive designed to foster local production, the offset has encouraged the production of high-budget, internationalized local blockbusters which draw upon a combination of national and international creative inputs, including Alex Proyas's science fiction movie *Knowing* (see the review in this collection) and the action film *Killer Elite* (Gary McKendry, 2011). While both of these movies are regarded as Australian, with mixed local and international creative input, it could be argued that they are aesthetically and stylistically undifferentiated from typical Hollywood movies.

As Sean McMullen (2010: 228) observed in the first edition of this directory,

> the health of Australian [science fiction film] depends upon how one identifies it. Apply strict criteria about scripting, settings, funding and stars, and it seems in a very bad state. Merely count [the science fiction] movies shot in Australia and the prospects could not be better.

As McMullen suggests in terms of the latter, numerous international science fiction films have been produced in Australia since the late 1950s. Melbourne was the setting for an early post-apocalyptic film, *On the Beach* (Stanley Kramer, 1959), based on Nevil Shute's 1957 novel by the same name. A Hollywood movie shot in Australia, the film was remade for Australian television by Southern Star Productions in 2000. Directed by Russell Mulcahy, the remake is more pessimistic than the earlier film in its observations of human behaviour and psychology after a nuclear war. *On the Beach* (both the film and the television series) is unusual in that Melbourne is identified as Melbourne, and not as a generic future North American city, as was the case with Sydney and *The Matrix*.

Since the late 1990s, several popular and commercially successful international science fiction movies have been filmed in Australia with Australian crews and actors, including *The Matrix*, *The Matrix Reloaded* (Andy and Lana Wachowski, 2003), *Ghost Rider* (Mark Steven Johnson, 2007), *Star Wars: Episode II: Attack of the Clones* (George Lucas, 2002) and *Star Wars: Episode III: Revenge of the Sith* (George Lucas, 2005). There are many other international examples. *Fortress* (Stuart Gordon, 1992) used Queensland locations and studio facilities on the Gold Coast for its story about a couple imprisoned after trying to escape from the United States into Canada to avoid a punitive law limiting childbirth. *Pitch Black* (David Twohy, 2000), a movie revolving around survivors of a crash-landing on a desert planet who are hunted by flesh-eating creatures, was filmed in various locations in Queensland and South Australia. The action-science fiction film *Stealth* (Rob Cohen, 2005) was shot in the Blue Mountains National Park west of Sydney, and in South Australia's Flinders Ranges.

This essay, however, is concerned with locally sourced science fiction movies; that is, films produced locally, led by Australian key creatives (directors, screenwriters and producers) and local production companies with a degree of creative control, wholly or partially financed domestically, and officially recognized as 'local productions' by government screen agencies, namely Screen Australia and its predecessor, the Australian Film Commission. While we acknowledge that in the case of high-end films and co-productions the distinction between the local and international can be unclear, shifting discussion away from international science fiction movies filmed in Australia (and the question of local input) to focus upon local science fiction production, provides a less impressive but more accurate picture of local production. In particular, it reveals that unlike local horror cinema – with an ongoing stream of production and established themes, tropes and iconography – Australia has no sustained tradition of science fiction film production. Furthermore, Australia does not have sustained periods of production where the 'science' in science fiction is taken seriously. Rather, Australian films with science fiction 'content' are mostly films which are more appropriately classified as belonging to a genre other than science fiction. The look or visual style – *mise-en-scène* and production design codes and conventions – and the futuristic settings and locations contribute to, but do not define, the science fiction genre.

At its most 'intellectual' science fiction explores social, cultural and moral themes and meanings in ways not necessarily possible in other film genres. By definition, science fiction should have some science in it; it is a genre that looks at a possible future, extrapolating from the science we know. It is a genre that engages with ideas and possibilities of future developments. Creating and communicating fictional stories premised on science is a form of speculative storytelling that tends to result in stories predisposed to 'hard' science with contemporary relevancy (for example cloning, genetic engineering, the theory of time travel and worm holes). The wonder and fear of 'science' is present in most 'hard' science fiction.

Science fiction is a genre that can readily be combined with other genres such as horror and thriller. This generic hybridization tends to facilitate films developed to elicit emotional rather than intellectual responses from audiences. The hybrid action-science fiction-exploitation thriller *The Chain Reaction* and the horror-science fiction *Daybreakers* are examples. 'Soft' science fiction films often employ science fiction settings and science itself as a pretext for themes associated with other genres. In the horror-science fiction hybrid *Daybreakers*, after humans become vampires as a result of a virus, a non-scientific cure is discovered. Although some scenes and sequences do exhibit a futuristic look (gleaming metal and shiny surfaces in rooms and labs, for example), this does not translate into a science-based narrative. Instead, the search for a cure devolves into action-thriller chases and melodramatic encounters between characters. In the cerebral Australian film *Zone 39* (John Tatoulis, 1996), the wife of a soldier and security expert dies, leaving him emotionally traumatized. A low-budget film, it envisages a desolate future where the world's environment is ravaged and where two global factions are at war. The movie is primarily a psychological drama rather than a science fiction film as it deals more with coming to terms with isolation and death than with scientific explanations or discourses related to a future global environment.

In the late 1980s, Hemdale Films sought to cash in on the international appeal of science fiction. *The Time Guardian* was an attempt at producing a local science fiction film with international ambitions. The 'science' in the film was rather implausible and, as such, was more in tune with 'soft' science fiction. In soft science fiction, there is only a very loose connection to actual scientific methods and findings. Nevertheless, as the international science fiction-space opera epic *Star Wars: Episode IV: A New Hope* (George Lucas, 1977) demonstrated, soft science fiction does not preclude audience engagement. Unfortunately, *The Time Guardian*'s story of a time-travelling city being pursued by semi-humans did not engage Australian or international audiences.

There have been two notable examples of 'experimental' science fiction films that do not fit comfortably into the hard science fiction category, both directed by Rolf de Heer: *Incident at Raven's Gate* (1988) and *Epsilon* (1995). *Incident* at Raven's Gate (aka Encounter at Raven's Gate) is a film with an 'arthouse' appeal, claiming a link to science fiction through a storyline in which a farming property, Raven's Gate, comes under the influence of an alien force. De Heer's next 'experimental' film, Epsilon (aka Alien Visitor), is essentially an extended conversation conducted in the outback between an alien (in the form of a human female) and a human (Australian) male.

National production systems like Australia can produce their own style of science fiction. This is evident in two films where science fiction has fragile links with comedy or satire (Dead End Drive-In [Brian Trenchard-Smith, 1986] and As Time Goes By [Barry Peak, 1988]). Dead End Drive-In, based loosely on Peter Carey's 1974 short story 'Crabs', envisions a future in which economic and environmental disasters have resulted in social collapse. Authorities construct an electrified fence around a drive-in cinema to imprison unemployed young people, some of whom have become violent 'car boys'. Action sequences rather than 'science' define the film. While Dead End Drive-In was not well received by Australian audiences it has achieved cult status, and was praised by Quentin Tarantino in the documentary Not Quite Hollywood: The Wild, Untold Story of Ozploitation! (Mark Hartley, 2008).

In As Time Goes By, two women drive Mike Taggart into the outback so he can go surfing. After an argument, the women leave Mike near the town of Dingo. Fifty miles west of Dingo, Mike meets the green-skinned Joe Bogart who claims to be a time-travelling alien needing help to recover a lost power capsule in order to travel back in time and prevent the Japanese from winning the Second World War. The film quickly descends into screwball comedy as eccentric outback characters mistake Mike for the alien. As Time Goes By has now largely faded into obscurity.

Despite Australia's poor track record in science fiction production, as outlined above, science fiction films from overseas produced in Australia have achieved worldwide box office success. This raises the question of why Australian producers continue to shy away from science fiction films. Reasons put forward for this lack of engagement with the genre range from the inability to meet audience expectations, to industry and government funding bodies not wanting to take financial risks (see for example Moran and Veith 2006). However, when compared to the science fiction films produced by other countries, these reasons prove to be unsatisfactory.

Claims that a science fiction film needs a large budget demonstrate a lack of understanding of the genre as effective science fiction films do not always require large budgets. Science fiction's classic 'What if?' question tends to demand a compelling idea to drive and motivate a film's narrative. In recent internationally successful low-budget 'hard' and 'soft' science fiction films, the idea has been more important than high-budget visual spectacle or expensive internationally recognizable actors. The British 'hard' science fiction film Moon (Duncan Jones, 2009) deals with human cloning, while the 'soft' South African science fiction movie District 9 (Neill Blomkamp, 2009) is based on aliens coming to earth as refugees. Both films canvas ideas that attracted critical praise and engaged mainstream audiences.

For skittish Australian investors, the funding model of the hybrid genre film Iron Sky (2012) – a very 'soft' science fiction film – might suggest how future science fiction genre (and cross-genre) film productions could be financed in Australia. Before being released in 2012, Iron Sky's €7.5 million budget was raised by German, Finnish and Australian investors, with a portion also sourced through online crowd funding. While this film is another in a line of cross-genre international co-productions, online crowd funding may go some way to alleviate the nervousness Australian investors feel when asked to fund science fiction films.

Another reason given for the lack of science fiction production in Australia is that the genre tends to attract cult audiences and a strong fan base. Consequently, the expectation is that these audiences will typically have a strong understanding of the genre and therefore have high expectations for a science fiction movie. It is indeed the case that hard science fiction may not be immediately accessible to uninitiated mainstream audiences. Nevertheless, the continued success of *Dark City* in DVD and Blu-ray formats does indicate audiences not versed in science fiction will watch hard science fiction. Yet there still remains the anomaly that *Dark City* has not led to more of this kind of science fiction film being produced (or even co-produced) in Australia.

While there has been a strong commitment to Australian horror film production targeting international markets in the last ten years (see for example Ryan 2010a), this has not been the case with science fiction films. Although a number of talented Australian science fiction novelists have a substantial international following, there may need to be a shift in Australian film culture before these writers are tapped by Australian film producers for science fiction themes and ideas. Making a science fiction film anywhere in the world is a challenge. Perhaps, therefore, it is not surprising that local Australian film-makers and screenwriters continue to be wary of science fiction.

Peter Schembri and Mark David Ryan

References

Helms, Michael (1998) '*Dark City*' [interview with Andrew Mason and Alex Proyas], *Cinema Papers*, 124, pp. 18–21.

McMullen, Sean (2010) 'Science fiction and Fantasy', in Ben Goldsmith and Geoff Lealand (eds), *Directory of World Cinema: Australian and New Zealand*, Bristol: Intellect, pp. 224–35.

Moran, Albert and Vieth, Errol (2006) *Film in Australia: An introduction*, Cambridge, UK: Cambridge University Press.

Ryan, Mark David (2010) 'Australian Cinema's Dark Sun: The Boom in Australian Horror Film Production', *Studies in Australasian Cinema*, 4: 1, pp. 23–41.

Dark City

Country of Origin:

Australia/USA

Studio/Distributor:

New Line Cinema

Director:

Alex Proyas

Producer:

Andrew Mason

Screenwriters:

Alex Proyas
Lem Dobbs
David S Goyer

Cinematographer:

Dariusz Wolski

Production Designers:

George Liddle
Patrick Tatopoulos

Composer:

Trevor Jones

Editor:

Dov Hoenig

Duration:

100 minutes (theatrical cut);
112 min (director's cut)

Genre:

Science fiction

Cast:

Rufus Sewell
William Hurt
Kiefer Sutherland
Jennifer Connelly
Richard O'Brien
Ian Richardson
Bruce Spence
Colin Friels

Format:

35mm

Year:

1998

Synopsis

John Murdoch regains consciousness in a hotel bathtub but has lost his memory. He finds a bloody knife and a dead woman in the hotel room. Accused of being a serial killer who has committed similar murders, he goes on the run and learns his real name. Pursued by police inspector Frank Bumstead and by an alien race called the Strangers, Murdoch discovers he has psychokinetic powers like the Strangers. Moving about a perpetually dark city, Murdoch witnesses the city's population becoming comatose at midnight. Murdoch tries to travel to Shell Beach, the town he recalls from childhood, but cannot find the way. With the help of a policeman, Bumstead, and a scientist, Dr Schreber, Murdoch eventually discovers the city's secret.

Critique

Visual style is everything in *Dark City*. Its stylistic qualities have contributed to the film's 'cult' status. Although recognizably the work of director Alex Proyas, the movie was a collaborative effort: co-written with Lem Dobbs and David Goyer. Goyer had written *The Crow: City of Angels* (Tim Pope, 1996), the sequel to Proyas's 1994 film *The Crow*. Andrew Mason, who supervised the visual effects, co-produced *Dark City* with Proyas. Production designers George Liddle and Patrick Tatopolous constructed the studio sets for a film with no external shooting. Developments in digital technology enabled Proyas to construct an alternative world while bringing down production costs. Yet it would be a grave error to claim that this is a film with more style than substance.

Proyas is well versed in genres of the fantastic. The movie is a recombination of generic elements derived from 'hard' science fiction, fantasy, Gothic horror, classic noir and neo-noir, and detective and thriller movies. There is also a dash of sardonic humour thrown in for good measure. It is a potent mix that renders the film unfathomable to some. This was probably the case when New Line Cinema, the American studio financially underwriting the movie, ordered a recut just before its theatrical release. There is now a Director's Cut (released in 2008) that removes the opening narration and renders the film as enigmatic as Proyas originally intended. Moreover, *Dark City* is not identifiable as 'an Australian movie' and is very much an international picture. Indeed, the film contains no distinct on-screen cultural markers (other than some secondary characters speaking with Australian accents). *Dark City*'s continued appeal is as a cross-genre non-mainstream non-blockbuster arthouse production that transcends national boundaries.

Proyas had demonstrated an attraction to post-apocalyptic themes and impressive production design while a student at the Australian Film, Television and Radio School. His 1981 student film *Strange Residues* explores territory similar to *Dark City* in its story of strange beings from another planet manipulating the dreams of men. Proyas and his production team on *Dark City* were heavily influenced by Fritz Lang's 1927 *Metropolis*, a movie that applied the visual style of German expressionism to what we now call 'science fiction'. Lang's visual style and speculative approach to cinematically representing science had an impact on Proyas and many other science fiction movie directors. When Lang left Germany for Hollywood to escape the rise of Nazism, he started a new career as a director of *films noir*. And classic *noir* styles and themes are present in *Dark City* as well: a man loses his memory, there is a dead woman, he is the main suspect, he goes on the run; all shot with low-key, high-contrast lighting. Neo-*noir* elements that have found their way into more recent 'puzzle' films, with their questioning of memory and identity, and their questions about who – in the end – can claim to be innocent, are also present in *Dark City*. We can almost imagine New Line Cinema's reactions upon seeing the rough cut of the movie: instead of reacting favourably to the 'What if ...?' speculations that drive the best science fiction, they most likely responded with a 'What the ...'

The 'What if ...?' factor is there in the studio cut, but it is harder to find than in the director's cut. What if aliens carted away a group of humans, placed them in an artificial environment and conducted experiments on them? What if what makes us human and what shapes our identities are our memories, and what if those memories can be altered and shifted? How these and similar questions are represented in *Dark City* demonstrates the power of visual storytelling and of cross-genre influences in more contemporary *intellectual* science fiction films.

Peter Schembri

Daybreakers

Country of Origin:

Australia/USA

Studio/Distributor:

Lionsgate Films
Pictures in Paradise
Furst Films

Directors:

Michael Spierig
Peter Spierig

Producers:

Chris Brown
Bryan Furst
Sean Furst

Screenwriters:

Michael Spierig
Peter Spierig

Director of Photography:

Ben Nott

Synopsis

It is 2019, ten years after a plague turns most humans into vampires. Human blood is in short supply. The shortage is causing panic in the vampire population. Charles Bromley, CEO of pharmaceutical company Bromley Marks – the largest supplier of human blood in the United States – is intent on developing a viable blood substitute. When a cure that can transform vampires back into humans is discovered, Bromley and the corporation do whatever it takes to prevent the cure from being made public.

Critique

Daybreakers is the second film directed by twin brothers Michael and Peter Spierig, following the cult success of their low-budget zombie movie *Undead* released in 2003. The film earned over US$51 million at the worldwide box office and received generally positive critical reviews. While *Daybreakers*, like *Undead*, was shot in Queensland, the film does not look or feel particularly Australian. The setting is a futuristic, non-specific American city, and most of the cast have American accents. Australian members of the cast mimic American accents with varying levels of proficiency. As this suggests, North America was the intended market for this film.

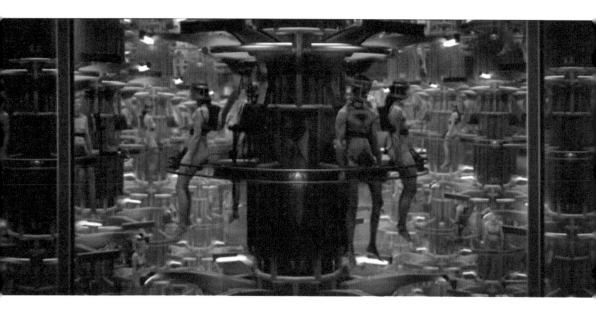

Daybreakers (Michael and
Peter Spierig, 2009)

Production Designer:

George Liddle

Composer:

Christopher Gordon

Editor:

Matt Villa

Duration:

98 minutes

Genres:

Horror
Science fiction
Action
Thriller

Cast:

Ethan Hawke
Willem Dafoe
Sam Neill
Claudia Karvan
Michael Dorman
Isabel Lucas

Format:

35mm

Year:

2009

Daybreakers took US$30 million at the US box office (by far its most lucrative market), suggesting that this strategy was successful for its producers.

In terms of genre, *Daybreakers* is a hybrid. A narrative revolving around vampires naturally skews it towards the horror genre; and the film is indeed an unashamed B-movie. Nevertheless, *Daybreakers* is part adventure, part thriller and part science fiction. The film's futuristic setting and production design are largely responsible for the narrative's science fiction trappings. George Liddle's production design creates the stylistic and stylish atmosphere of the film: the greyish glass and steel architecture of the city; the cafes where cups of coffee come with a splash of blood instead of milk; the corporation's blood farm where naked, comatose humans are held within metallic structures (reminiscent of *The Matrix* [Andy and Lana Wachowski, 1999]) and are connected to tubes that extract their blood. In terms of the vampire subgenre, *Daybreakers* is an inventive movie in the way in which it envisions how technology provides coping strategies for vampires with an aversion to sunlight. The city has vast underground walkways; above ground there are enclosed connecting bridges between skyscrapers; houses and buildings have automatic shutters that lower during daylight hours; and cars are fitted with shutters and video cameras so they can be driven during the day (as well as UV warning systems).

Vampirism comes with rules and conventions most audiences would quickly recognize and, indeed, *Daybreakers* tends to work more effectively as a horror film than as science fiction. For the most part, the vampires in *Daybreakers* follow the main codes and conventions of the vampire subgenre. The whole vampire world is active at night – as was common for pre-*Twilight* (Catherine Hardwicke, 2008) vampires – and vampires are incinerated by sunlight, while a stake through the heart obliterates them. Arguably the science fiction qualities provide the film with any number of metaphorical and allegorical readings, from corporate greed and rapacious businessmen, to plundering the world's dwindling natural resources, to the mechanization of livestock farming. And in the tradition of tech *noir* science fiction movies, it is the film's science fiction 'look' that provides the film with its visual style. In the end, *Daybreakers* may be more style than substance, but it is what it is: an unpretentious B-movie that competently combines horror codes and conventions with science fiction-inspired production design.

Peter Schembri

Iron Sky

Country of Origin:

Finland/Germany/Australia

Studio/Distributor:

Blind Spot Pictures
New Holland Pictures
27 Films Production

Director:

Timo Vuorensola

Producers:

Tero Kaukomaa
Oliver Damian
Cathy Overett
Mark Overett
Samuli Torssonen

Screenwriters:

Michael Kalesniko
Timo Vuorensola

Director of Photography:

Mika Orasmaa

Production Designer:

Ulrika von Vegesack

Composer:

Laibach

Editor:

Suresh Ayyar

Duration:

93 minutes

Synopsis

In 2018, astronauts are sent to the moon by the president of the United States of America as a publicity stunt to breathe life into her re-election bid. However, ever since the end of the Second World War, Nazis, who escaped to the dark side of the moon by spaceship, have been mining Helium-3 fuel and plotting an assault on earth to institute the next Reich. Inadvertently the astronauts provide the vital component that the Nazis need to fuel the 'Götterdämmerung' – a gargantuan spacecraft capable of destroying planets. When the Nazis attack earth, a full-scale space war ensues.

Critique

There is a tradition of alternate history films in cinema – *It Happened Here* (Kevin Brownlow and Andrew Mollo, 1965) and *Inglourious Basterds* (Quentin Tarantino, 2009) among others – and the concept of space Nazis is a particularly seductive science fiction premise. *Iron Sky* opens with a number of promising sequences from blonde-haired, Aryan schoolchildren, dressed in military uniforms chanting 'Heil Hitler' in a lunar bunker, to impressive establishing shots of the Nazi moon base and Helium-3 mine. However, beyond the movie's initial set-up, *Iron Sky* is a poorly executed, gimmick-laden movie, which never fulfils its potential. Though the movie contains a handful of clunky cinematic references to the classic film *Dr. Strangelove or: How I Learned to Stop Worrying and Love the Bomb* (Stanley Kubrick, 1964), and even an Internet meme based on the movie *Downfall* (Oliver Hirschbiegel, 2004), *Iron Sky* fails to draw on the history of science fiction in any meaningful way. Indeed, the movie's blueprint could have been sketched from the rich vein of science fiction as political critique in a similar way to *District 9* (Neill Blomkamp, 2009) which revolves around alien eviction from a slum as an allegory for apartheid; and *Daybreakers* (Michael and Peter Spierig, 2009), a futurist story about vampires and their dwindling

Genres:

Science fiction
Comedy

Cast:

Julia Dietze
Christopher Kirby
Götz Otto
Peta Sergeant
Stephanie Paul
Udo Kier

Format:

35 mm
D-Cinema

Year:

2012

blood reserves as a comment on contemporary society's dependency upon petroleum. Furthermore, Duncan Jones's cult film *Moon* (2009) showed that visually inventive and thought-provoking science fiction can be crafted exceptionally well on a low budget (utilizing a character-based plot, suspense and physical sets and effects over CGI and special effects). *Iron Sky*'s film-makers, however, were evidently unable to decide whether they were making a comedy, satire, dystopian parable or a straight-laced fantasy flick. In terms of comedy, the US president (Stephanie Paul) is a parody of the 2008 Republican Party vice presidential nominee, Sarah Palin, and alludes to what might have happened had she become president; the story mocks the efficiency of the United Nations Security Council; and makes fun of Nazism. But overall, these jokes are one-dimensional, kitsch and mostly lame. While the film has a plethora of ideas at the visual level (the CGI spaceships; the *mise-en-scène* of the moon base and space Nazi costumes; and the special effects for the battle sequences are impressive), at a story level, very few of the key ideas and themes are fully developed.

Iron Sky's patchwork low-budget production and unconventional funding sources may be partly responsible for the film's confused generic personality and underdeveloped script. The film makes most sense as a study in new co-production and financing models, and as an example of the uneasy place of the science fiction genre within Australian cinema. Like many Australian fantasy or science fiction movies (such as Alex Proyas's 1998 film *Dark City*, and *Daybreakers*), *Iron Sky* was an international co-production between Finland, Germany and Australia. Unlike *Dark City* and *Daybreakers*, however, which were written and directed by Australians Alex Proyas, and Michael and Peter Spierig respectively, *Iron Sky* was an internationally sourced story spearheaded by Finnish national Samuli Torssonen and written with international collaborators. The majority of the key cast and crew are from overseas, although a good portion of the film's principal photography – including scenes set in the moonbase and spaceship interiors – was shot at the Village Roadshow Studios on the Gold Coast. In terms of creative talent and heads of department, two of the movie's producers, the editor and local actors Christopher Kirby, Peta Sergeant and Stephanie Paul are Australian and played leading roles. Furthermore, the state-based government funding agency Screen Queensland invested AU$350,000 into the movie which resulted in an estimated 130 jobs for local cast and crew members, and AU$3.6 million in expenditure into the state's economy (Nash 2012).

Iron Sky was also financed by a large body of fan-investors mobilized by social media and cultivated since the early 1990s when visual effects director Samuli Torssonen began a series of Star Trek parodies. The film's screenplay would have benefited from a tighter edit and keener studio oversight; though at the time of writing, it remains unclear how rigorous script development is to be in the brave new world of direct crowd-sourced funding. Developments in special effects and digital photography (the film was shot on a Red digital camera) provided the film-makers with the final pieces of their low-budget production puzzle. For this reason, style rather than substance is *Iron Sky*'s strength, and the film clearly makes good use of the abundant Australian production talent (in production management, the art department and visual effects) that could spur on more local films in the genre. Even though a lush, neo-*noir* aesthetic could not save *Iron Sky*, its low production and marketing budget, Do-It-Yourself ambition and excellent digital effects may well inspire more independent Australian film-makers to explore the possibilities of the science fiction genre.

Lauren Carroll Harris

References

Nash, Cara (2012) '*Iron Sky* to Open Gold Coast Film Festival', *Film Ink*, 28 February, http://www.filmink.com.au/news/iron-sky-to-open-gold-coast-film-festival/ Accessed 30 September 2013.

Knowing

Country of Origin:

UK/USA/Australia

Studio/Distributor:

Escape Artists
Goldcrest Pictures
Kaplan/Perrone Entertainment
Wintergreen Productions

Director:

Alex Proyas

Producers:

Todd Black
Jason Blumenthal
Alex Proyas
Steve Tisch

Screenwriters:

Ryne Douglas Pearson
Juliet Snowden
Stiles White

Director of Photography:

Simon Duggan

Production Designer:

Steven Jones-Evans

Composer:

Marco Beltrami

Editor:

Richard Learoyd

Duration:

121 minutes

Synopsis

In 1959, a time capsule is to be buried at the William Dawes Elementary school in Lexington, Massachusetts. While the students draw pictures to place in the capsule, Lucinda – whose idea this was – fills her page with number sequences. Fifty years later, the class of 2009 open the capsule. Massachusetts Institute of Technology astrophysicist John Koestler deciphers Lucinda's page of numbers, and realizes that they represent dates predicting every major global catastrophe in the last 50 years as well as future events, their geographical coordinates and the number of dead. Disturbingly, the final date predicts an approaching disaster that will wipe out the world's population. John's son Caleb and Lucinda's granddaughter Abby hold the key to the future of human civilization.

Critique

Directed by Alex Proyas, *Knowing* is an action-packed science fiction disaster movie.

A well-known Australian director who has worked in Hollywood, Proyas has developed an international reputation for stylized fantasy and science fiction movies, including the neo-Gothic movie *The Crow* (1994), the complex science fiction film *Dark City* (1998) and the adaptation of Isaac Asimov's sci-fi classic *I, Robot* (2004) which earned almost US$350 million theatrically worldwide. *Knowing* was produced for US$50 million and relies heavily upon special effects (including a visually impressive sequence of the world being destroyed) and high-octane action sequences (including a notable plane crash). *Knowing*'s cast included Australian actors, Rose Byrne and Ben Mendelsohn, and American actor Nicolas Cage. While *Knowing* received typically poor critical reviews, the movie performed well at the box office earning over US$183 million worldwide.

Controversy surrounded the movie during its production in Australia. A film with strong creative, stylistic and financial

Genres:

Science fiction
Action

Cast:

Nicolas Cage
Chandler Canterbury
Rose Byrne
Lara Robinson
Ben Mendelsohn
Nadia Townsend

Format:

35 mm
D-Cinema

Year:

2009

input from Hollywood, *Knowing* was one of the first local 'blockbusters' to receive funding through the Producer Offset. The offset, implemented in 2007, is an incentive designed to foster commercially-driven Australian production (as opposed to cultural films without commercial imperatives) (Ryan 2012) and provides Australian producers with a 40 per cent rebate on eligible film expenditure. Individual projects are assessed on whether a film meets criteria defining 'Australian content' and provisions regarding domestic production expenditure, namely: creative control (production company/studio), creative input, location of production and the Significant Australian Content (SAC) test (at the time, to determine whether or not the content was significantly Australian in terms of subject matter and whether the amount of Australian creative input involved in the script was adequate). Not long after the incentive's inception in 2008, George Miller's Hollywood blockbuster then in development, *Justice League of America* (still in development at the time of writing), was controversially refused provisional certification for the Producer Offset by Screen Australia on grounds that the movie failed to pass the SAC test, despite the fact the production had commercial potential and would have been directed by an Australian. At the time, this decision positioned the offset as a cultural production incentive.

Knowing was Screen Australia's next critical decision. Despite being filmed in Australia, and directed and co-written by Proyas, *Knowing* could have been viewed by proponents of localism vis-à-vis internationalism as a Hollywood movie helmed by an Australian, with partial Australian creative input but significant Hollywood control, attempting to gain access to a generous 40 per cent rebate aimed at stimulating 'local' production. Following *Knowing*'s release, the film-makers were surprised to receive notification that the movie had qualified for the Producer Offset as 'the film had previously been denied the offset, presumably because it wasn't considered Australian enough' (Bodey 2010). As a commentator for *The Australian* newspaper wrote,

> in a farcical situation […] the Australian director and producers of the film *Knowing*, Alex Proyas and Topher Dow, were unaware that their film had finally qualified for the federal government's 40 per cent producer offset, a subsidy that could pay for up to $20 million of the film's budget. (Bodey 2010)

Yet the movie is now officially regarded as Australian by Screen Australia. Following this decision, a number of similar films with strong international creative input have been funded under the offset, including *Legend of the Guardians: The Owls of Ga'Hoole* (2010) directed by American Zack Snyder, based on a book series written by US author Kathryn Lasky, and produced by local animation and visual effects company Animal Logic with a strong Australian cast.

Despite an intriguing premise and some impressive sequences, *Knowing* is laced with *clichés*. The depiction of Lucinda as a pale, creepy girl with black hair as well as the scene in which she scratches into the door are strikingly similar to the iconography of *The Ring* (Gore Verbinski, 2002) and its sequel *The Ring 2* (Hideo Nakata, 2005). Although Proyas's signature pessimistic tone (prominent in *The Crow* and *Dark City*) is present in the film, predictable train/ plane crashes, end of days prophecies, apocalyptic hysteria, possessed children and blonde aliens (reminiscent of Ridley Scott's 1982 film *Blade Runner*) are all derivative of countless science fiction and apocalyptic disaster movies.

Knowing's ending is poorly conceived and grossly undeveloped. For most of the narrative, Proyas attempts to build suspense and mystery. Yet the alien twist is glaringly obvious and anti-climatic. The question of why the aliens are on earth, and why they save the 'chosen ones' is poorly explained, other than to preserve humanity. But most of the human race is left to die. This – perhaps inadvertently – suggests that the human race should be wiped, and humanity needs to start over. This idea, however, is never foregrounded in the narrative. Moreover, when Abby and Caleb leave earth their spaceship is joined by other craft departing the atmosphere which suggests that numerous others were chosen to continue the human population. Caleb and Abby each take with them a rabbit given to them by the aliens. But it is never explained if the rabbits came from the alien planet, or whether animals were also saved from earth. Have other animals also been saved, or have only children and rabbits been chosen to restore life from earth after the disaster? As this suggests, the motivation for, and explanation of, the alien twist and the salvation of humanity are thin and opaque. Overall, the movie is somewhat entertaining without being ground-breaking; but it is slow, clichéd and fails to be entirely engaging.

Mark David Ryan

Reference

Bodey, Michael (2010) 'Lack of Clarity Offsets Benefits', *The Australian*, 27 January, http://www.theaustralian.com.au/arts/ lack-of-clarity-offsets-benefits/story-e6frg8n6-1225823745715. Accessed 5 April 2013.
Ryan, Mark David (2012) 'A Silver Bullet for Australian Cinema? Genre Movies and the Audience Debate', *Studies in Australasian Cinema*, 6: 2, pp. 141–57.

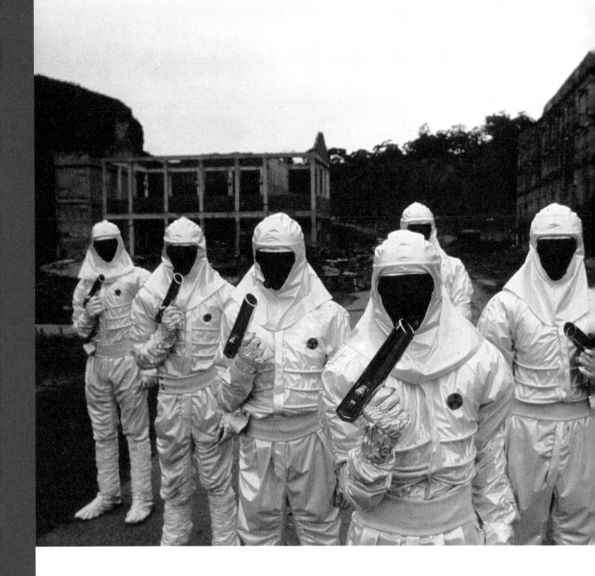

THRILLER

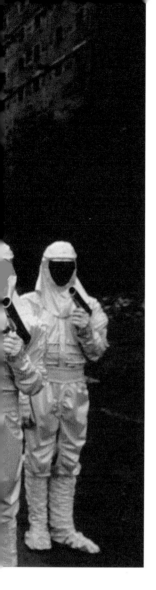

The Chain Reaction
(Ian Barry, 1980).
© Kobal Collection

Shifts in genre definitions and classifications over time are very much a part of a living art form such as cinema. Films that today we might identify as bearing some of the hallmarks of the thriller, but which were not understood as such at the time of release, have been made in Australia since the earliest days of narrative cinema. *The Story of the Kelly Gang* (Charles Tait, 1906) contains some of the thriller's stock elements: crime, conspiracy, suspense, a chase, heroes and villains. The fact that these elements are not exclusive to the thriller underscores the point that genres change, evolve and often overlap. While contemporary reportage attests that *The Story of the Kelly Gang* thrilled audiences, it was not named as a 'thriller' at the time. Even so, a genealogy of the thriller can be traced through Australian film history, despite quiescent periods.

Even in those periods in which the thriller was a prominent feature of Australian cinema, critical work on the genre here is relatively thin on the ground. For example, although Scott Murray (1994: 97) asserts that the genre was a 'main staple of the 10BA era' (i.e. the 1980s), importantly he fails to define the term, assuming perhaps that it is widely understood and agreed upon when this is not necessarily the case in Australia, just as it is not overseas. Taking up Jerry Palmer's (1978) argument that the thriller can be reduced to just two essential elements (a hero and a conspiracy), Paul Cobley proposes that 'the threat of conspiracy [is] the thriller's prime mover' (Cobley 2000: 3). This rings especially true for the political thriller as I will expand on below. Cobley argues that 'the notion of conspiracy is so wide and accommodating that it *enables* an expansive range of diverse texts' (Cobley 2000: 3).

It is precisely the expansiveness of the thriller that leads Martin Rubin to argue that it is perhaps best understood as a 'metagenre' rather than a genre because '[t]he range of stories that have been called thrillers is simply too broad' to be contained by a single generic label or set of codes and conventions (Rubin 1999: 4). In a similar vein, David Bordwell and Kristin Thompson observe that like comedy the thriller is 'a very broad category, virtually an umbrella genre' (Bordwell and Thompson 2003: 112). Other critics argue that the thriller is not a genre at all; Barry Keith Grant suggests it is 'a term that is more appropriately used to describe tone and [...] too vague as a generic category' (Grant 1995: 503). Tom Ryall counters that, like comedies and horror films, thrillers were, and continue to be, identified in terms of the feelings that they induce in audiences (Ryall 1998). Rubin concurs, arguing that the thriller 'stresses *sensations* more than sensitivity', with suspense being 'one of the primary ingredients' (Rubin 1999: 6). This point is taken up by Virginia Luzón Aguado (2002) in her analysis of the psychothriller, in which she argues that

> [t]he most characteristic feature of the thriller would [...] seem to be the psychological effect that unremitting relentless suspense produces on the audience through the delayed resolution of action, rather than elements that we could identify as generic features in terms of iconography, plot or formal structure. (2002: 165)

This expansiveness, coupled with the thriller's principal feature being the sensation induced in audiences rather than readily agreed upon generic codes and conventions, may be the reason why few of the books in the Directory of World Cinema series contain essays specifically on thrillers despite the fact that, like comedy or drama, they feature in the cinema of all film-producing countries.

Australian films labelled as thrillers either in advertising or by reviewers at the time of release date back at least to *Face at the Window* (the first film produced by theatrical entrepreneur DB O'Connor, directed by Charles Villiers in 1919). In a review in April 1920, the Launceston *Examiner* described this story of a master criminal in Paris, which bears more than a passing resemblance to Louis Feuillade's Fantômas series, as 'a stock thriller'. Contemporary advertising for the film promised 'the most sensational "thriller" that ever faced an audience or thrilled thousands on the screen!' Appearances like this of the term 'thriller' in Australian press coverage in the early twentieth century mirror to some extent Mark Jancovich's (2009) findings about the use of the terms 'horror' and 'thriller' in the American press in the 1940s. Jancovich not only notes that the two were used interchangeably, but also that 'thriller'

> was not used to describe a particular *type* of film but rather to describe films that featured a particular quality [...] 'Thrillers' were simply *thrilling* films – films that 'thrilled' audiences – but this reference to 'thrills' connoted something more than simply mere 'excitement' or 'suspense'. (2009: 158, original emphasis)

Indeed 'thriller' was used quite loosely to describe films that today might be classified as action or horror: in its review of *The Shadow of Lightning Ridge* (Wilfred Lucas, 1920) the Adelaide newspaper *The Register* referred to stunts performed by the legendary Australian actor and athlete Snowy Baker as 'thrillers'; and in an account of the decision to ban the Efftee short *The Haunted Barn* (EA Dietrich-Derrick, 1931) for its depiction of wailing winds that the Victorian state censor thought would frighten children, the Perth *Sunday Times* described the film as 'mystery thriller'. Pike and Cooper (1998 [1980]:155), by contrast, note that the film was temporarily banned 'for its alleged horror content'.

The connection (and distinction) between horror and suspense films also forms the basis of Brian McFarlane's contribution to one of the first book-length critiques of Australian cinema after the revival, *The New Australian Cinema* (Murray 1980). Despite McFarlane's opening gambit that 'Horror and suspense have not been major elements in the Australian film renaissance of the 1970s' (McFarlane 1980: 61), he provides a lengthy and detailed survey of the genres in the first decade of the revival, paying particular attention to films such as *The Cars That Ate Paris* (Peter Weir, 1974), *Patrick* (Richard Franklin, 1978) and *Long Weekend* (Colin Eggleston, 1978) all of which are now considered to be exemplars of the Australian Gothic (see Rayner, this volume). By 2006, Albert Moran and Errol Vieth had much more material to work with, and consequently devote separate chapters to horror and 'the suspense thriller' in their book on Australian film genres (2006: 157–71).

Drawing on Charles Derry's typology of suspense thrillers originally developed in a book on the films of Alfred Hitchcock, Moran and Vieth identify eight types of

Australian suspense thriller. The erotic thriller, or 'Thriller of Murderous Passions' is exemplified in Moran and Vieth's study, erroneously in my view, by *Dead Calm* (Phillip Noyce, 1989); better examples would include *The Monkey's Mask* (Samantha Lang, 2000) and *In the Cut* (Jane Campion, 2003). The Australian archetype of the 'Thriller of Acquired Identity' is Robert Connolly's *The Bank* (2001), in which a software developer takes a job with the bank that caused his father's ruin with the intention of unleashing malicious code that will paralyse it. A more recent example is Daniel Nettheim's *The Hunter* (2011) in which an American mercenary (Willem Dafoe) hired by a biotech company poses as a naturalist in order to capture a Tasmanian tiger (long thought to be extinct in the wild) and harvest its genes. In the 'psychotraumatic thriller', a victim's past trauma is exploited by others for gain. Moran and Vieth suggest Frank Shields's *Hostage: The Christine Maresch Story* (1983), in which a woman is forced by her psychotic husband to commit a series of robberies; a contemporary example is Kieran Darcy-Smith's *Wish You Were Here* (2012), in which a young Australian couple are harassed by a crime syndicate following a holiday tragedy in Cambodia. The 'thriller of moral confrontation' is at base the clash between 'good' and 'evil' characters. Noyce's *Dead Calm* is an obvious candidate, with John and Rae Ingram (Sam Neill and Nicole Kidman) confronted by Billy Zane's psychopath Hughie Warriner. Moran and Vieth cite the little-known feature *Running from the Guns* (John Dixon, 1987) as the Australian example of Derry's self-explanatory 'innocent-on-the-run thriller'. More widely seen examples would include Bill Bennett's *Kiss or Kill* (1997) – although the lovers-on-the-run are far from innocent – and Craig Lahiff's *Heaven's Burning* (1997) in which a runaway Japanese bride is caught up in the aftermath of a bank robbery gone wrong. Lahiff returned to the theme again in 2011's *Swerve*, in which a man's decision to take a bag of cash he finds by the side of the road to the police in a small country town is the catalyst for a series of unfortunate events. (Lahiff's rarely seen 1989 feature *Fever*, incidentally, begins with the same plot device, although the story takes a somewhat different course.) The race against the clock that defines the 'thriller of time' is a common device in many films and genres; Australian examples include Ian Barry's sci-fi thriller *The Chain Reaction* (1980) about a nuclear waste spillage, and the comedy-thriller *Two Hands* (Gregor Jordan, 1999), in which low-level gangster Jimmy (Heath Ledger) loses $10,000 of his boss's money and must find a way to pay it back or face the wrath of the mob. The 'thriller of place' restricts its drama to a few key settings, and again illustrates the tendency for genre-blending, with films that could be classified as horror providing prime Australian examples. *Bait* (Kimble Rendall, 2012) is set in a flooded supermarket following a tsunami, with the unfortunate surviving shoppers menaced by sharks. In *Long Weekend*, a city couple's beach holiday turns into a nightmare as nature takes its revenge.

The last category is the 'political thriller'. Despite Australian film-makers' longstanding interest in Australian history and dramatizations of real events, and despite a wealth of potential subjects, political thrillers have featured occasionally, but perhaps not in the numbers that might be expected given the rich subject matter in Australian history and mythology. Politicians and politics have, by contrast, been regular targets of Australian comedies from Raymond Longford's second adaptation of Steele Rudd's Dad and Dave stories, *Rudd's New Selection* (1921) to PJ Hogan's *Mental* (2012). Corrupt politicians feature in satirical comedies including *Muriel's Wedding* (PJ Hogan, 1994) and *A Sting in the Tail* (Eugene Schlusser, 1989), but these in no way could be claimed to be political thrillers. That said, there are some notable examples of thrillers built around a core conspiracy involving police corruption (such as Esben Storm's *Deadly* [1992]; Tony Martin's *Bad Eggs* [2003]; and the Australian western *Red Hill* [Patrick Hughes, 2010]). Other notable Australian thrillers feature political cover-ups (Terry Ohlsson's *Scobie Malone* [1975]), revolutionary plots (Arthur Shirley's *The Sealed Room* [1926]; Esben Storm's *With Prejudice* [1982]), corrupt corporate dealings (*The Bank*) and international intrigues and scandals (Peter Weir's *The Year of Living Dangerously* [1982]; John Duigan's *Far East* [1982]; Robert Connolly's *Balibo* [2009]). Thrillers about the politics and consequences of nuclear accidents or nuclear war date back to Stanley Kramer's 1960 adaptation of Nevil Shute's novel *On the Beach*, which was followed ten years later by Giorgio Mangiamele's *Beyond Reason* (1970), in which staff and patients at a mental hospital take refuge in a basement following a nuclear attack. Another decade on, *The Chain Reaction* took up the theme anew. In a different vein is Gary L Keady's *Sons of Steel* (1989), more of a science fiction comedy than a thriller, which features a rock singer/peace activist who travels back in time to prevent a nuclear disaster. Perhaps the best of this cycle was *Ground Zero* (Michael Pattinson and Bruce Myles, 1987), which centres on a conspiracy and cover-up around the 1950s British nuclear tests in the South Australian outback.

The relative dearth of political thrillers makes it even more surprising and noteworthy that two lightly fictionalized versions of the same story, albeit made in wildly different styles, were released within months of each other in 1981 and 1982. Both *The Killing of Angel Street* (Donald Crombie, 1981) and *Heatwave* (Phillip Noyce, 1982) are thrillers, though only the former can properly be described as a political thriller since the latter eschews the suggestion of political machinations and (unusually in Australian films) treats the property developer character sympathetically, at least until the final shot. Both films take as their subject the contentious redevelopment of inner Sydney in the 1970s, which pitted property developers and incumbent politicians against local residents and the New South Wales branch of one of the major construction unions. And both reference the mysterious disappearance of anti-development campaigner and newspaper publisher Juanita Nielsen in 1975. Of the two films, *Angel Street* is much more overtly concerned with the issue of corruption and collusion between developers, the police and the government, set against the background of the 'green bans' under which residents' action groups opposed to development were supported by the New South Wales Builders Labourers Federation (NSWBLF). For several years in the early to mid-1970s the NSWBLF barred its members from working on construction sites that its leaders deemed ecologically or socially harmful. *Angel Street*'s key creatives held a widely shared certainty that Nielsen's disappearance and the harassment of residents were the result of a conspiracy that reached from the murky criminal underworld of Kings Cross right up to the highest levels of government – a belief that was reinforced by the several warnings they received to drop the project before it went into production (see Goldsmith 2012).

Ben Goldsmith

References

Aguado, Virginia Luzón (2002) 'Film Genre and Its Vicissitudes: The Case of the Psychothriller', *Atlantis*, 24: 2, pp. 163–72.

Bordwell, David and Kristin Thompson (2003) *Film Art: An Introduction*, 7th edn, Boston: McGraw Hill.

Cobley, Paul (2000) *The American Thriller: Generic Innovation and Social Change in the 1970s*, Basingstoke and New York: Palgrave.

Goldsmith, Ben (2012) 'The Killing of Angel Street', *Metro*, 174, pp. 70–81.

Grant, Barry Keith (ed.) (1995) *Film Genre Reader II*, Austin: University of Texas Press.

Jancovich, Mark (2009) '"Thrills and Chills": Horror, The Woman's Film, and the Origins of *Film Noir*', *New Review of Film and Television Studies*, 7: 2, pp. 157–71.

McFarlane, Brian (1980) 'Horror and Suspense', in Scott Murray (ed.), *The New Australian Cinema*, West Melbourne: Nelson.

Moran, Albert and Vieth, Errol (2006) *Film in Australia: An introduction*, Cambridge, UK: Cambridge University Press.

Murray, Scott (ed.) (1980) *The New Australian Cinema*, West Melbourne: Thomas Nelson.

Murray, Scott (ed.) (1994) *Australian Cinema*, North Sydney: Allen and Unwin, in association with the Australian Film Commission.

Palmer, Jerry (1978) *Thrillers: Genesis and Structure of a Popular Genre*, London: Edward Arnold.

Pike, Andrew and Cooper, Ross (1998 [1980]) *Australian Film, 1900–1977: A Guide to Feature Film Production*, Melbourne: Oxford University Press.

Rubin, Martin (1999) *Thrillers*, Cambridge: Cambridge University Press.

Ryall, Tom (1998) 'Genre and Hollywood', in John Hill and Pamela Church Gibson (eds), *The Oxford Guide to Film Studies*, Oxford: Oxford University Press, pp. 327–38.

Balibo

Country of Origin:

Australia

Studio/Distributor:

Balibo Films

Director:

Robert Connolly

Producers:

John Maynard
Rebecca Williamson

Balibo
(Robert Connolly, 2009)

Synopsis

In present-day East Timor, Juliana is interviewed by the East Timorese Commission for Reception, Truth and Reconciliation about the Indonesian invasion of October-December 1975 and the subsequent twenty-four year occupation. In Darwin in 1975, East Timorese Secretary of Foreign Affairs, José Ramos-Horta offers the job of head of the East Timor news agency to veteran journalist Roger East. Initially reluctant, East takes up the offer in order to investigate the fate of five missing Australian television journalists, believed killed by Indonesian troops. East's quest is intercut with the story of the missing journalists. With Horta and later resistance fighter Sabika as his guides, East retraces the journalists' journey to the small town of Balibo on the border of the Indonesian territory of West Timor. In the present day, Juliana recalls what happened after the invasion when East attempted to report his findings in Balibo.

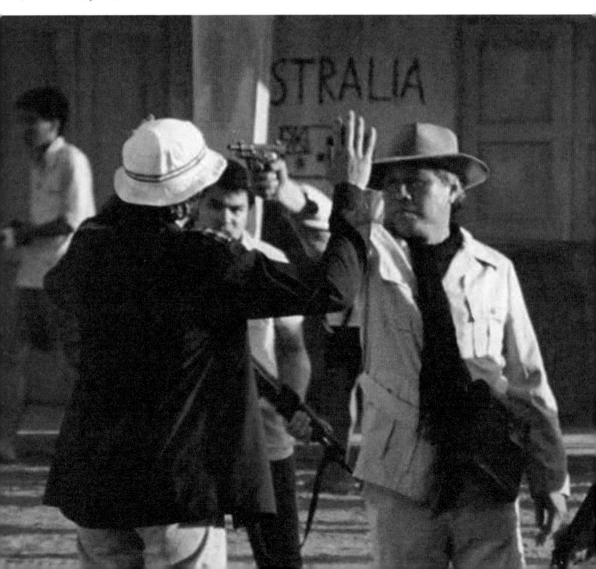

Screenwriters:

David Williamson
Robert Connolly, based on the
book *Cover Up: The Inside
Story of the Balibo Five* by Jill
Jolliffe (2001)

Cinematographer:

Tristan Milani

Production Designer:

Robert Cousins

Composer:

Marcello De Francisci
Lisa Gerrard

Editor:

Nick Meyers

Genre:

Political thriller

Duration:

111 minutes

Cast:

Anthony LaPaglia
Oscar Isaac
Damon Gameau
Thomas Wright
Mark Leonard Winter
Gyton Grantley
Nathan Phillips
Bea Viegas
Anamaria Barreto
Simon Stone
José da Costa

Format:

35mm

Year:

2009

Critique

Balibo is not only a film about the deaths of six Australian
journalists and a decades-long official cover-up, it is also a story
about a pivotal event in the history of East Timor, as well as a
reflection on the history of the often fraught relationship between
Australia and Indonesia. The geopolitical context for the film is
complex and not particularly well understood, hence the frequent
use of on-screen titles or cards to provide critical background
information. The 'Carnation Revolution' that led to the fall of the
fascist dictatorship in Portugal in 1974 also ended 400 years of
colonial rule of Portuguese Timor (now East Timor, or Timor Leste).
Indonesia, with the backing of the United States and Australia,
began a campaign to destabilize the country and foment civil war.
The group of Australian journalists later dubbed the Balibo Five
were reporting on these covert Indonesian operations when they
were killed in October 1975. The invasion of the capital, Dili, on 7
December 1975, inaugurated 24 years of Indonesian rule.

The deaths of the Balibo Five (Channel 9 reporter Malcolm
Rennie and cameraman Brian Peters, and reporter Greg Shackleton,
cameraman Gary Cunningham and soundman Tony Stewart from
Channel 7 in Melbourne) were widely reported at the time; the
execution of Roger East (Anthony LaPaglia) by the Indonesian
military in Dili on 8 December was less well known. Successive
Australian and Indonesian governments claimed for many
years that the Balibo Five had been killed in crossfire between
Indonesian troops and fighters loyal to the Revolutionary Front
for an Independent East Timor, FRETILIN. In 2007, a New South
Wales coronial inquest in to the death of cameraman Brian Peters
(Thomas Wright) concluded that there was strong evidence that
the killings had been ordered by the overall commander of the
Indonesian forces, and that the first shot had been fired by Yunus
Yosfiah, later commander of the Indonesian military and Minister of
Information under President Habibie (1998–99). In 2009, the year
in which the film *Balibo* was released, the Australian Federal Police
commenced a war crimes inquiry. Despite the testimony of a former
Indonesian officer who came forward in 2009 to claim that the
journalists had indeed been executed, the Indonesian government
has been reluctant to assist the inquiry. *Balibo* was banned in
Indonesia shortly before it was due to be screened at the 2009
Jakarta International Film Festival.

Balibo is a powerful and deeply moving film about a series of
events that continue to resonate and, shockingly, remain unresolved.
While several scenes and conversations are necessarily speculative,
the film-makers drew on testimonies collected by the East Timorese
Commission for Reception, Truth and Reconciliation, and evidence
presented to the 2007 coronial inquest into the death of Brian
Peters, as well as extensive interviews and conversations with the
men's families, friends and colleagues. The film mixes actual footage
shot by the ill-fated journalists and other historical documentary film
with painstaking recreations of their reports and other key scenes,
many of which were shot in the original locations. Several of the
Timorese cast members had personal experience of the events

depicted in the film which weaves together three stories: that of Juliana (Bea Viegas/Ana Rosa Mendoça), who stands in for the people of East Timor; the last days of the Balibo Five; and Roger East's investigation of their deaths that leads to his own unfortunate demise. The scenes featuring the five young journalists were shot with 16 mm lenses and film stock similar to that which would have been used at the time so that they resemble 1970s news reports. The look of these scenes both enhances the impression of historical fidelity, and helps to differentiate them from the other interwoven story strands. It is a testament to the talents and storytelling abilities of director Robert Connolly, cinematographer Tristan Milani and editor Nick Meyers, that the complex structure, requiring constant intercutting between the three stories, never becomes confusing or alienating.

Along with the emotionally charged scenes in which the six journalists are murdered, one brief scene in the film carries particular dramatic weight. Reaching Balibo at night after a journey fraught with danger at every turn, Roger East is taken to the house in which several of the Balibo Five were killed. The beam of his torch picks out blood spatters on the walls and floor. The film cuts to the moments after the killings, when the journalists' bodies and equipment were piled up and burnt, then cuts back to East's story. His guide, Komandante Sabika (José da Costa), picks up a handful of ashes from the middle of the room and pours them into East's outstretched palm. This symbolic gesture recalls the celebrated moment in the Northern Territory in August 1975 when Prime Minister Gough Whitlam poured a handful of earth into the hand of Indigenous elder, Vincent Lingiari, to symbolize the return of the land to its traditional owners. This is a pivotal moment in the history of the struggle for Indigenous land rights in Australia, and one for which Whitlam received enormous praise. The equivalent scene in *Balibo* silently damns Whitlam, the prime minister at the time of the journalists' deaths; his government's failure to make an official protest to the Indonesians over the Balibo incident sealed Roger East's own fate, as the Indonesian military took this as a sign that the Australian government placed greater weight on maintaining good relations with Indonesia than on the lives of its journalists and citizens.

Ben Goldsmith

Dead Calm

Country of Origin:
Australia
Studio/Distributor:
Kennedy Miller
Director:
Phillip Noyce

Synopsis

Naval captain John Ingram returns from duty, expecting to be met by his wife Rae and toddler son. But on the way to the train station they have been involved in a car crash which kills the boy and leaves Rae with minor physical injuries and major psychological trauma. Recovering later on their yacht, the *Saracen*, they spot a sinking black schooner, the *Orpheus*. A lone man, Hughie, rows towards them in a dinghy. He claims that the several others on board with him all died of food poisoning. John finds Hughie's story suspicious, and decides to board the *Orpheus* while Hughie rests. What John

Screenwriter:

Terry Hayes, based on the novel *Dead Calm* by Charles Williams (1963)

Producers:

George Miller
Terry Hayes
Doug Mitchell

Director of Photography:

Dean Semler

Production Designer:

Graham 'Grace' Walker

Composer:

Graeme Revell

Editor:

Richard Francis-Bruce

Duration:

96 minutes

Genre:

Thriller

Cast:

Nicole Kidman
Sam Neill
Billy Zane

Format:

35mm

Year:

1989

finds there confirms his suspicions, but also places him and Rae in mortal danger.

Critique

Filmed in the Great Barrier Reef's Whitsunday Passage, this adaptation of Texan hardboiled writer Charles Williams's 1963 novel of the same name, is one of the most memorable films in the latter years of the Australian New Wave. In adapting the novel, screenwriter Terry Hayes and director Phillip Noyce succeed where Orson Welles had failed; Welles never finished his version, entitled 'The Deep'. Noyce uses a small cast in the confined space of a boat to craft a thriller that has much in common with Roman Polanski's *Knife in the Water* (1962), also about a husband, wife and a stranger who they pick up at sea.

 Dead Calm contains several gruesome and macabre scenes. Only a few minutes in, the Ingrams' toddler son flies through a windscreen. The Tokens's 'The Lion Sleeps Tonight' (1961), one of several popular, diegetic songs in the film, plays while Rae (Nicole Kidman) adds tranquilizers to Hughie's (Billy Zane) lemonade. Rae accidentally harpoons her own dog through a closed door. Hughie shampoos an unsuspecting Rae's hair with his bruised, bloody hands. And John (Sam Neill) shoots a flare into Hughie's mouth.

 Noyce's previous work in the thriller genre included *Backroads* (1977) and some episodes for American-Canadian mystery anthology series *The Hitchhiker* (Corazon Productions, HBO, 1983–91). *Dead Calm* confirmed that Noyce could make stylish, sexy thrillers, and he would later tackle *Sliver* (1993), *Salt* (2010) and the Jack Ryan films starring Harrison Ford, *Patriot Games* (1992) and *Clear and Present Danger* (1994). *Dead Calm*'s thriller elements were certainly emphasized in the film's marketing, as evident in its tagline: 'A Voyage Into Fear'. *Dead Calm* even includes elements of the slasher film, including the monster who refuses to die. Just as Michael Myers comes back from certain death in *Halloween* (John Carpenter, 1978), Noyce throws in one last scare with Hughie's chilling return and grisly demise in a final scene that was actually filmed at the request of Warner Brothers several months after production ended, but was derided by critics. Graeme Revell's score, notable for its pulsating, heavy breathing sounds, heightens the film's suspenseful moments and won the Australian Film Institute Award. While a mild success at the international box office, *Dead Calm* found its main audience on home video and television, particularly after Kidman's stardom. She garnered enough attention from her performance to land her first Hollywood role in *Days of Thunder* (Tony Scott, 1990), while *Dead Calm* was also Billy Zane's first major role.

Zachary Ingle

Ground Zero

Country of Origin:

Australia

Studio/Distributor:

Ground Zero Productions
BDB Production and
Distribution
Burrowes Film Group

Directors:

Michael Pattinson
Bruce Myles

Producer:

Michael Pattinson

Screenwriters:

Mac Gudgeon
Jan Sardi

Cinematographer:

Steve Dobson

Production Designer:

Brian Thomson

Composer:

Tom Bähler
Chris Neal

Editor:

David Pulbrook

Genre:

Political thriller

Duration:

96 minutes

Cast:

Colin Friels
Jack Thompson
Donald Pleasence
Natalie Bate
Bob Maza
Burnum Burnum (credited as
Burnham Burnham)
Peter Sardi

Format:

35mm

Year:

1987

Synopsis

In the Australian outback, men in radiation suits exhume a British aeroplane from the desert. In Melbourne, classified documents are stolen from the Royal Commission investigating the British atomic tests in Australia in the 1950s and 1960s. Returning home, cinematographer Harvey disturbs two burglars and is knocked unconscious. The burglars steal some home movies shot by his father Carl, who had worked as a news cameraman and documentary film-maker, and who disappeared in 1954. Harvey goes to the offices of the Australian Security Intelligence Organisation. He is apprehended, and interviewed by Trebilcock who gives Harvey information about his father's work at the time of the atomic tests. Harvey resolves to discover the truth about his father's fate. At the Royal Commission hearings, Australian army veterans and Indigenous witnesses contradict British experts' claims that no Indigenous people were killed by the fallout from the tests. Harvey contacts a mysterious British army veteran, Prosper Gaffney, who claims that the Royal Commission is a whitewash. Harvey learns more about his father and makes a discovery that could change the course of the Royal Commission's investigation.

Critique

While the murder of film-maker Carl Denton (Peter Sardi) that animates the plot of *Ground Zero* is fictional, the implication that there was a conspiracy to cover-up the effects of the British atomic tests of the 1950s and 1960s on human and environmental health would have rung true for many Australians in the 1980s. Many of the details of the tests were covered by secrecy provisions, but even before the Royal Commission into British Nuclear Tests in Australia was held in 1984–85 stories had long circulated not only about high rates of death and disease arising from the tests, but also about the inadequacy of preparations and subsequent attempts to clean up the sites. Scenes in the film that depict the hearings of the Royal Commission draw on evidence presented at the time: one of the Indigenous witnesses describes what was known as the 'Black Mist Incident', when many fell sick following the passing of a radioactive cloud over Indigenous settlements near the test site at Emu Field; other witnesses describe unexpected wind changes that deposited radioactive fallout beyond the anticipated areas, thus affecting many more people than those directly involved in the tests; and the recurring background reports of illness and disability stand in for thousands of reports of adverse health impacts on civilians and military personnel that were claimed to be the direct result of the tests. A closing title lists the names of 118 Australian veterans who were involved in the tests in some form, either observing the blasts, remediating the sites or servicing military equipment including aeroplanes, who had died of cancer up to 1987. The title goes on to note that while there are no death or injury statistics for the Indigenous population of the affected areas, 'Estimates have placed the Aboriginal dead at thousands'. Ultimately the film ends in

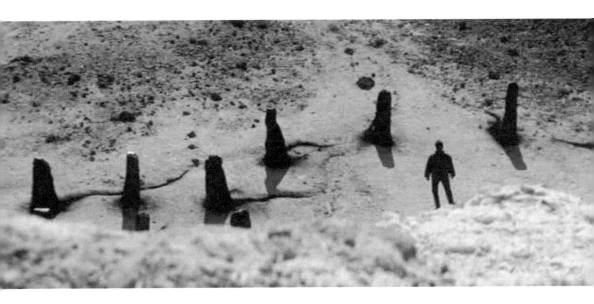

Ground Zero (Michael Pattinson
and Bruce Myles, 1987)

familiar Australian fashion, with the hero frustrated and defeated by forces beyond their control, the moral victory a hollow consolation as the conspiracy remains unproven.

At the time of the film's release in 1987, a year before the Bicentenary, issues around the historical and contemporary treatment of Aboriginal people, and relations between Britain and Australia, were very much at the forefront of the mind for many Australians. *Ground Zero* plays into these debates in several ways, to a great extent successfully using the political thriller genre to ensure that public interest in the issue of the atomic tests and their fallout remained high. But the narrative decision to focus the story on a non-Indigenous observer and only indirectly address the impact on Pitjantjatjara and Yankunytjatjara people – many of whom were moved off traditional lands and prevented from returning, while many others died or experienced adverse health effects as a result of exposure to the tests – reduces its political clout. The film also falls rather too easily into the lazy, but popular, Australian nationalist discourse of British bastardry and culpability. Although the depiction of the involvement and motivations of the Australian intelligence agency ASIO (Australian Security Intelligence Organisation) is appropriately ambivalent and suggests that the local political establishment had significant interest in the suppression of certain details, the clear villains of the piece are all British. While official British–Australian relations had certainly changed in the years between the tests and the Royal Commission, such characterization conveniently ignores the enthusiasm with which Australian politicians in the 1950s greeted the prospect of assisting the British to become a nuclear power.

The revelation of the 'lost' footage in the final scene depicting an abandoned medical facility and a room full of body bags containing the corpses of Indigenous people, reinforces the themes of the image as historical record and the special power of documentary imagery that run through the film. At the ASIO offices, Harvey (Colin Friels) catches sight of one of his assailants on a surveillance camera, which leads him to Trebilcock (Jack Thompson) and the initial revelations about his father's death. Men fight and die over the film of the army base. This footage is the crux of the film; Harvey chases it in archives and in the outback, returning to Melbourne convinced that even though (at that point) he has not seen the complete film, it is the key evidence necessary to prove the cover-up. The footage transforms and defines Harvey, in stark contrast to his well-paid work in television advertising, which is trivialized both by Harvey himself, and by the makers of *Ground Zero*; an early scene depicts Harvey at work making a chaotic and surreal hot-dog commercial, his focus easily distracted by attractive onlookers. This work is also contrasted with television news reporting, which both through Harvey's estranged wife Pat's (Natalie Bate) role as a journalist and through the news programs that play in the background of many scenes provide leads and information that advance Harvey's investigation. Then in the last scene the missing sequence is projected across Harvey's face as he explains what has happened in a telephone call to his son.

Ground Zero was nominated for nine Australian Film Institute (AFI) Awards in 1987, winning three: Best Cinematography (Steve Dobson), Best Production Design (Brian Thomson) and Best Sound (Gary Wilkins, Mark Wasiutak, Livia Ruzic, Craig Carter and Roger Savage). Burnum Burnum (credited here as Burnham Burnham), who plays Charlie, an Indigenous man blinded by one of the atomic blasts, subsequently gained international notoriety when he planted the Indigenous flag under the white cliffs of Dover and claimed possession of England 'on behalf of the Aboriginal crown of Australia' on 26 January 1988, the day of the Australian Bicentenary. Donald Pleasence gives his last and most restrained performance in an Australian film following memorable turns as 'Doc' Tydon in *Wake in Fright* (Ted Koetcheff, 1971), Count Plasma in *Barry McKenzie Holds His Own* (Bruce Beresford, 1974) and Gibbie in the ill-fated *Race for the Yankee Zephyr* (David Hemmings, 1981). Pleasence received his only AFI nomination (Best Supporting Actor) for his role as Prosper Gaffney, but lost out to Ben Mendelsohn (Trevor in John Duigan's *The Year My Voice Broke* [1987]).

Ben Goldsmith

The Chain Reaction

Country of Origin:

Australia

Synopsis

An earth tremor causes a spillage of nuclear waste at a remote disposal facility operated by the Western Atomic Longterm Dumping Organisation (WALDO). One scientist, Heinrich, is exposed to radiation. WALDO's on-site medical team tell him he has only three more days to live. Resisting their desire to 'monitor' him and prevent

Studio/Distributor:

Palm Beach Pictures

Director:

Ian Barry

Producer:

David Elfick

Screenwriter:

Ian Barry

Cinematographer:

Russell Boyd

Production Designer:

Graham Walker

Composer:

Andrew Thomas Wilson

Editor:

Tim Wellburn

Duration:

92 minutes

Genre:

Thriller

Cast:

Steve Bisley
Arna-Maria Winchester
Ross Thompson
Ralph Cotterill
Hugh Keays-Byrne

Format:

35mm

Year:

1980

word of the spill leaking out, Heinrich escapes. Settling into their country house for the night, Larry and Carmel Stilson are disturbed by Heinrich's appearance at the window. Heinrich collapses. When he awakes, he has lost his memory. WALDO operatives arrive in the area to monitor the spill. Larry is arrested, but manages to escape from police custody, only to discover that he and Carmel have been contaminated. Refusing to acquiesce to WALDO's attempts to silence them, they race against time to make news of the spill public.

Critique

Recounting the enthusiasm with which an audience of children greeted *The Chain Reaction* on its release in 1980, film critic Sandra Hall described the film as 'probably the world's first nuclear western' (Hall 1985: 172). By this, Hall meant that despite its supposedly serious subject matter, the film rapidly and happily descends into the kind of knockabout two-dimensional genre fare that once was a staple of Saturdays at the movies. There are civic-minded goodies and sadistic baddies, a dying amnesiac, a shady corporation bent on covering up a potential catastrophe, two fast-paced car chases, regular doses of nudity and plenty of bad jokes and (often unintentionally) laughable dialogue. With its aspirations to genre and associations with *Mad Max* (George Miller, 1979), the film was unusual for its time, preceding by several years the efflorescence of genre films in the 10BA period.

The Chain Reaction was Ian Barry's first film as writer and director. He had worked as a television editor in the early 1970s, before his first big break editing and sound editing the cult Australian film *Stone* (Sandy Harbutt, 1974). He has since worked extensively directing telemovies and television series, many in Queensland where Barry has become a leading member of the industry based on the Gold Coast. He has directed several other films since *The Chain Reaction*, mostly thrillers, often mixing American and Japanese actors and Australian locations: *Minnamurra* (1989), also known as *Wrangler*, a historical outback melodrama starring Jeff Fahey; *Crime Broker* (1993), a thriller starring Jacqueline Bisset and Masaya Kotô; *The Seventh Floor* (1994), a thriller starring Brooke Shields and Masaya Kotô; *Blackwater Trail* (1995), a psychological thriller starring Judd Nelson; *Joey* (1997), a children's film with Ed Begley Jr and *Robo Warriors* (1997), a low-budget sci-fi thriller made in the Philippines.

While *The Chain Reaction* is capably put together, the director's ambition was frustrated by the Australian Film Commission's last-minute decision to cut the budget by almost one-third to AU$450,000. The crew then experienced a series of misfortunes in the shoot, including several (unplanned) car crashes, a close encounter with a drunken local who drove his car through the set at speed four times, an outbreak of gastro, a hepatitis scare and the director's fall from a semi-trailer. Coupled with the many night scenes at the remote location – Glen Davis, a former oil-shale mine and processing plant 200 km north-west of Sydney – the first-time director's difficulties in keeping to schedule were compounded, leading to the decision to pass responsibility for shooting the major stunts and car chase scenes to producer David Elfick and his old university friend and Associate Producer, *Mad Max* director George Miller. Miller and the car-chase scenes were not the only connections to *Mad Max*. The two films also shared the actors Steve Bisley (Larry), Hugh Keays-Byrne (Eagle), Roger Ward (Moose) and David Bracks (a spray painter), with Mel Gibson making a cameo appearance as a mechanic in Stilson's garage.

The film's themes of the risks of nuclear industry and the problems of waste disposal were topical at the time, just a year after both the accident at the Three Mile Island nuclear power plant in Pennsylvania, and the release of *The China Syndrome* (James Bridges, 1979) which, like *The Chain Reaction*, dealt with the cover-up of an accident at a nuclear facility. And the theme resonates today, as Australia prepares to expand uranium mining and begin exports to India while questions remain over responsibility for waste disposal.

In the film, however, the theme is clumsily handled, and the viewer who attempts to follow the story is left with many unanswered questions. Performances are mixed: Bisley's impassioned displays of shirtless machismo and extraordinary hair are markers of their time; Ross Thompson (Heinrich) seems to have modelled his expressions and accent on Klaus Kinski; while Keays-Byrne is difficult to take seriously in a role that makes very little sense. And yet the film was good enough to convince Warner Bros. to purchase global rights at Cannes, and to receive six Australian Film Institute (AFI) Award nominations.

Ben Goldsmith

Reference

Hall, Sandra (1985) *Critical Business: The New Australian Cinema in Review*, Adelaide: Rigby.

The Hunter

Country of Origin:

Australia

Studio/Distributor:

Porchlight Films
Madman Entertainment

Director:

Daniel Nettheim

Producer:

Vincent Sheehan

Screenwriter:

Alice Addison, based on the book *The Hunter* by Julia Leigh (1999)

Cinematographer:

Robert Humphreys

Synopsis

Martin David is hired by a mysterious biotech company named Red Leaf to investigate rumoured sightings of the long presumed extinct thylacine – or Tasmanian tiger – in a remote plateau of the central highlands of Tasmania. His instructions are to capture then harvest tissue and organ samples for genetic information. Posing as a naturalist he is billeted at the foot of the mountain plateau with single mother Lucy Armstrong and her two young children Sass and Bike. On arriving, Martin finds the household neglected, the children unsupervised and the mother somnolent and drug dependent, grieving over the disappearance of her husband, Jarrah Armstrong. Using the Armstrong homestead as his base camp, Martin takes regular twelve-day incursions into the high country, setting vicious steel traps and makeshift snares using the entrails of animals he slaughters. On each return, he becomes more emotionally drawn into the travails of the family as Lucy and the two children struggle to reassemble their lives without husband or father. As he becomes closer to finding his quarry the hunter becomes the hunted.

Production Designer:

Stephen Jones-Evans

Composers:

Andrew Lancaster
Michael Lira
Matteo Zingales

Editor:

Roland Gallois

Duration:

102 minutes

Genre:

Eco thriller

Cast:

Willem Dafoe
Frances O'Connor
Sam Neill
Morgana Davies
Finn Woodlock
Marc Watson-Paul

Format:

35mm

Year:

2011

Critique

David Nettheim's film *The Hunter* is based on Julia Leigh's debut novel of the same name published to national and international acclaim in 1999. Identified by literary critic D'Aeth (2002) as an ecological novel, the book challenges human centred orthodoxies of Australian environmental writing by explicitly resisting conventional eco-fantasy themes. In the book the main character is a mysterious, morally ambiguous figure who is confronted with many narrative possibilities for redemption: his immersive experience within the magnificent natural environment of Tasmania hints of potential in the awakening of an environmental sensibility; his encounters with family and potential romance on each return to his base camp offers possibilities for a similar emotional epiphany that would encourage him to question his misguided quest. These expectations, however, are never met. In the book, the family is destroyed through accidental fire, and Martin David pedantically follows through on his commissioned objective to destroy the last remaining thylacine leaving the reader with a heightened sense of irrevocable loss.

Addison's screenplay (for which she won a Queensland Premier's Literary Award) transforms this narrative into an eco-thriller, foregrounding the political realities of contemporary Tasmania, though according to Addison, 'there was no intention of making an environmental statement' (Wilson 2011). Whereas in the book, environmental activists appear briefly as ciphers revealing the discursive limitations of 'new age' ideologies, in the film the heated antagonism between the logging community and environmental activists adds to narrative suspense, discord and uncertainty with the main character forced to navigate between warring factions. As a thriller, this film is about unresolved tensions, criminal acts and betrayal. Martin (Willem Dafoe) finds the murdered body of the missing father and husband (Marc Watson-Paul), but fails to report his find thereby forestalling any form of closure for the grieving family. On returning from a long stay in the bush he finds that Lucy (Frances O'Connor) and her daughter (Morgana Davies) have died in a fire he later confirms was deliberately lit by the mercenary sent in to replace him. Neighbour Jack Mindy (Sam Neill) unwittingly causes Lucy Armstrong and her daughter's death by jealously reporting to Red Leaf Martin's growing attachment to the family. But ultimately this film is about the criminal act of species extinction that takes place in the bounded protected space of a nature reserve, first by Martin who remorselessly slaughters the local wildlife, but ultimately by a sinister corporation that is never held to account for its criminality. Even though he has a growing respect for the quarry he seeks, Martin is still compelled to execute the last remaining thylacine to put an end to Red Leaf's murderous pursuit, removing all traces of its DNA by cremating the body.

The moody expanse of a silent landscape adds to the sense of creeping menace, suggesting a wilderness that while remote, beautiful and mysterious is nonetheless a contested space. Along its borders greenie activists remain ever vigilant against encroaching logging activities. University researchers make regular incursions to monitor local environmental conditions including the pandemic of disease in Tasmanian devils. National Parks and Wildlife personnel hope to prove and protect the thylacine's existence, yet human predators stalk the bush (and each other) setting up vicious steel traps, trip snares and motion detectors that capture movements of both animal and human. Unlike the book, the film's main character does have his moments of redemption. Willem Dafoe's character is clearly amazed by the breadth and scale of the landscape on emerging onto the plateau. He develops a reverent respect for the thylacine as the last remaining survivor of her species and is emotionally distraught by his part in her destruction. Despite his natural reticence he establishes a relationship with the grieving widow and her two children; in the end renouncing his association with Red Leaf (thereby repudiating an emotionally detached life as a mercenary) to assume guardianship of the orphaned boy (Finn Woodlock).

The film was nominated for fourteen Australian Academy of Cinema and Television Arts Awards in 2012, winning two: Best Cinematography for Robert Humphreys, and Best Original Music Score for Matteo Zingales, Michael Lira and Andrew Lancaster.

Susan Ward

References

D'Aeth, Tony Hughes (2002) 'Australian Writing, Deep Ecology And Julia Leigh's The Hunter', Journal of the Association for the Study of Australian Literature, 1, pp. 19–31. http://www.nla. gov.au/openpublish/index.php/jasal/article/viewArticle/14/. Accessed 19 November 2012.

Wilson Jake (2011) 'Solitary Soul of the South', Sydney Morning Herald, 8 October, http://smh.com.au/entertainment/movies/ solitary-soul-of-the-south-20111007-1ld94.html. Accessed 23 November 2012.

The Killing of Angel Street

Country of Origin:

Australia

Studio/Distributor:

Forest Home Films

Director:

Donald Crombie

Producer:

Anthony Buckley

Screenwriters:

Evan Jones

Synopsis

Jessica returns to her family home in inner-Sydney to find thugs loitering on the half-demolished street, and her father BC Simmonds in gaol following a protest by residents. Following her father's release, Jessica decides to stay with her brother Alan and his wife in their posh house in the suburbs. BC dies in a mysterious house fire that is blamed on faulty electrical wiring. Old resident Riley tells Jessica that BC was murdered, linking the death to the (real life) disappearance of activist Juanita Nielsen, and alleging collusion between politicians, the developers and the police. Before he can give a sworn statement, Riley is kidnapped and beaten by the street thugs. The intimidation of residents gathers pace. Communist union official Elliott organizes for Jessica to appear on a local current affairs television program to tell the residents' story, but the intimidation continues with deadly results.

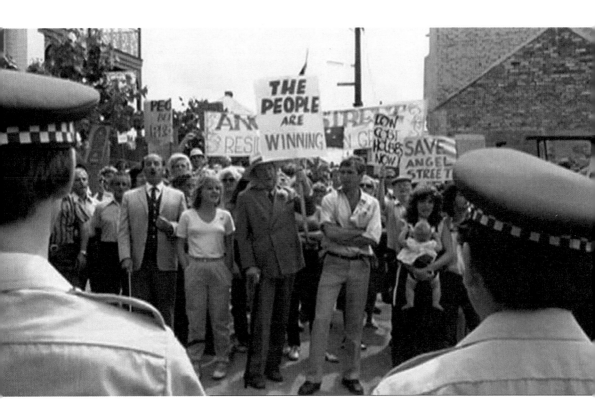

The Killing of Angel Street
(Donald Crombie, 1981)

Michael Craig
Cecil Holmes, from an original
unpublished story by Michael
Craig
Cinematographer:
Peter James
Production Designer:
David Copping
Composer:
Brian May
Editor:
Tim Wellburn
Genre:
Political thriller
Duration:
96 minutes
Cast:
Liz Alexander

Critique

The production of *The Killing of Angel Street* was almost as eventful
as the film itself (Goldsmith 2012). Prominent figures including
the head of the New South Wales Film Corporation, a senior
government minister, and an investigative journalist warned the
producers off the project because of its parallels with the unsolved
disappearance of anti-development campaigner and newspaper
publisher Juanita Nielsen in 1975. As many suspected, and as a
1983 coronial inquest confirmed, it was likely that Nielsen had
been murdered to silence her and end the long-running campaign
against the redevelopment of Victoria Street in Sydney's Kings
Cross. Michael Craig's first draft explicitly made the connection in
its original title, 'The Juanita Factor', but after multiple rewrites by
several writers, the story evolved and fiction prevailed. The project
was retitled 'Not in the Public Interest', and then 'Hot Property',
before Buckley and Crombie settled on *The Killing of Angel Street*.
    Crombie and Buckley's creative partnership had begun in 1971
at the Commonwealth Film Unit, the Australian government's
documentary film production arm later renamed Film Australia.
Crombie had joined the CFU in the 1960s, making a series of
films as writer, producer and director that display his longstanding

John Hargreaves
Reg Lye
David Downer
Caz Lederman
Alexander Archdale
Brendon Lunney
Allen Bickford
Gordon McDougall
Norman Kaye

Format:

35mm

Year:

1981

interest in social issue-driven film-making and social-realist style. Buckley produced two of Crombie's three feature films prior to *The Killing of Angel Street* (*Caddie* [1976] and *The Irishman* [1978]); *Angel Street* was the second film produced by their company Forest Home Films.

After a dogged pursuit, Crombie initially secured the reclusive English actress Julie Christie for the lead role of Jessica Simmonds early in 1980. The deal fell through following protests about the employment of an international star to Actors Equity led by Crombie's then agent, Hilary Linstead. Unbeknownst to Crombie, Linstead was preparing to produce Phillip Noyce's feature film *Heatwave* (1982), which like *Angel Street* drew inspiration from the story of Juanita Nielsen and the redevelopment of Kings Cross. Crombie's second choice for the role of Jessica, Helen Morse (who had played the eponymous lead in Crombie's earlier feature *Caddie*), then withdrew just before the start of production. The subsequent casting of Liz Alexander triggered further changes; Crombie decided that Bill Hunter, who had originally been cast in the role of union official Elliott when Christie was still attached to the project, was no longer right for the part. Hunter did not take the news well, and never spoke to Crombie again.

The role of Elliott (John Hargreaves), the Communist building union official, was fleshed out by veteran film-maker and fellow traveller, Cecil Holmes. Holmes, the film's third writer after Craig and the English dramatist Evan Jones, drew on his own history of involvement in labour struggles and on his first-hand knowledge of the Kings Cross saga to tease out parallels with the environmental activism of the New South Wales Builders Labourers Federation in the 1970s. The union had instigated the world's first 'green bans' in areas including Kings Cross, Woolloomooloo and the Rocks, under which the union's members refused to work on projects that were deemed socially or environmentally harmful (Burgmann and Burgmann 1998).

The Killing of Angel Street opened to mixed critical reviews in October 1981 after a distinctly lacklustre marketing campaign by the Greater Union Organisation. For reasons the film-makers are yet to learn, the film was pulled from cinemas after only three weeks despite rising attendances and growing popular buzz. *Angel Street* did achieve some success overseas, winning a Jury Prize at the 1982 Berlin Film Festival. It was subsequently released theatrically in Germany and the United States.

Ben Goldsmith

References

Burgmann, Meredity and Burgmann, Verity (1998) *Green Bans, Red Union: Environmental Activism and the New South Wales Builders Labourers' Federation*, Sydney: University of New South Wales Press.

Goldsmith, Ben (2012) 'The Killing of Angel Street', *Metro*, 174, pp. 70–81.

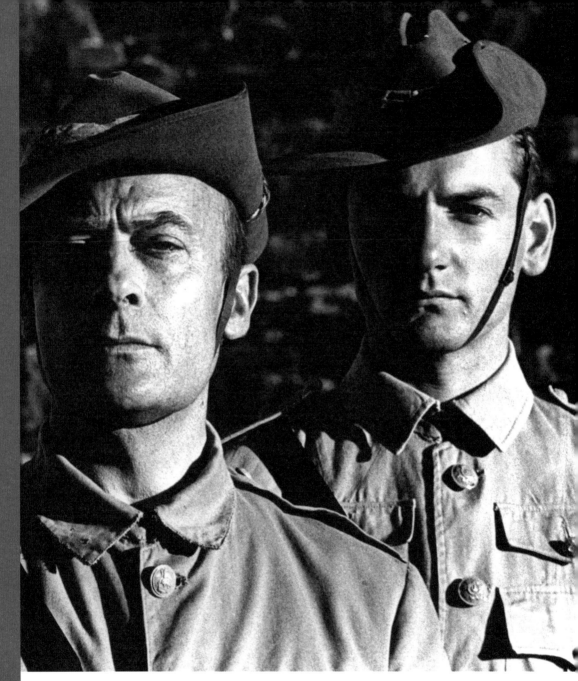

WAR

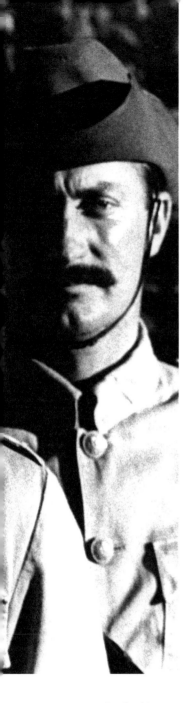

Breaker Morant
(Bruce Beresford, 1980).
© Kobal Collection

The revival of Australian cinema which began in the late 1960s, gaining momentum throughout the 1970s and flourishing during the 1980s, saw a heavy emphasis on period films, which allowed Australian film-makers and audiences to explore the significance of their past in the light of a revived and modified nationalism that both fuelled and fed off the new cinema. This nationalism threw off the traditional emotional ties to Britain, and celebrated an aggressively jingoistic national identity through a reinterpretation of Australia's history.

Among the stories at the heart of Australian national history is that of Anzac, an acronym derived from the Australian and New Zealand Army Corps, which came to be loosely applied to the Australian military as a whole. The Australian army's performance at Gallipoli and on the Western Front in France and Belgium in the First World War formed the basis of a national mythology that evolved, shedding most of its divisive characteristics, into what is now the most powerful unifying national story, with many commentators describing it as a kind of new secular state religion.

It is hardly surprising, then, that it forms a definable theme in the body of modern Australian cinema. Four Anzac-related war films, three of them significant, were released between 1979 and 1982, with scattered offerings after that. However, it is impossible to separate the discussion of Anzac cinema from television during this period, as they coalesced into a single public narrative, alongside other public discourse such as books, news and political rhetoric. This combination of Anzac cinema and television represents an unprecedented concentration on screening the Anzac story to the nation, unmatched even by the Anzac productions of the Great War itself (see Reynaud 2010). The myth broadly celebrates the virtues of egalitarian Australians whose natural qualities of resourcefulness and mateship fostered by life in the bush made them inherently the best fighters in the world, although often unsoldierly in attitude and spirit. Often this is juxtaposed against the hide-bound hierarchical British military, long on spit-and-polish soldiering and short on practical effectiveness.

The Anzac myth's obsession with the First World War is best demonstrated in the eight television mini-series of the 1980s, but is also reflected in the movies; three films have been set during the First World War in the last thirty years – *Gallipoli* (Peter Weir, 1981), *The Lighthorsemen* (Simon Wincer, 1987) and *Beneath Hill 60* (Jeremy Sims, 2010). The Second World War has always played second fiddle to the Great War in Anzac mythology, with a mix of cinematic and television representations. Five films make some reference to the Second World War, though in fact only two, *Attack Force Z* (Tim Burstall, 1982) and *Kokoda* (Alister Grierson, 2006), really elaborate the Anzac story. In the others, the war is only part of a more complex story, with perspectives that transcend the purely Anzac (*Blood Oath* [aka *Prisoners of the Sun*, Stephen Wallace, 1990]; *Paradise Road* [Bruce Beresford, 1997]; *Australia* [Baz Luhrmann, 2008]). These films may still advance key Anzac themes – *Blood Oath* for example, although focusing on the prosecution of Japanese war criminals immediately after the war, tells the story of how the low-level innocent die while the high-level criminals escape justice because of the sordid political machinations of governments, though in this case it is the Americans rather than the British, while *Australia* ambitiously aims to be *the* quintessential Australian epic in theme and content. The remaining two films, alongside *Gallipoli*, are the key cinematic representations of Australia at war: *The Odd Angry Shot* (Tom M Jeffrey, 1979), set during the Vietnam War, and *Breaker Morant* (Bruce Beresford, 1980), which depicts events during the Boer War.

The facile clichés of larrikin Australian bushmen finding mateship in the trenches, and dying heroically as victims of the stupidity of British generals, or succeeding despite them, is best exemplified in *Breaker Morant*, *Gallipoli* and the television mini-series *Anzacs* (Burrowes-Dixon Company/Nine Network Australia, Nine Network, 1985). Among the earliest of the recent swag of productions, and as triumphs of their arts, these pay largely uncritical homage to the Anzac myth. They came at a time when audiences were most receptive to populist nationalistic fare, and their immature self-congratulatory tone captured public attention in ways unmatched since then. In particular *Gallipoli* and *Anzacs* have achieved iconic status as encapsulations and definitions of the modern version of the Anzac myth. They reached huge audiences at the time of their release in the early and mid-1980s, arguably doing more to update and propagate the modernized Anzac story than any other medium or text. So dominant were these productions that other film and television productions, both contemporary and in later decades, were often seen and interpreted within their frame of reference, even when others might have challenged some of the easy assumptions of both the Anzac myth and the iconic productions.

Furthermore, both of these productions have remained seminal texts in Australian Anzac culture, with strong video and DVD sales indicating their ongoing popularity and influence as definers and disseminators of the Anzac story. Online popular reviews of the DVDs, posted well into the 2000s, are overwhelmingly positive about the representations of Anzac in *Gallipoli* and *Anzacs*, while other less idealized productions such as the television mini-series *1915* (ABC/Lionheart Television International, ABC [Australia], 1982) are unfavourably compared to them. There is no arguing with the fact that the most commercially successful productions have been those that offered a narrowly heroic interpretation of Anzac. What sustains their appeal is their ability to articulate a version of Anzac that still resonates with popular audiences, because it most closely accords with the heroic and tragic valorization of Anzac that continues in the media, with increasing force and fewer dissident voices. In other words, their ideological stand renders them still relevant and potent for today's Australians.

A testimony to how completely these two productions encapsulate popular sentiment about Anzac, even thirty or more years after their production, is that only one new major Great War film has been made (*Beneath Hill 60*), despite the growing popularity of Anzac Day. For the Anzac myth has continued from strength to strength in Australian popular imagination, its annual celebration taking on more and more ritual and dogma as the last of the original Anzacs slipped into history. The once-predicted death of Anzac Day has failed to materialize; instead an even more robust memorialization has emerged, heavily supported by various institutions from parliaments, the school curriculum, the Australian War Memorial in Canberra, the Returned and Services League (RSL) and the extensive news coverage given to the annual celebrations. With the centenary of the Anzac landings at Gallipoli just around the corner, the publishing industry is in overdrive with a plethora of books released over the last few years, and many more slated to come.

Yet there is irony in that the popular obsession for all things Anzac seems not to have touched film and television drama producers. It is as if audiences have tired of cinematic representations of Anzac. The glut of period productions in general, and Anzac productions in particular, saw the whole genre in steep decline post-1990. The Anzac myth, having averaged at least one drama production for large or small screen per year during the decade of the 1980s, made only occasional appearances on the big and small screen in more than twenty years following. Between 1990 and 2012, the Great War, once a staple of Anzac cinema, made just one screen appearance, and the Second World War just three. The films mostly returned respectable box-office receipts, but failed to have the same kind of impact as the productions of the 1980s. A similar absence from television adds further mystery to the question of why the screen version of Anzac should be so unappealing in a climate of increased reverence and interest in all other things Anzac. There is however a mini-series titled *Gallipoli* in pre-production at the time of writing. The mini-series will be screened as part of the Anzac centenary commemorations in 2015. The mini-series is promised to be 'the definitive dramatization of the battle that shaped the Anzac legend' (Channel Nine, 2013). It is highly likely to take a celebratory and reverential approach in keeping with the majority of publications, productions and events planned for that year.

Yet there is much more that can be said about Anzac. Among the multitude of books on the topic are texts that are challenging the easy myth-making of populist literature, though these largely appeal to a limited, often academic, audience and are still to have much impact on popular ones (Rieff 2011; Lake and Reynolds 2010; Stockings 2010). The same is true of cinematic attempts to broaden the Anzac story. While the most popular and best-remembered of the Anzac movies and television programmes have been on the whole narrow, others, particularly on television, were not so. But it is interesting that both audiences and critics of the 1980s tended to read virtually all the productions as being monosemic. Thomson (1994: 196) and Beaumont (1995: xix) are two who have tarred the 1980s productions with the same brush. Having established the characteristics of the myth, the cinema has proved unequal to the challenge of modifying it in any meaningful way, even when films attempted to offer variant versions of the myth.

There is a need to take issue with sweeping assessments that place all productions in the same category, which have the potential to perpetuate a new myth: that all Australian Anzac productions of the 1980s (and indeed of all ages) are ideologically more or less the same. Perhaps some of these assessments are like the first great mythologizer of Anzac, journalist and official Great War historian CEW Bean, in their tendency to work contradictory themes into a unitary thesis. As with Bean, the problem is not so much what they have included but what they have overlooked and ignored. There are films and programmes from this era that are fully deserving of the judgements passed by various critics of being simplistic and uncritical purveyors of the Anzac myth. However, the fact that all have been tarred with the same brush suggests that viewers tend to bring their own agendas to the viewing process, reacting according to expectation rather than the actual content of the programme.

For there have been some productions that are subtle, divergent and even revisionist, more among television productions than in cinema, but still significant. Far from being uniform in outlook, uncritical and comforting, some of the productions can rate as being quite the opposite, offering potentially powerful voices and images which broaden the range of representations and offer more mature interpretations of Anzac, recognizing that Australian soldiers had genuine failings as well as virtues, and that they are not the only ones who exhibit the qualities often held to be unique to the Anzac. Some of the cinematic revisions and broadenings have included *The Lighthorsemen*, *Blood Oath* and *Paradise Road*. In particular the latter two take Australian eyes off the narrow celebration of the Anzac legend and suggest that there are other aspects of the wars worth focusing on. The fact that Australian directors can imagine a war film containing at least some Australian presence without feeling obliged to tell yet another Anzac story is encouraging, although it also raises the unanswerable question of what exactly an *Australian* film is. A case could be made that *Paradise Road* at least is not an Australian film, despite the presence of Australian financing, crew and cast, as its themes have little to do with national cinematic concerns. Nevertheless, these productions need to be revisited and watched with fresh eyes, to see how conventional representations of the Anzac myth have been challenged, broadened and enriched at a time when a populist and simplistic version often made no alternative seem possible. Indeed, as the myth increasingly becomes an unchallengeable canonical doctrine, we would do well to remember and to celebrate the productions that dared to ask questions of one of Australia's most sacred stories.

Daniel Reynaud

References

Beaumont, Joan (ed.) (1995) *Australia's War, 1914–18*, Sydney: Allen & Unwin.
Channel Nine (2013) 'Gallipoli Coming Soon on Nine', http://channelnine.ninemsn. com.au/article.aspx?id=8575307 Accessed 7 May 2013.
Lake, Marilyn and Reynolds, Henry (eds) (2010) *What's Wrong with Anzac: The Militarisation of Australian History*, Sydney: University of New South Wales Press.
Reynaud, Daniel (2010) 'War', in Ben Goldsmith and Geoff Lealand (eds), *Directory of World Cinema: Australia and New Zealand*, Bristol: Intellect, pp. 102–13.
Rieff, David (2011) *Against Remembrance*, Carlton, Victoria: Melbourne University Press.
Stockings, Craig (ed.) (2010) *Zombie Myths of Australian Military History*, Sydney: University of New South Wales Press.
Thomson, Alistair (1994) *Anzac Memories: Living with the Legend*, Melbourne: Oxford University Press.

Beneath Hill 60

Country of Origin:

Australia

Studio/Distributor:

Lucky Country Productions
The Silence Productions

Director:

Jeremy Sims

Producer:

Bill Leimbach

Screenwriter:

David Roach

Director of Photography:

Toby Oliver

Production Designer:

Clayton Jauncey

Composer:

Cezary Skubiszewski

Editor:

Dany Cooper

Synopsis

Oliver Woodward, an experienced mining engineer, falls in love with his boss's young daughter at the outbreak of the First World War. He eventually joins the Australian Imperial Force, commanding a tunnelling unit. At first working on the Somme, then later transferred to Flanders, Woodward is involved in several operations, during which his mettle, and the mettle of his men, is tested repeatedly. In Flanders they are involved in a deadly underground war of mining and counter-mining, with losses on both sides. Woodward's task is to protect and preserve a massive mine dug under Hill 60 at Messines, which he does with ingenuity and courage. When the mine is due to be detonated, Woodward knows that the detonation will kill one of his own men who is trapped underground. The film ends with a brief look at the post-war fates of the survivors.

Critique

Beneath Hill 60 has many virtues, and a few faults. It is a story worth telling, based on the diary of a tunnelling officer in France in the First World War, thus giving Australian audiences a much-needed account of the Western Front to counter the national obsession with Gallipoli. The compelling drama of the miners working in cramped conditions, constantly at risk of cave-ins and counter-mining is effectively captured in the claustrophobic cinematography (even

Beneath Hill 60
(Jeremy Sims, 2010)

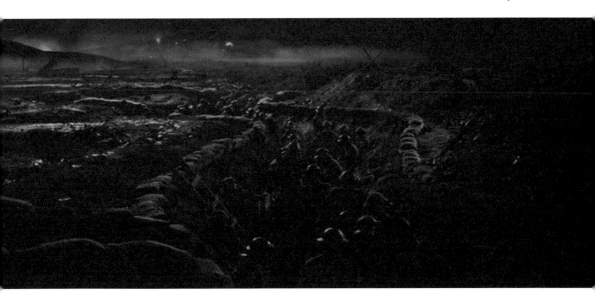

Duration:

123 minutes

Genre:

War

Cast:

Brendan Cowell
Alan Dukes
Harrison Gilbertson
Gyton Grantley
Anthony Hayes
Chris Haywood
Isabella Heathcote
Steve Le Marquand

Format:

35mm

Year:

2010

if the tunnels are not as small as the original ones, for cinematic reasons). Overall, the story follows the arc of history and gives a fair impression of the real events. The acting, on the whole is competent and at times excellent, and the script manages to avoid overworking the Anzac myth and its attendant mateship. Flashbacks contrast the war with pre-war civilian existence, allowing the tension of the war-time episodes to be leavened with lighter material.

The weaknesses are few, but they are significant. The script has too much heavy-handed expository dialogue, and fails to eliminate some of the worst clichés of Australian war cinema: the criminally stupid senior officers, the heroic death of a soldier moments from safety after having guided his mates into refuge, the fearful soldier who redeems himself by a noble death, and the inevitable deaths of soldiers who speak of their post-war hopes and aspirations. Once the slow start is overcome, the film moves along briskly, but its character development is sometimes weak. On the other hand, there are many fine moments in the film: the highlight being how the director encourages the audience to identify with a German miner, who is then killed when the Australians set off a counter-mine. The schoolboy expressions of joy by the Australians are poignantly counterpoised by the audience's awareness of the tragedy of the occasion.

While this is not a great Australian war film, it is a good one. In both its story and its execution, it offers a wider representation of Anzac, capable of being interpreted narrowly, but also having sufficient nuance to sustain a gentle revision of the Anzac legend.

Daniel Reynaud

Blood Oath (aka Prisoners of the Sun)

Country of Origin:

Australia

Studio/Distributor:

Blood Oath Productions
Siege
Sovereign Pictures
Village Roadshow Pictures

Director:

Stephen Wallace

Producers:

Charles Waterstreet
Denis Whitburn

Synopsis

Captain Cooper, a military lawyer, is collecting evidence for war crimes trials of the Japanese at Ambon in the Dutch East Indies (now Indonesia) in 1946. A mass grave of executed Australian prisoners is unearthed, but the Japanese commanders, Baron Takahashi and Captain Ikeuchi, deny knowledge and responsibility. Cooper is frustrated as both the Australian and American higher authorities are uncooperative. Australian soldiers who may have witnessed atrocities are repatriated before he can interview them, and those still there are off limits because of their fragile physical and emotional state. American authorities constantly block his attempts to obtain records from the Japanese archives, claiming they have been destroyed. Cooper prosecutes Takahashi, but the lack of evidence means he is acquitted and returned to Japan to help the US government of occupation. With the covert help of nursing sister Littell, and a Christian Japanese officer, Lt Tanaka, new evidence comes to light.

Screenwriters:

Denis Whitburn

Brian A Williams

Director of Photography:

Russell Boyd

Production Designer:

Bernard Hides

Composer:

David McHugh

Editor:

Nicholas Beauman

Duration:

109 minutes

Genre:

War

Cast:

Bryan Brown

George Takei

Terry O'Quinn

John Bach

Toshi Shioya

John Clarke

Deborah Unger

Tetsu Watanabe

Russell Crowe

Format:

35mm

Year:

1990

Critique

Released in some countries as *Prisoners of the Sun*, *Blood Oath* is evidence that Australian directors can make war films that are not about the Anzac myth, despite having enough elements to permit yet another glorification of Australian virtue over those of others (in this case the Americans). The film borrows the standard dramatic advantages of a courtroom drama, which can make the plot feel a little predictable, when the high-level criminals escape and the low-ranking innocent are shot. Cooper's (Bryan Brown) passion for finding those responsible for killing Australian prisoners spills over into confronting scenes between himself and several Japanese officers, the American minder (Terry O'Quinn) sent to ensure that Takahashi (George Takei) is not convicted, his own Australian commander (John Bach) following repatriation orders, and nursing Sister Littell (Deborah Unger) determined to protect the health of her fragile patients.

The acting is almost consistently good, the tension is maintained, and the action, often told in flashback, is vigorous and uncompromising, making for challenging viewing at times. The film has many opportunities to moralize, but largely refuses the temptation (a speech or two by Cooper notwithstanding). In the end, Takahashi is revealed as having been guilty, but remains untouchable by the court, Ikeuchi (Tetsu Watanabe) upholds his honour in the eyes of the Japanese and escapes a judicial execution, and the morally-upright Tanaka (Toshi Shioya) becomes the victim of politics gone wrong, facing up to his death with dignity. This is a powerful story that director Stephen Wallace largely allows to make its own point. It was a modest performer at the box office and possibly remains best known today as Russell Crowe's debut film performance, in a minor role.

Daniel Reynaud

Breaker Morant

Country of Origin:

Australia

Studio/Distributor:

South Australian Film

Corporation

Director:

Bruce Beresford

Producer:

Matt Carroll

Screenwriters:

Bruce Beresford

Synopsis

Three Australian officers in an irregular unit, Lieutenants Harry 'Breaker' Morant, Peter Handcock and George Witton, are on trial for the murder of civilian prisoners during the Boer War. They are allocated an inexperienced defence counsel, Major JF Thomas, who has limited time and resources to defend them. As the trial unfolds, the case is told in flashbacks, as the unit responded to guerrilla tactics by the Boers with increasingly forceful action. Several prisoners in civilian clothes and a German missionary are executed after the popular Captain Hunt is killed. Despite his inexperience, Major Thomas conducts a spirited defence that exposes the trial as a hypocritical political showpiece designed to mollify German anger over the atrocities, deflecting the complicity of British commander Lord Kitchener by making scapegoats of the Australian irregulars.

David Stephens

Jonathan Hardy, adapted from the play 'Breaker' Morant by Kenneth Ross (1979)

Director of Photography:

Donald McAlpine

Production Designer:

David Copping

Editor:

William Anderson

Duration:

104 minutes

Genre:

War

Cast:

Edward Woodward
Jack Thompson
Bryan Brown
Lewis Fitz-Gerald
John Waters
Charles 'Bud' Tingwell
Terence Donovan
Vincent Ball
Chris Haywood
Alan Cassell

Format:

35mm

Year:

1980

Critique

Breaker Morant was the first film of the era to peddle the updated Anzac legend, revised to suit the taste of this aggressively nationalistic period. The film offered a proto-Anzac interpretation of its Boer War story. The film constructed a dichotomy between the Australian and the British characters, with the large part of the fault lying on the side of the British, although it could have been worse, as director Bruce Beresford rejected earlier versions of the script that were even more anti-British. On the whole it is a fine film, with nuances in its presentation, but it was the overt attack on the criminal incompetence and prejudice of the British that struck a resonant chord with Australian audiences at the time. This film, and its successors, was the final step in an evolutionary thread of the Anzac legend in cinema, which had begun in 1915 with representations of the ideal Anzac as being as British as possible, moving to the interwar representations of different-but-equal (Reynaud 2010). From the late 1960s the Anzac legend in cinema painted the enemy as noble opponents, akin to respected opponents on a sports field, and the British as the real enemy: stupid, bound by class prejudice and incapable of comprehending the rough diamond that was the typical Australian soldier.

The film is not as simplistic as it may first appear. The character development is well executed, with convincing and engaging performances from the leads, and the film is sufficiently complex to prevent the major participants from becoming clichés in the Anzac myth. It explores successfully the nature of the pressures which occur in wartime which lead men to commit atrocities.

While not a huge commercial success, *Breaker Morant* is an important artistic milestone in Australian cinema. It helped establish Beresford's reputation internationally, and its artistic merit was a hallmark of the Australian New Wave. In tackling the story of Morant, it reignited the fires of controversy that still surround his story, with rumblings in the press and in parliament even in 2013.

Daniel Reynaud

Reference

Reynaud, Daniel (2010) 'War', in Ben Goldsmith and Geoff Lealand (eds), *Directory of World Cinema: Australia and New Zealand*, Bristol: Intellect, pp. 102–13.

Gallipoli

Country of Origin:

Australia

Studio/Distributor:

Associated R & R Films

Synopsis

Two young Western Australian men, the innocent stockman Archy and more worldly-wise railway worker Frank, meet at a sprint event, then decide to enlist, taking a hazardous train and foot journey across the desert to Perth. Archy joins the Light Horse, while Frank is forced to settle for the infantry, with three railway mates. In Egypt the pair meet again, and are involved in larrikin confrontations with the locals and

Director:

Peter Weir

Producers:

Robert Stigwood
Patricia Lovell

Screenwriter:

David Williamson, from a story
by Peter Weir

Director of Photography:

Russell Boyd

Art Director:

Herbert Pinter

Composer:

Brian May

Editor:

William Anderson

Duration:

106 minutes

Genre:

War

Cast:

Mel Gibson
Mark Lee
Bill Hunter
Harold Hopkins
Bill Kerr
Robert Grubb

Format:

35mm

Year:

1981

with disapproving British officers. Frank transfers to the Light Horse. On Gallipoli in August, Frank's friends are caught up in the attack on Lone Pine, while the next day the Light Horse launch a diversionary attack on the Nek to help the British offensive at Suvla Bay. The first two waves of Light Horsemen are cut down in a mistimed attack that allows the Turks time to set up between the artillery bombardment and the launch of the attack. The commanding officer is ordered to continue the attack despite the massacre.

Critique

The trouble with writing about *Gallipoli* is, what is there new to say? No Australian film has been so dissected and analysed. It is without doubt the definitive representation of Anzac of the period, and has had an enormous and lasting impact on Australian audiences. It invoked a massive response, both at the box office and in critical writing – there are more than two hundred books and articles which discuss the film, and it is not merely *the* Anzac film of the period but a contender for *the* Australian film of the period. It won critical acclaim for its artistic merit, but the more insightful writers also noted its thematic limitations, and it fully deserved the critical observations that it merely retells the myth, albeit in a powerful and effective manner.

As the first cinematic representation of the Gallipoli campaign since 1916 and certainly the most influential of the new generation of Anzac films, its mythic presentation seemed to fix responses by both audiences and critics to later productions. It portrayed the Anzacs as good-natured, simple larrikin bushmen, bound by egalitarian mateship and practical idealism, who became the tragic victims of the pompous and unimaginative British. It became the benchmark for what was to be considered a true or valid representation, and for many Australians, it has been probably the single most influential source of information about the campaign. A history lecturer in the 1990s lamented to the author that she could not get her students to read about Gallipoli: they already 'knew' what happened because they had seen the film. It remains a paradox: a film of undoubted artistic merit, but of questionable history.

Daniel Reynaud

Kokoda (aka Kokoda: 39ᵗʰ Battalion)

Country of Origin:

Australia

Studio/Distributor:

GFN Productions

Synopsis

In August 1942 around the village of Isurava in the highlands of New Guinea (now Papua New Guinea), a squad of soldiers from the 39ᵗʰ Battalion (militia) which has been cut off by the Japanese advance, lose their officer and the only non-commissioned officer. Under stress, one soldier panics, while two more witness the brutal murder of a comrade captured by the Japanese. Leadership falls to the most enterprising, Jack, and the squad attempt to rejoin the Australian positions at Isurava, which are already under Japanese attack.

Director:

Alister Grierson

Producers:

Catriona Hughes

Leesa Kahn

Screenwriters:

Alister Grierson

John Lonie

Director of Photography:

Jules O'Loughlin

Production Designer:

Nicholas McCallum

Composer:

John Gray

Editor:

Adrian Rostirolla

Duration:

95 minutes

Genre:

War

Cast:

Jack Finsterer

Travis McMahon

Simon Stone

Luke Ford

Steve Le Marquand

Tom Budge

William McInnes

Format:

35mm

Year:

2006

Critique

In just its second ever appearance on the big screen (it features in the second half of Charles Chauvel's 1944 feature *The Rats of Tobruk*) the Battle of Kokoda is one that has grown in stature in modern Australian consciousness. Perhaps the most important battle fought by Australians in the Second World War, Kokoda draws more media coverage each Anzac Day and Kokoda Track tourist walks are increasingly popular. The film convincingly captures the claustrophobic character of jungle warfare, as the enemy is only glimpsed in snatches through the undergrowth while maintaining an ever-menacing presence.

As a representation of the Anzac legend, the film is restrained, choosing to tell the story in a relatively straightforward way, representing a variety of responses from the soldiers, and accurately capturing some of the tensions between the Chockos (militia) and the Australian Imperial Force. Even the Colonel's (William McInnes) speech at the end is moderate compared to the usual propaganda piece characteristic of so many war films. Unfortunately it still feels forced, a pat speech to summarize what we should have learnt for ourselves from the actual story.

The biggest weakness of the film is that character development is slight: it is only once the squad is reduced to half a dozen men that time is spent on building up individual identities. The impact of the battle scenes is undermined as a result. The realistic confusion of the battle means that we do not know what any particular character is doing, and hence have little emotional attachment to the survival of particular individuals. Instead, we have a series of detached noble actions and heroic endurance. The end result is that the impact, while worthy, is muted and emotionally remote.

Daniel Reynaud

Paradise Road

Country of Origin:

Australia

Studio/Distributor:

Village Roadshow Pictures

Samson Productions

Planet Pictures

YTC Motion Picture

Investments

Synopsis

In Singapore in early 1942, the fashionable crowd dancing at Raffles Hotel is shattered by the news that the Japanese have broken through the island's defences. They flee to the docks, but a ship full of evacuees is sunk by Japanese aircraft. The survivors are brutally herded into a camp for women and children. They endure abuse, particularly from a violent guard and a Kempeitei officer. They also disagree among themselves, the blend of various classes and races (British, Dutch, Australian, American, German-Jewish, Asian) leading to cliques and occasional scuffles. Two inmates, Adrienne Pargiter and Daisy Drummond, form an unlikely partnership based on shared

Director:

Bruce Beresford

Producers:

Greg Coote
Sue Milliken

Screenwriters:

David Giles
Martin Meader
Bruce Beresford

Director of Photography:

Peter James

Production Designer:

Herbert Pinter

Composer:

Ross Edwards

Editor:

Tim Wellburn

Duration:

100 minutes (original release);
122 minutes (director's cut,
2000)

Genre:

War

Cast:

Glenn Close
Frances McDormand
Pauline Collins
Cate Blanchett
Jennifer Ehler
Wendy Hughes
Clyde Kusatsu

Format:

35mm

Year:

1997

musical expertise and secretly form a vocal ensemble to perform orchestral works. The performances charm the guards, who permit the assemblies. However, violence and death continue, and late in the war the inmates are moved to a remote location, where several key choir members succumb to starvation, disease and despair.

Critique

Paradise Road provides further evidence that Australian producers can make war films about themes other than Anzac, although there is an Australian presence in the story. The ensemble cast generally deliver fine performances in this cat-and mouse story. The characters are well defined, even if some steer close to stereotypes, and there are enough little touches of personality and acutely-observed detail to prevent it lapsing into sentimentalism. The Japanese guards are predictably brutal, but again, there are hints of humanity behind the faces. One prisoner exchanges admiring glances with one of the young guards, while the brutal guard Sergeant 'The Snake' Tomiashi (Clyde Kusatsu), surprises when he takes Pargiter (Glenn Close) at gunpoint deep into the jungle, in order to sing to her for her approval.

While the women and their vocal orchestra pull off a moral victory over the brutal Japanese, the tragedy of death, both violently immediate and gradual, ensures genuine pathos, as the choir is whittled down to a point where it cannot continue. The plot of the story is not overwritten, as the film chooses to reveal more than preach, and it reaches no great victorious ending, for by the end of the war, some of the main characters have died. There is merely a sense of relief when the Japanese guards announce the end of the war and march out. In that sense it lacks the characteristic polemic of Anzac war cinema, for it appears to have little agenda apart from merely telling the story.

Daniel Reynaud

The Lighthorsemen

Country of Origin:

Australia

Studio/Distributor:

Picture Show Productions

Synopsis

Four young men, Frank, Chiller, Scotty and Tas, are in the Australian Light Horse in Palestine in 1917. Frank dies of wounds and is replaced in the section by Dave, a soldier who finds himself unable to fire at the enemy, and so is transferred to the Medical Corps. The section has to help Major Meinertzhagen, an apparently foppish British intelligence officer, drop false information to deceive the Turks. In between actions, Dave forms a romantic attachment with an Australian nurse, Anne. The British move to attack Beersheba,

RKO Pictures

Director:

Simon Wincer

Producers:

Ian Jones
Simon Wincer

Screenwriter:

Ian Jones

Cinematographer:

Dean Semler

Production Designer:

Bernard Hides

Composer:

Mario Millo

Editor:

Adrian Carr

Duration:

131 minutes

Genre:

War

Cast:

Gary Sweet
Tim McKenzie
Jon Blake
John Walton
Peter Phelps
Anthony Andrews
Sigrid Thornton
Bill Kerr

Format:

35mm

Year:

1987

but the German advisor supporting the Turks will not believe that this is more than a diversionary attack. The battle reaches a crucial moment where a quick victory is required or the British will have to retreat for lack of water. General Chauvel orders the Light Horse to charge. Not all of the mates will survive this pivotal battle.

Critique

The Lighthorsemen was a labour of love for writer Ian Jones, who has made a speciality of Australian legends, having written extensively on the Kelly gang for both screen and print. The film is his tribute to the Light Horse, and tries earnestly to be both faithful history and good cinema, and manages to fall somewhere between the two.

Not as crass as *Anzacs*, nor as stylistic and energetic as *Gallipoli*, *The Lighthorsemen* gives an unconvincing tweak to most of the Anzac stereotypes, but the unsentimental, pragmatic bushman is sentimentalized in the best tradition of the Anzac myth. Particularly underwhelming is the romantic relationship between the main character Dave (Peter Phelps) and the nurse Anne (Sigrid Thornton). Dave's inability to shoot his fellow men, and consequent transfer to the stretcher-bearers, is more in tune with the attitudes of the 1980s than of 1917, but still falls flat. At least one Englishman, the intelligence officer Meinertzhagen (Anthony Andrews), is given an honourable part, as his ridiculous English ways are merely the cover for an incisive and practical mind.

There is too much stagey exposition from unlikely sources to ensure that the audience is as historically informed as possible. It is beautifully filmed, however, as was characteristic of Australian period films. In particular the charge at the end of the film is powerful, reminiscent of the impressive scene in *Forty Thousand Horsemen* (Charles Chauvel, 1940). It is difficult to tell whether the film's modest returns were due to audience weariness with Anzac stereotypes or with the lacklustre qualities of the film as a piece of entertainment. It is handsome in many ways, and cloying in many others. In effect, the combination ensured that the film was neither a flop nor a success.

Daniel Reynaud

The Odd Angry Shot

Country of Origin:

Australia

Studio/Distributor:

Samson Productions

Synopsis

A young recruit, Bill, celebrates his birthday immediately before being flown out to Vietnam with the Special Air Service. While there, he experiences the boredom and the mateship, then the fear and terror of short, sharp actions, the first being a mortar attack on his base, while the others revolve around patrols in the jungle. On one patrol, a soldier loses both feet. Others are killed in a successful battle for a bridge, which once captured, they are ordered to abandon. The intensity of the patrols is set against the practical

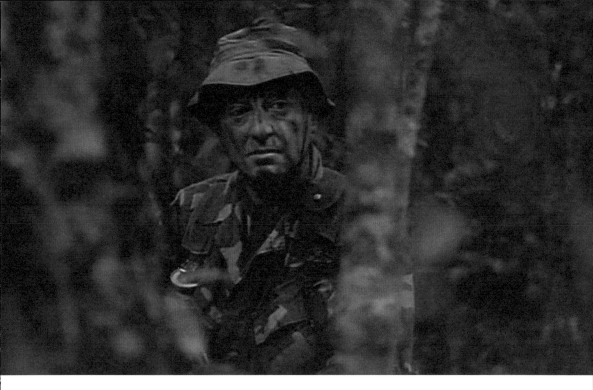

The Odd Angry Shot
(Tom M Jeffrey, 1979)

Director:

Tom M Jeffrey

Producers:

Tom M Jeffrey
Sue Milliken

Screenwriter:

Tom Jeffrey, based on the
novel *The Odd Angry Shot* by
William Nagle (1975)

Director of Photography:

Don McAlpine

Production Designer:

Bernard Hides

Composer:

Michael Carlos

Editor:

Brian Kavanagh

Duration:

92 minutes

jokes and the personal dramas of the soldiers. Bill's girlfriend breaks up with him, another soldier loses his mother and girlfriend in an accident, while another reveals his artistic background and painful divorce that led him to join the army. Bill is eventually rotated home, where he and his mate refuse to acknowledge that they have served in Vietnam in order to avoid having to discuss it with civilians who are ignorant of the experience of the war.

Critique

Made while the recent conflict in Vietnam was still a vivid memory, *The Odd Angry Shot* is both a chronological and ideological precursor to the Great War films of the following decade, and an interesting comparison to the American Vietnam war movies of the 1970s. *Coming Home* (Hal Ashby, 1978), *The Deer Hunter* (Michael Cimino, 1978) and *Apocalypse Now* (Francis Ford Coppola, 1979) were largely disillusioned, anti-heroic and epic. *The Odd Angry Shot* shares some of these elements, speaking to some extent of the angst which this war provoked both in the soldiers who were involved and in certain civilian responses in Australia. However, it leans towards the low-key rather than the epic, and tends to minimize its anti-war sentiment in favour of an emphasis on mateship. Some of the dialogue and acting has not aged well,

Genre:

War

Cast:

Tony Barry
Graeme Blundell
Bryan Brown
Ian Gilmour
John Hargreaves
John Jarratt
Graham Kennedy
Richard Moir
Graham Rouse

Format:

35mm

Year:

1979

making the mateship theme feel rather stagey at times. However, it mixes nicely the various stresses on the soldiers and the ways in which they relieve them. The families' grief addressed in the story emphasizes that sometimes a soldier finds domestic tragedy more difficult to manage than loss in battle.

The film points the way in which many of the war films and television programs of the 1980s would portray Australians at war: critical of war at the higher level, while depoliticizing it at the level of the ordinary soldier, and restoring the Anzac image as the ideal or archetypical Australian man. Yet at the same time *The Odd Angry Shot* points to more contemporary concerns, just as American Vietnam movies of the era did; the politics and myth-making were living issues, with the war in very recent memory and its veterans alive but still largely silent and invisible in Australia's remembrance of war, for the film does not sit easily in the glorification of Australian military history. Perhaps the conflict was, and is still, too recent to be easily integrated into the national myth-making of Anzac.

Daniel Reynaud

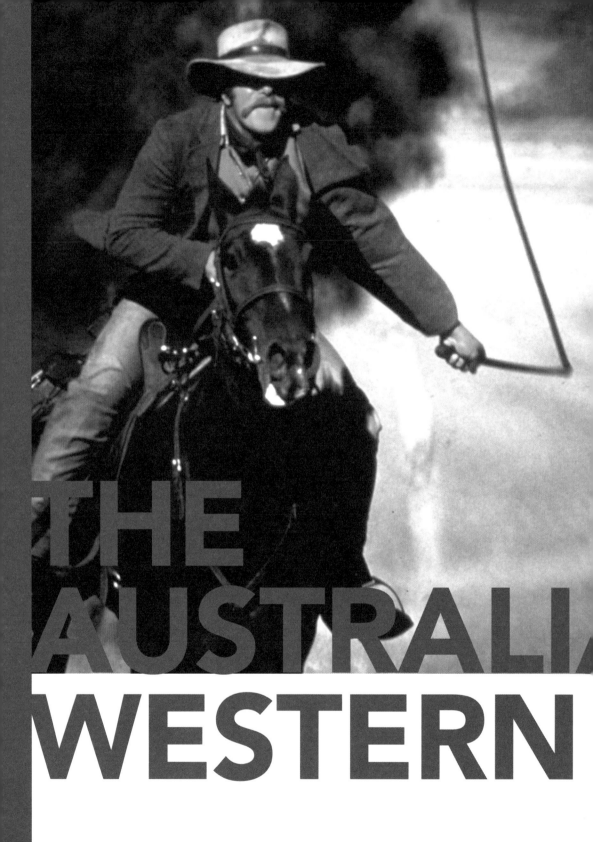

THE AUSTRALIA
WESTERN

The Man from Snowy River
(George Miller, 1982).
© Kobal Collection

The Australian western is a genre identifiable throughout the history of Australian cinema. Indeed, the genre has played a pivotal role in the development and evolution of the industry and has attracted some of Australia's most prolific film-makers and performers, among them Charles Chauvel, Ken G Hall, Rolf de Heer, Chips Rafferty, Jack Thompson and Geoffrey Rush.

The prototypes of the Australian western are the early bushranger films, starting with the very first Australian feature-length narrative film, *The Story of the Kelly Gang* (Charles Tait, 1906). Many others followed: at least nineteen films that contained the adventures of bushrangers were released before the outbreak of the First World War in 1914. These outback adventures of anti-heroes, forging their place in the new world, contain a certain similarity to, but evolved almost entirely independently from, the American western. As William Routt argues, 'there would have been bushranger films if there had been no westerns and I am pretty sure that they would have looked very much the same as they actually looked' (Routt 2003). These early films commonly featured bushrangers travelling away from the oppression and persecution of civilization (usually the British) into the dangerous yet welcoming landscape. Of course, once Hollywood cinema had spread across the globe, the influence of the American frontier genre on Australia's equivalent was inevitable, but the majority of the films that fall under the umbrella of Australian western contain echoes of both their parents – bushrangers *and* cowboys.

From distinctly Australian narratives of survival in the outback like *Bitter Springs* (Ralph Smart, 1950) and revisionist re-imaginings of our cinematic and social past like *Lucky Country* (Kriv Stenders, 2009); to strange cross-cultural hybrids like *The Sundowners* (Fred Zinnemann, 1960) or *Ned Kelly* (Tony Richardson, 1970), the Australian western has taken many forms. For all the variety within the genre, the films contain traits that mark them as proudly Australian and distinct from their American counterparts. In particular, a complex, combative and yet cautionary relationship with the uniquely Australian landscape and the ongoing struggles around what it takes to survive within that landscape are constants.

Unlike the spaghetti (Italian), sauerkraut (German) or kimchi (South Korean) westerns, the Australian western is not a cinematic response to the myth of America. For Peter Limbrick, one of the core elements of this dialogue is a constantly evolving exploration of the relationships between colonial powers, settlers and Indigenous peoples within this settler society (Limbrick 2007: 70). Taking a lead from Limbrick, and although acknowledging the American western as a stylistic point of reference, the Australian western is engaged in a dialogue with Australia's own myths and history. For example, *The Tracker* (Rolf de Heer, 2002) is a resonant and haunting exploration of the relationship between settlers and Indigenous people and the clash between cultures in an outback setting. Other bushranger films explore the dynamic between the colonizers (typically portrayed as British) and the settlers (typically portrayed as Australian). *Captain Thunderbolt* (Cecil Holmes, 1953) with its anti-authoritarian, left leaning hero, is a standout example. In another permutation, *Morris West's The Naked Country* (Tim Burstall, 1985) contrasts the ways in which Indigenous and non-Indigenous Australians navigate the land in the guise of an outback revenge story. *The Man from Snowy River* (George Miller, 1982) suggests that the settler characters – Jim Craig (Tom Burlinson) or Clancy of the Overflow (Jack Thompson) – have an understanding of the land and an ability to communicate with it that outsiders – the American Harrison (Kirk Douglas) in particular – could never obtain.

These overlaps and interactions can be found germinating in earlier incarnations. In Charles Chauvel's *Greenhide* (1926), which took place in a 'land of slumberous strength,' hard working station hands on horseback fight off cattle duffers. *The Squatter's Daughter* (Ken G Hall, 1933) and *Rangle River* (Clarence G Badger, 1936) both portray strong women of the bush fending off rival station owners. In *The Overlanders* (Harry Watt, 1946), Chips Rafferty – arguably the most iconic Australian western star – droves cattle across the country accompanied by, in his words, 'just plain cattlemen – hard yakka and hard tucker'. There are no gun-slinging heroes on this frontier.

The Overlanders has become one of the most iconic Australian westerns; revered French critic André Bazin described it as 'excellent' (Bazin 1974: 142). And yet it was directed and produced by Englishmen, Harry Watt and Michael Balcon. This does not, however, compromise its Australian spirit and outlook. For Tom O'Regan, *The Overlanders* is one of the few international films filmed in Australia that have successfully been accepted by the Australian public as one of their own 'imaginings' (O'Regan 1996: 56).

A large number of the more American-style westerns made in Australia have not been received as warmly. Films like *The Kangaroo Kid* (Lesley Selander, 1950), *Kangaroo: The Australian Story* (Lewis Milestone, 1952) or *Adam's Woman* (Philip Leacock, 1970) are all American westerns in style and substance, except for a smattering of gum trees and – as spelled out by some of their titles – the presence of kangaroos. These films merely substitute Arkalooa for Arizona rather than tell an Australian story. It becomes clear that it is not because films are set *in* Australia that they are part of the genre, it is because they are *about* Australia and the Australian outback experience. The differences in narrative and visual representation between Australian and American westerns are in part due to the fact that the Australian outback is never conquered on-screen like the West of the American imagination. The movement through the Australian landscape by settlers is not a form of liberation as it is in America. As Ross Gibson argues, 'there was never, in the myths of frontier America, the Australian sense of the forestalled reward, never a sense that the entire continent was cruelly tantalizing the settlers, simultaneously withholding and offering'(Gibson 1992: 12). In the Australian western, the landscape is survived, explored, rustled, ranged and settled – but never conquered. There is rarely a sense of manifest destiny, or the ever expanding frontier that are common themes in American westerns. Rather Australian westerns are stories of survival and endurance.

It is the distinct attitude towards landscape and the interactions between colonizers, settlers and Indigenous peoples that defines the Australian western. In *Mad Dog Morgan* (Philippe Mora, 1976), the violent outlaw only truly understands how the world works when he is surrounded by the dangers of the bush; civilization is what drives him mad. In *Red Hill* (Patrick Hughes, 2010), an

Indigenous gunslinger rides into town to avenge his family's death and to right the wrongs of colonial (and contemporary) racism. The list goes on. Drawing upon those characteristics shaped by Australia's convict heritage, the nation's origin as a British colony displaced in a vast, isolated, primordial continent, and coloured slightly by tropes from the American western, the genre stands distinct and defiant against a bush horizon. Though it has gone by many names – Wallaby, Witchetty, Bush or Meat-Pie western – the Australian western is the only label that truly encapsulates the genre.

Daniel Eisenberg

References

Bazin, A. (1974) *What is Cinema?: Essays*, Berkeley: University of California Press.
Gibson, Ross (1992) *South of the West*, Indianapolis: Indiana University Press.
Limbrick, Peter (2007) 'The Australian Western, or A Settler Colonial Cinema Par Excellence', *Cinema Journal*, 46, pp. 68–95.
O'Regan, Tom (1996) *Australian National Cinema*, London and New York: Routledge.
Routt, WD (2003), 'Bush Westerns? The Lost Genre' [lecture delivered at the Australian Centre for the Moving Image], Melbourne, 3 February, http://www.routt.net/Bill/BushWesterns.htm. Accessed 12 September 2012.

Lucky Country (aka Dark Frontier)

Country of Origin:

Australia

Studio/Distributor:

Footprint Films
Smoking Gun Productions

Director:

Kriv Stenders

Producer:

Kristian Moliere

Screenwriter:

Andy Cox

Director of Photography:

Jules O'Loughlin

Production Designer:

Lisa Stonham

Composer:

Tom Schutzinger

Editor:

Gabriella Muir

Duration:

96 minutes

Genre:

Australian western

Cast:

Aden Young
Toby Wallace
Hanna Mangan-Lawrence
Pip Miller
Neil Pigot
Eamon Farren
Helmut Bakaitis

Format:

35mm

Year:

2009

Synopsis

It is 1902, a year after the federation of the previously self-governing Australian colonies into a single nation. Nat lives on an isolated, run down farm somewhere in the harsh Australian bush with his two children, Tom who is wiser than his youth suggests, and Sarah who just wants to leave this unforgiving place. After Nat falls on a rusty nail, the children take over more of the chores, and life becomes more difficult. The struggling family's world changes dramatically with the arrival of three strangers, led by the kind, yet gruff, Henry. As the youngest of the men, Jimmy, recovers from illness, Carver and Henry start to help out around the farm. But as Nat's mind becomes increasingly unhinged, and stories of found gold begin to circulate, tensions grow.

Critique

Donald Horne's 1964 book *The Lucky Country* was an indictment of the country he called home. The title was meant ironically. Since then, however, the phrase has often been used jingoistically to sing the praises of Australia. Stenders's film actively re-invokes Horne's original intent. The film opens with Tom (Toby Wallace) reading aloud to his father (Aden Young) – 'what Australia means to me'. He describes a land for the homeless, the childless, those who need this earth to call their own. The camera pulls back, first to reveal his loving father looking on approvingly, and then out to the landscape. On a cold blue night, ghostly gums surround the weathered wooden building, as the warmth of the homestead radiates from the window, a stereotypical depiction of that idealistic Australia. The movie's title appears and the illusion, the myth, is quickly dispersed – Nat falls clumsily and impales his hand on a rusty nail in a rubbish tip. This infirmity will force him to welcome Henry (Pip Miller) and his men on to the property and, because of their actions, cost the life of his daughter (Hanna Mangan Lawrence), the lives of all three of the men and, from the tetanus caused by the nail itself, his own life. This is what Australia ends up meaning to Tom – greed, sickness, suffering and death.

This dark tone is complemented by the eerie way the landscape is shot. The farm can barely sustain the family and instead of the dusty, dry outback that is traditionally the setting of a struggling homestead, *Lucky Country* is set in a wet, cold tract of bush land; one that is just as unforgiving and uncaring. As the plot draws its characters down into the darkness of human nature, the cinematography follows suit, framing the characters within the cold, sharp landscape. Bruce Isaacs suggests that 'the land seems to have a life of its own, a sense of being that watches over the destruction wrought upon, and by, the intruders' (Isaacs 2009: 40). Isaacs is referring to Henry, Carver (Neil Pigot) and Jimmy (Eamon Farren) as the intruders but the cinematography suggests that all the characters are intruders of some kind, entering a landscape to which they do not belong. This is driven home in the closing moments of the film when, after Tom escapes his ordeal, one of the men from the nearby work site brings him to Connolly (Helmut Bakaitis). He asks Tom what his dream is, since all men have one. It is made explicit that Tom no longer dreams of this New Australia since as soon as he answers, the camera cuts to him burning down the farm. The one cinematic space that even hinted at a place to call home is burnt to the ground, Tom cleansing the land of civilization, of home, of new Australia. By morning all the men of the camp have gone in search of the suggestion of gold that Tom brought with him. As they pan in the river, the trees and sky glare down upon them, watching and waiting for their next self-inflicted disaster.

Stenders's vision of colonial Australia is a dark one, and yet it sits comfortably among contemporary Australian westerns. The land in this film has a power, and is treated and shot as such. In the back and forth between civilization and the land that is constantly played out in the genre, the landscape almost always triumphs or, at least, it is never beaten – just survived. The bush cares so little for these people that it leaves them to destroy themselves. Maybe the country is lucky after all, since it will go on, with or without its intruders.

Daniel Eisenberg

References

Isaacs, Bruce (2009) 'The Birth of a Nation: Living on the Land in *Lucky Country' Metro*, 161, pp. 36–40.

The Man from Snowy River

Country of Origin:

Australia

Studio/Distributor:

Cambridge Productions
Michael Edgley International
Snowy River Investment

Director:

George Miller

Producer:

Geoff Burrowes

Screenwriters:

John Dixon
Fred Cul Cullen, based on the poem 'The Man from Snowy River' by AB 'Banjo' Paterson, first published in the *Bulletin*, April 1890.

Synopsis

Jim Craig lives with his father on a farm high in the Snowy Mountains. After his father is killed in an unfortunate accident Jim decides, after some encouragement from old friend Spur, to leave the farm and make his own way in the world. He descends from the mountains and takes up work on the station of the big-money American, Harrison. Though the other station hands do not take too kindly to this Mountains boy, he is quickly smitten with the boss's lively daughter, Jessica. When Harrison's prize colt escapes, led off by the wild brumbies that cost Jim's father his life, all the men spring into action to track them down. They even call in Clancy of the Overflow, the best stockman in all the land. But as the brumbies push further up into the Snowy, there is only one man who can ride down the brumbies.

Critique

The Man from Snowy River contains one of the most iconic scenes in Australian film history. In a long, sweeping shot, a mob of wild brumbies gallop across a verdant hillside. Riders spur their horses on, trying to catch the Colt from Old Regret who leads them. But one figure separates from the pack. Jim Craig (Tom Burlinson), holding tightly to the reins of a weedy brown horse, urges his mount

Director of Photography:

Keith Wagstaff

Art Director:

Leslie Binns

Composer:

Bruce Rowland

Editor:

Adrian Carr

Duration:

100 minutes

Genre:

Australian western

Cast:

Tom Burlinson
Sigrid Thornton
Kirk Douglas
Jack Thompson
Tony Bonner
Terence Donovan

Format:

35 mm

Year:

1982

onward. The mob reaches a seemingly vertical edge, and charges over it. The camera captures it from below, sweating, sinewy beasts thundering overhead. All the men stop suddenly, even the legendary Clancy (Jack Thompson), and the camera pulls up and away. But the boy on the weedy horse breaks through the crowd and jumps over the edge. A bugle sounds, the camera slows, the angle tilts and Jim rides straight down the mountain. The horse's hooves beat like drums, nostrils flare and the wind whips around the boy's face. He has become the Man from Snowy River. In this scene Banjo Paterson's poem, with it strong imagery of horsemanship, the high country of New South Wales and mythic Australian masculinity, leaps off the screen.

George Miller's film is the oldest in the top ten highest grossing Australian films of all time. Its success inspired a sequel, *The Man from Snowy River II* (Geoff Burrowes, 1988) and a television series, *Snowy River: The Macgregor Saga* (Becker Entertainment/ Family Channel/MTM Enterprises/Pro Films, Nine Network, 1993), albeit with diminishing returns. The iconography of the poem, as represented in the *mise-en-scène* of the film, appeared in the opening ceremony of the 2000 Sydney Olympic Games and even spawned a live-action Arena Spectacular. The film turned the poem into an entertainment industry built around Australian stereotypes that films such as *Wake in Fright* (Ted Kotcheff, 1971) and its New Wave contemporaries have tried to debunk.

Miller's film is at least conscious of its almost anachronistic tone and embraces it whole-heartily, with Bruce Roland's bombastic score and multiple sweeping, dramatic long-shots across the expansive vistas of Australia. The performances are also pushed to melodramatic levels – Tom Burlinson is overly naive and full of enthusiasm, Sigrid Thornton plays Jessica as such a stereotypical 'outback woman' she could have stepped out of a Charles Chauvel or Ken G Hall film, and Jack Thompson is as square-jawed and laconic as possible. However, the casting of Kirk Douglas, primarily in his role as Harrison, speaks to the film's desire to smuggle its old-fashioned ideals of Australia to a wider audience – by masking it in the trappings of an American western. Harrison embodies the frontier spirit of the Old West, wanting to push ever onward into the landscape, conquering as he goes. The cinematography too, though shooting the Australian bush, is certainly more in line with the bold panoramas typically used to shoot Arizona than the harsh outback of other Australian westerns. Even Edward Buscombe lists this film as an example of a western (Buscombe 1993: 63). Although this creates an uneasy tone throughout, since *The Man* is an Australian film in its setting and ideals (dated as they are) cloaked in the stylistic and narrative beats of an American genre, its longevity and success show that the strategy worked.

Yet at its core the film contains a restlessness, a desperation to prove that the Australia described so lovingly by Paterson was not just a myth; it was (could have been, could still be) a real place. Paterson even appears in the film as a character, watching the plot unfold, trying to suggest to the viewer that the narrative is based on true events that Paterson himself observed and immortalized in verse. But that is not the case. *The Man from Snowy River* was just a poem that conjured up a mythic ideal of Australia and its past, one that this film successfully recreates on the silver screen.

Daniel Eisenberg

References

Buscombe, Edward (1993) *The BFI Companion to the Western*, London: BFI.

The Overlanders

Country of Origin:

UK/Australia

Studio/Distributor:

Ealing Studios

Director:

Harry Watt

Producers:

Michael Balcon
Ralph Smart

Screenwriter:

Harry Watt

Cinematographer:

Osmond Borradaile

Composer:

John Ireland

Editor:

EM Inman Hunter

Duration:

91 minutes

Genre:

Australian western

Cast:

Chips Rafferty
John Nugent Hayward
Daphne Campbell
Jean Blue
John Fernside
Clyde Combo

Format:

35 mm

Synopsis

During the Second World War, Australia's north is threatened by the possibility of Japanese invasion. The Australian government orders a 'scorched earth policy'. In Western Australia, drover Dan McAlpine is instructed to shoot his 1,000 head of cattle. Seeing this as only waste and destruction he decides to drove them overland to Queensland, across 2,600 km of dangerous terrain. He assembles an unlikely mob to help out on the drove: 'Corky' Corkindale an Irish drinker and gambler, Sinbad a Scottish sailor far from the coast, cattle man Bill Parsons, his family and two Indigenous stockmen, Jacky and Nipper. Two brothers also join them, but desert the drove – along with twenty horses – very swiftly, fearing the harsh landscape. McAlpine leads the party across the country, fording a crocodile-infested river leading to the drought-ravaged interior. Fearing for the cattle in the dry conditions, McAlpine decides to lead them over a dangerous mountain path to get them to water swiftly. Despite the desertion of some of the group, injuries to other, and cattle stampedes, they push on towards the Queensland coast.

Critique

In 1943, the Australian Government was keen to draw attention to the contributions of the Australian war effort – particularly on the home front – and asked the British Ministry of Information if they could improve the coverage of Australia in British propaganda. The ministry sent director Harry Watt to Australia, with support from Ealing Studios head Michael Balcon, as an official war correspondent. Watt had a long history in documentary film and had played a crucial part in the boom of the 1930s, most notably as one of the creators of the iconic documentary on the British postal service, *Night Mail* (Harry Watt and Basil Wright, 1936).

While scouting for ideas, Watt encountered the story of a massive head of cattle that had been driven from Western Australia to Queensland to avoid Japanese attacks. He soon realized that he had found his narrative. Though some crew were imported from Ealing Studios, the majority of those involved were Australians. Combining all this with the assembled series of archetypical Australian characters anchored around the grounded, 'hard yakka' Chips Rafferty (Dan McAlpine), Watt had the perfect cinematic blueprint from which to highlight the Australian effort and spirit.

Year:

1946

The subsequent popularity of the film can be attributed, in part, to its authentic imagery and its engagement with Australian concerns contained within an identifiably Australian narrative, which also struck a chord overseas. The film appeared in many international top ten lists in the year of its release (Pike and Cooper 1998 [1980]: 204).

Watt's documentary background is evident throughout the film. He shot everything on location, travelling the famous drover's trail with cast and crew behind him. The sweeping aerial shots do not try to romanticize the landscape. They simply show the long tracts of dry land that stretch to the horizon and beyond. When the camera closes in on a dried up waterhole or twisted gum, the distinct lines and shapes of these spaces are etched on the screen. The kinetic energy of the push across the crocodile filled river is enthralling – the dramatic tension is heightened by the fact the cast all actually forded the river in the sequence. The various stampedes and rushes of cattle are also full of action, excitement and danger. Watt frames even the smaller moments in natural light and lets characters speak – Rafferty most notably – with unaffected Australian accents.

The narrative also plays out more like a documentary than a high plains adventure. The difficulties encountered are not rogue gunslingers, bloodthirsty natives or marauding wild beasts. Instead it is the landscape itself that provides the obstacles: poison weeds, dry water holes, muddy bogs. The challenges presented in *The Overlanders* are everyday hardships rather than extraordinary events. Equally, these challenges are overcome not by feats of strength or grand individual heroics, but by ingenuity, hard work and team spirit. When they lose the horses, they manage to trap and calm some wild brumbies. When the mountain trail is blocked, Jacky (Clyde Combo) and Mary (Daphne Campbell) work together to clear the path and keep the cattle moving. This particular scene also highlights another distinct feature of the film, everyone, regardless of gender or skin colour or social standing, works together on the drove. Through Watt's documentarian lens, this dream of equality certainly seems possible – at least out there on the dry plains of inland Australia. Inevitably the film does become caught up in an idealistic and jingoistic view of Australian culture and society. Its initial purpose was just that. But it also shows the landscape honestly, and clearly sets the Australian western apart from its American cousins.

Daniel Eisenberg

Reference

Pike, Andrew and Cooper, Ross (1998 [1980]) *Australian Film, 1900–1977: A Guide to Feature Film Production*, Melbourne: Oxford University Press.

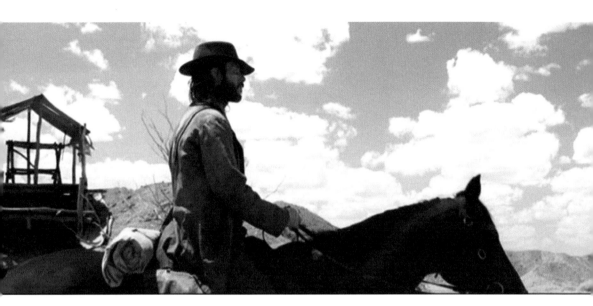

The Proposition
(John Hillcoat, 2005)

The Proposition

Country of Origin:

Australia/UK

Studio/Distributor:

Surefire Film Productions
Autonomous
Jackie O Productions
Pictures in Paradise

Director:

John Hillcoat

Producers:

Chris Brown
Chiara Menage
Jackie O'Sullivan
Cat Villiers

Screenwriter:

Nick Cave

Director of Photography:

Benoît Delhomme

Production Designer:

Chris Kennedy

Synopsis

In far north Queensland at the end of the nineteenth century, Captain Stanley offers Charlie, a notorious outlaw and middle brother of the Burns gang, a choice. Either he seeks out and kills his older brother Arthur within nine days or his younger brother Mikey will hang. As Charlie ventures into the sun bleached Australian outback in search of his brother, Stanley tries to balance his domestic life with his fragile wife Martha, his role as an officer of the law among disloyal men, and the threatening presence of landowner Eden Fletcher who demands Mikey's blood. Charlie is torn between loyalty to his elder brother and horror at the acts that Arthur has committed. As civilization crumbles around Stanley, the threat posed by Arthur and his gang grows ever greater.

Critique

The Proposition is not an easy film to watch. For many viewers an Aboriginal man's head exploding from a shotgun blast, a spear bursting gorily through a shoulder, the brutal rape of a female protagonist and a graphic flogging are enough to make the stomach churn. But the violence, though key to Cave's and Hillcoat's vision of colonial Australia, is just window dressing to the decay and darkness that is stitched into the fabric of the film. *The Proposition* is a film that strives to reveal truths about Australia's past; debunk romanticized stories of wild colonial boys and men from snowy rivers

Composer:

Nick Cave
Warren Ellis

Editor:

Jon Gregory

Duration:

104 minutes

Genre:

Australian western

Cast:

Guy Pearce
Ray Winstone
Emily Watson
Danny Huston
John Hurt
David Wenham
David Gulpilil
Tom E Lewis

Format:

35 mm

Year:

2005

who tame the landscape; and, instead, show the blood, sweat, flies and brutality of the Australian frontier. In an American western, there is a constant tension between the wilderness and civilization, pulling the characters (and the audience) toward one and then the other. In *The Proposition*, characters are pushed away from both; each indignity and horror in one setting is countered by one in the other. For example, the misogyny, racism and disloyalty of the bounty hunter Jellon Lamb (John Hurt) at a remote outpost in the wilderness is matched, if not surpassed, by similar traits in the policemen and civilians in town. The aggression and then murder of Aboriginal people in the outback is matched by the humiliation of the captured Indigenous men at the hands of the police. The servitude of Jacko (David Gulpilil) is equally as upsetting as the brutality of Two Bob (Tom E Lewis). It seems on this frontier there is no better way, no safe space to escape to. Both civilization and the wilderness are damned. The movie's brutal climax runs the two worlds into each other. The primal outback, represented by the wild outlaw Arthur (Danny Huston), tears down the trappings of society that the Stanleys have built around them. The Stanleys' homestead is an eyesore, a blemish of civilization out of place in the natural world.

As the camera lingers on the homestead, the inherent contradictions of the film bubble to the surface. For all its harsh and unrelenting darkness, the film is shot and scored beautifully. The sharp, blood-red sunsets over almost surreal landscapes, the attention to detail in the *mise-en-scène* and particularly the sets of the Stanleys' home and the bar where Jellon waits all bring a texture and richness to the image. Unsurprisingly, given Nick Cave – an iconic Australian musician and writer – holds both pen and plectrum, the words spoken and songs sung are deep and sombre, yet rousing, elegiac and affecting. The inherent tension and overlap of the darkness and the beauty in the work of Cave translates perfectly to an Australian western. The Australian mythic ballads which Cave emulates in his narrative rhythm and soundtrack cannot escape the decay that lies insidiously in wait as Australia's past is interrogated. The film most certainly is a heightened version of reality, and does push the boundaries between violence, darkness, beauty and art. But *The Proposition* is a film that resonates; constantly pushing the viewer to and between extremes.

Daniel Eisenberg

Red Hill

Country of Origin:

Australia

Studio/Distributor:

Destination Films
Hughes House Films

Synopsis

On his first day on duty at the small, isolated town of Red Hill, policeman Shane Cooper loses his gun, rides his first horse, learns about the panther living in the surrounding national park, and is caught up in the panic over a prison escapee who has sworn to take revenge on the town. The escapee is a local Aboriginal man, Jimmy Conway, who had been imprisoned for killing his wife. Conway disables the town's communications tower, and proceeds

Wildheart Films
Wolf Creek Films
McMahon International
Productions

Director:

Patrick Hughes

Producers:

Patrick Hughes
Al Clark

Screenwriter:

Patrick Hughes

Cinematographer:

Tim Hudson

Production Designer:

Enzo Iacono

Composer:

Dmitri Golovko

Editor:

Patrick Hughes

Genre:

Australian western

Duration:

94 minutes

to eliminate the posse one by one. As Shane learns more about the case and the town's treatment of Conway, he is forced to question his loyalties and the lengths he will go to in order to enforce the law.

Critique

After winning the Tropfest short film competition in 2001 with his film *The Lighter*, Victorian College of the Arts graduate Patrick Hughes went on to a successful career in advertising – he won a Gold Lion at the Cannes International Advertising Festival in 2009 – before returning to film-making to write, co-produce, direct and edit this highly impressive, low-budget genre film. With support from leading industry figures Al Clark (producer of *The Adventures of Priscilla: Queen of the Desert* [Stephan Elliott, 1994]) and Greg McLean (whose horror film *Wolf Creek* [2005] is credited by some with kickstarting investors' and agencies' interest in genre films), Hughes raised the finance to shoot the film privately, before receiving completion funding from Screen Australia. After a successful screening at the 60th Berlin International Film Festival in February 2010, local and US distribution rights were sold to Sony Pictures Releasing.

Red Hill hits all the classic western marks: a sheriff (Steve Bisley) is shaved by a swarthy barber (Christopher Davis) in an old gold-mining town; lawmen and cowboys gallop across stunning landscape; grizzled, weather-beaten mountain men prepare to defend their town from a fearsome foe; a taciturn, wronged man (Tom E Lewis) returns to avenge an ancient crime; in a shootout on the dusty main street, gunmen hide behind barrels down side alleys,

Red Hill (Patrick Hughes, 2010)

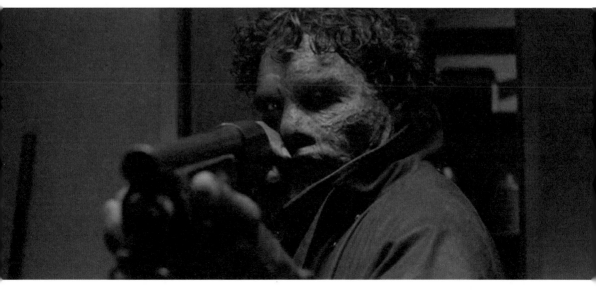

Cast:

Ryan Kwanten
Steve Bisley
Tom E Lewis
Claire van der Boom
Kevin Harrington
Richard Sutherland
Cliff Ellen
Jada Alberts
Christopher Davis

Format:

35 mm

Year:

2010

and fall to their deaths from rooftops. And yet despite the bizarre criticism of one reviewer who claimed that 'the one thing that cripples the film is that it's written, shot and produced by people who *think* generically' (Hoskins 2010: 14), this is far from being simply a 'textbook western' (13) transported to the modern-day Victorian high country.

Both implicitly and explicitly, *Red Hill* engages, sometimes problematically, with Australian historical and contemporary issues in ways that invite critique and discussion. It should not be dismissed as an entertaining but ultimately insignificant genre film. Jimmy Conway's story opens up the questions of frontier violence, contemporary racism and the silences in local history, as well as issues around environmental protection and the economic future of once-thriving rural towns. There is also the nominal connection between Tom E Lewis's character in *Red Hill* and the character he played in *The Chant of Jimmie Blacksmith* (Fred Schepisi, 1978), although the differences between these characters and narratives are more remarkable than their similarities. We first encounter Old Bill, the police inspector, giving a speech at a town hall meeting in which he passionately denounces environmentalists for causing the demise of the town's mining and timber industries, and to rapturous applause pledges not to let the town die. It is eventually revealed that Bill and what appears to be every other man in the town conspired to murder Conway's wife Ellin (Jada Alberts), and to frame Jimmy for her murder, in order to punish Conway for revealing the location of a sacred Indigenous burial site that stopped a proposed railway development. The townspeople justify their actions to themselves as being in what they see as the best interests of their town; they are motivated by desire to ensure its survival and future prosperity. That is, they are motivated by a sense of *community*, albeit one which deliberately and violently excludes Indigenous Australians.

The film is also very much concerned with 'the law', or rather competing systems of law, codes of behaviour, custom, culture and tradition. This is apparent in the story of Jimmy Conway's encounters with Old Bill and the townsfolk, although the opposition between attitudes to law and history – faithfulness and custodianship on one hand, versus corruption and manipulation on the other – is only fully revealed towards the end of the film. The film's concern with competing attitudes to law is also apparent in the opposition between city cop Shane Cooper (Ryan Kwanten), and the town's Inspector, Old Bill, who seems to have been hewn from the mountains that overlook Red Hill. Cooper's preference for dialogue, negotiation and understanding over gunplay had earlier resulted in him being shot on duty by a young boy in the city. And finding himself several times in a Mexican standoff with Conway, and later with Old Bill, he cannot bring himself to pull the trigger. These events, and the fact that he has lost his gun at the start of the film, both signal his emasculation and illustrate how out of place he seems to be. How can he be a lawman – or a cowboy – without a gun? His wife (Claire van der Boom) underscores this connection: when Shane briefly returns home in the middle of the action to retrieve his weapon, she bids him a sleepy farewell, 'Be careful, cowboy.' Inspector Bill, by contrast, epitomizes the law of the gun, believing himself to be not a servant of the law but its personification and expression. In the final climactic scene, as Shane finds himself once again in a Mexican standoff, Bill tells his would-be rescuers that Shane 'doesn't have the balls to pull the trigger'. Now complete, and in full possession of the facts behind Jimmy's rampage, Shane unblinkingly shoots the two horsemen dead.

Red Hill signposts its generic origins and proudly pays homage to the western's heritage in a variety of ways, most obviously in the name of its hero character. 'Shane Cooper' invokes both a classic of the genre (*Shane* [George Stevens, 1953]) and one of its most recognizable stars (Gary Cooper). The nod to Cooper is more particularly a nod to the storyline and to the character he plays in *High Noon* (Fred Zinnemann, 1952), although *Red Hill*'s Cooper is more the observer and mediator of the feud, while Old Bill is the object of the avenger's ire. *Red Hill* invokes a range of other westerns, from *High Plains Drifter* (Clint Eastwood, 1973), and *The Good, the Bad and the Ugly* (Sergio Leone, 1966), to more contemporary classics like *No Country for Old Men* (Ethan Coen and Joel Coen, 2007).

But it would be a mistake to write the film off either as a 'western-by-numbers' or as a derivative homage to an imported form. There is plenty of play in the film with the codes and conventions of the genre, albeit never too much to alienate general audiences or aficionados. And as briefly outlined above, there are multiple points of connection to Australian cinema, local issues and histories. Together, these mark the film out as much more than a shallow imitation of the American western.

Ben Goldsmith

Reference

Hoskins, Dave (2011) 'Familiar Territory: Red Hill Rides into Town', *Metro*, 167, pp. 12–15.

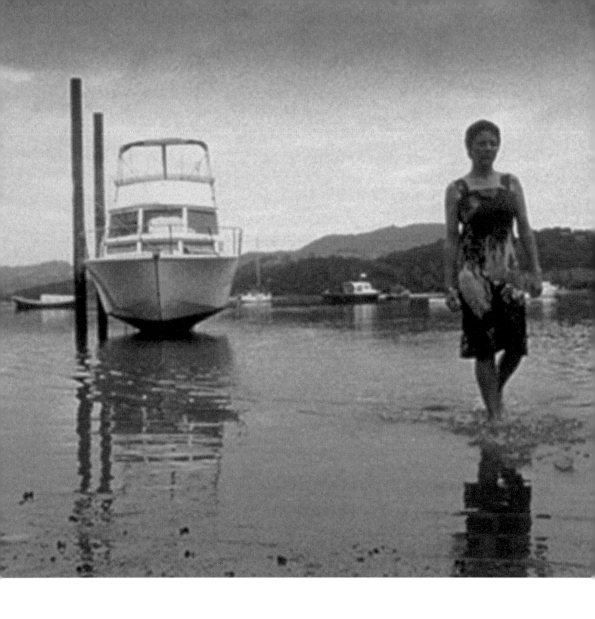

INTRODUCTION: TWO NATIONS UNITED?
AUSTRALIAN FILM AND NEW ZEALAND FILM

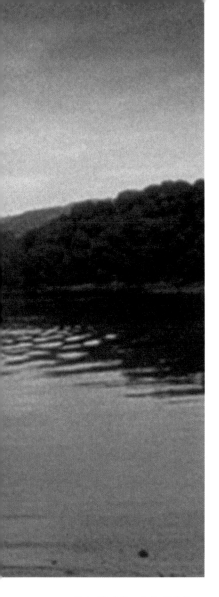

Rain (Christine Jeffs, 2011).
Image courtesy of the director.

It is four years since the first edition of this Directory devoted to the cinema of Australia and New Zealand appeared, and although the content in this second edition is new, some commonalities persist. Several reviewers of the first edition commented on the weighting given to the two countries, with the New Zealand contribution being significantly slimmer than the Australian contribution. This will once again characterize this new edition. This is inevitable, given the respective histories, scale and current populations of the two countries: 23 million Australians versus 4.4 million New Zealanders. But there are other possible explanations, such as far fewer New Zealand film scholars and academics.

Nevertheless, there has been some significant scholarship in recent years, such as the monumental Stark, Pivac and McDonald-edited *New Zealand Film: An Illustrated History* (Te Papa Press, 2011) and Dunleavy and Joyce, *New Zealand Film & Television: Institution, Industry and Cultural Change* (Intellect, 2011) and Sigley, *Transnational Film Culture in New Zealand* (Intellect, 2013). It is not the intention of this second edition of the Directory to replicate this work, but instead focus on other aspects of film in New Zealand.

Australia and New Zealand

Australia and New Zealand cling together as two countries at the furthermost ends of the earth, but with very different social and cultural trajectories. Geographically, Australia is a continent with human habitation largely clustered on its extensive coastline; New Zealand is an island nation, comparable in size to the United Kingdom, with over half of its population clustered in the upper half of the North Island. Colonial Australia treated its first inhabitants (both Aboriginals and transported convicts) very badly; after a period of accommodation, confrontation and warfare, New Zealand colonists reached a formal agreement with Maori (*tangata whenua*, or 'people of the land') through the Treaty of Waitangi, which remains the founding document of a bicultural country. Australia was originally shaped as a monocultural society but has rapidly moved towards multiculturalism, as a result of extensive immigration (particularly from Europe and

Asia); with the Treaty, New Zealand has long shaped itself as a bicultural society and has only lately begun to confront the possibilities of multiculturalism.

Economically the two countries have long had their hands in each others pockets; a situation intensified since the Closer Economic Relations (CER), a free trade agreement signed in 1983. Such economic connections have always operated in favour of the larger partner, with the current New Zealand landscape of retailing, media, banking and financial services largely Australian-owned. Australia is the most favoured destination for New Zealanders setting off overseas (as tourists, or to seek higher wages), whilst New Zealand is a top tourist destination for Australians. Sporting links also run deep. There is occasional talk of a closer political or constitutional relationship (such as New Zealand formally incorporated in the state structure of Australia) but there seems to be little enthusiasm for this, from either side.

Cao (2012: 240) has suggested that, 'One of the most popular and influential formulations of Australia is that of a nation caught between empires, namely, between the British Empire and the American Empire'. There are echoes of this experience in New Zealand's history but it is more complex: there is a third imperialist influence for New Zealand in the shape of Australia, as well as a particular local inflection in the relationship between Maori and colonizing forces. This has made the New Zealand historical experience similar to the Australian historical experience, but also remarkably different.

Film

How does this incomplete and often vexed relationship translate to film, and exchange of cultural products generally? In their joint contribution, Alfio Leotta and Tom O'Regan (a trans-Tasman collaboration, which follows this Introduction) argue that, 'New Zealand and Australian film are, and have always been, intimately connected', through the processes of cultural exchange and borrowings, the transfer of expertise, and shared cultural policies. Such connections are important but we need to acknowledge significant disconnections as well. It is instructive, for example, that Jane Campion is variously described as an 'Australian director' and a 'New Zealand director', just as her 1993 film *The Piano* is sometimes described as an Australian film and sometimes as a New Zealand film. Of course, this is a general problem in these days of transnational film and co-production deals, but it is also a particular inflection of the Australia–New Zealand relationship and a self-conscious nationalism.

There is also a long history of benign neglect or studied disinterest in both countries' cinema, with no special effort being put into the promotion and distribution of Australian films in New Zealand (with Australian films customarily included in general release patterns), and little attention to New Zealand films in Australia. There have been modest successes for New Zealand-produced films in Australia, such as *Boy* (Taika Waititi, 2010) and *Mt. Zion* (Tearapa Kahi, 2013), but they have been few. In respect of these two films, the sizeable New Zealand diaspora living in cities such as Sydney and Brisbane may well have made a significant contribution to the Australian box office. Likewise, New Zealand audiences have responded to more populist fare such as *The Castle* (1997) and *Red Dog* (2011), but numerous releases from both countries do not make it across the Tasman.

This is particularly ironic, given that film distribution and exhibition in New Zealand is owned or controlled by Australian-owned companies (such as Roadshow or Madman), or through Australian-based subsidiaries of US-based distributors.[1] There have been attempts to address this mutual neglect, or at least seek some reconsideration of an imbalance which sees far more cultural products flow from Australia to New Zealand, than from New Zealand to Australia. Project Blue Sky, an initiative headed by a number of New Zealand screen producers, led to the High Court of Australia decision of April 1998 permitting New Zealand television programmes to be under local content quotas (redefined as 'Australian' programmes) on Australian commercial networks. This somewhat curious decision resulted in early warnings about a flood of New Zealand programmes on Australian screens but such alarms had little foundation, for Australian-produced drama and reality TV continue to occupy primetime slots on New Zealand screens, for example, the drama series *Packed to the Rafters* (created by Bevan Lee, Seven Network, 2008–2013) and *Puberty Blues* (created by Kathy Lette & Gabrielle Carey, Channel Ten, 2012–2013) in the prime slot of Sunday 8.30 to 10.30pm on the dominant channel TV1 in May 2013. Meanwhile, the presence of New Zealand programmes on Australian screens remains minimal and off-peak.

Another more recent case with Australian and New Zealand participants from respective film industries concerned threats (real or perceived) to the New Zealand-based production of the Peter Jackson-directed *The Hobbit* trilogy in late 2010, when the Australian trade union Media, Entertainment and Arts Alliance (MEAA) and its representative Simon Whipp was positioned in the public discourse as villains in the saga. Leotta and O'Regan also refer to this incident in their contribution.

Peter Jackson echoed considerable popular sentiment when he damned Whipp in the following terms, 'I can't see beyond the ugly spectre of an Australian bully, using what he perceives as his weak Kiwi cousins to gain a foothold in this country's film industry' (quoted in Handel 2013: 6).[2]

This affair ended with Warner Bros. executives flying into the country for a meeting with Prime Minister John Key, 'to save the film', which resulted in quite extraordinary consequences. These included further tax incentives and advertising funds for the American corporation, and the emergency passage of anti-union legislation. The consequences of this case linger, leading to an even more welcoming environment for off-shore productions, increased tax incentives and benefits, and deep suspicions about Australian motivations in respect of the New Zealand film industry. This is despite more recent disclosures from official sources, which suggests that varieties of 'truth' were being constructed in the heat of debate, and that the actions of some participants (including Jackson) do not look very noble in retrospect.

Meanwhile, the trans-Tasman trade in audio-visual materials remains sporadic – and largely in Australian's favour, when it does occur. It is certainly true that the domestic film and television sector is extremely important for both countries. A recent PricewaterhouseCoopers (PwC) study of the New Zealand film and television industry in New Zealand, described it as a 'high-productivity and high-wage sector that accounts for a significant portion of national GDP and employment', and estimated that film contributed NZ$1,500 million to the total industry GDP of NZ$2,781 million in 2011 with 21,315 full-time employees (FTEs).[3]

Meanwhile, an August 2011 report by Access Economics for the Australian Federation Against Copyright Theft (AFACT) cited an AU$6.1 billion contribution to the Australian economy flowing from the Australian film and television industry.[4] Speaking at the official launch of this report, Australian actor Roy Billing declared,

> It would be hard to imagine what our society would be like without screen entertainment: In purely economic terms, it is a substantial contributor to our economy, as this report makes clear – but culturally, it's much more difficult to put a price on it. This is an important study for understanding how our business has grown, how many jobs it supports, and how we contribute to Australia's economic and cultural make-up.[5]

Certainly the financial value of their film and television industries is of great importance to both Australia and New Zealand but, as Billing suggests, there are also other significant cultural benefits – which include employment, opportunities to tell local stories, and opportunities to occupy a place in global entertainment flows. The summary figures above also tend to obscure the various components of screen production in both countries, which is characterized by a complex mix of film and television made primarily for indigenous (local) audiences, or films or television programmes which aspire to attract transnational audiences, or off-shore, globally-oriented productions which utilize the locations, expertise or post-production facilities of the host country.

This complexity evokes a question raised in the Introduction in the first edition of this Directory, that is, the difficulty in clarifying what a 'New Zealand film' might be in such circumstances. One possible example of how conditional and cautious one must be in assigning country of origin to a film (whether it be New Zealand or Australia) is the recent remake of *Evil Dead* (Fede Alvarez, 2013), which is officially assigned as a 'USA/ New Zealand' co-production because it used New Zealand locations and productions, and drew on the financial resources of the New Zealand Large Budget Screen Production Grant. In no other respects (theme, narratives, accent, acting, other creative input) can it be regarded as a New Zealand film.

Even though it produces a high volume of locally-produced features, Australian film is also subject to similar ambiguities resulting from the nature of global film production in the twenty-first century – especially the need to attract big budget, off-shore productions to its shores. Australian director Baz Luhrmann recently pointed to this, in his explanation as to why he shot his big budget, 3D adaptation of F Scott Fitzgerald's *The Great Gatsby* (2013) in Australia, rather than New York,

> I was instrumental in organizing the [tax] rebate in Australia with the previous prime minister. I met with him personally and said, 'Look, the issue here isn't how to give a rebate to stories set under gum trees. It's creativity, imagination—people who drive creativity by bringing other creators here and making major works, getting Australians to make their imaginations here, in their hometown'. (Dodes 2013)

Perspectives on New Zealand Film

Given the proliferation of *major* foreign-funded but locally-subsidized productions completed or underway in both countries, (*The Great Gatsby* in Australia; *The Hobbit: An Unexpected Journey* [Peter Jackson, 2012] and *Avatar 2* [James Cameron, 2016] in New Zealand), a default definition of *minor* could be the primary characteristic of more locally-initiated and produced film features. This is certainly the case in respect of the box office share for local films. With the eleven New Zealand-produced features released in 2013 gaining a very slight 2.6 per cent of that year's total box office.[6] Screen Australia reported a 3.5 per cent box office share for 15 Australian films released in the same year.[7]

A celebration of minor status does seem to be the focus in the following contributions, which centre on film-makers and films best known in their native country, but worthy of being more widely known. My fellow Australian editors have obviously had a much larger body of work to draw on, which has enabled them to sort their material into a greater number of themes or genres.

My strategy for this second edition has been to concentrate on a specific range of themes and several areas of neglect in New Zealand film scholarship, namely;

1. Innovative New Zealand film-makers – most particularly female film-makers such as Annie Goldson, Gaylene Preston and Yvonne Mackay. Marian Evans has provided a very useful list of female directors, whilst other writers address the particular work of such film-makers.

2. Film-makers and documentary directors whose work is motivated by political agendas, or addresses issues of human rights.

3. Emerging film-makers who are employing alternative means of creating, promoting and distributing low-budget features and documentaries.

4. New film-makers, who celebrate a changing New Zealand in respect of multiculturalism. Mandy Treagus on the Samoan feature *The Orator* (Tusi Tamasese, 2011) and Arezou Zalipour on Asian New Zealand film-makers provide good examples of such shifts in the New Zealand consciousness.

Geoff Lealand

References

Cao, Benito (2012) 'Beyond empire: Australian cinematic identity in the twenty-first century', *Studies in Australasian Cinema*, 6: 3.

Dodes, Rachel (2013) 'Jay-Z, 3-D and Jay Gatsby: The Interview: Baz Luhrmann', *Wall Street Journal*, 3 May, p. D4.

Handel, Jonathan with Pip Bulbeck (2013) *The New Zealand Hobbit Crisis: How Warner Bros. Bent a Government to its Will and Crushed an Attempt to Unionize 'The Hobbit'*, Los Angeles: Hollywood Analytics.

Notes

1. For detailed analysis, see Geoff Lealand, 'A Nation of Film-goers: Audiences, Exhibition and Distribution in New Zealand' in Albert Moran and Karina Aveyard (eds), *Watching Films: New Perspectives on Movie-going, Exhibition and Reception*, Bristol: Intellect, 2013.

2. Cited in Handel (2013), *The New Zealand Hobbit crisis: How Warner Bros. Bent a Government to Its Will and Crushed an Attempt to Unionize The Hobbit*. This small book, written by a contributing editor to the *Hollywood Reporter*, provides a detailed and balanced overview of the issues.

3. 'The economic contribution of the film and television industry in New Zealand: A statistical snapshot', PwC New Zealand, 2012. This report cites the total New Zealand GDP in 2011 as NZ$195 billion, with the film and television industry contributing 1.4 per cent.

4. http://www.afact.org.au/index.php/news/film_and_tv_industry_contributes_6.1_billion_to_australian_economy.

5. http://www.afact.org.au/index.php/news/film_and_tv_industry_contributes_6.1_billion_to_australian_economy. It should also be noted that Wikipedia/wiki/Roy Billing describes him as 'a New Zealand television actor, now based in Sydney, Australia'.

6. http://www.nzfilm.co.nz/sites/nzfc/files/NZ%20Feature%20Films%20Share%20of%20NZ%20/updated%20Jan%202014.pdf.

7. http://www.screenaustralia.gov.au/research/statistics/mrstfeatscin.aspx.

CROSSING THE DITCH:
TRANS-TASMAN FILM EXPATRIATES

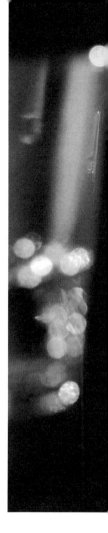

When Australian trade unionists were blamed for infiltrating the New Zealand film labour movement, and putting the production of Peter Jackson's *The Hobbit* (2012) at risk (Conor 2011), commentators overlooked the extent to which the New Zealand and Australian film industries are, and have always been, intimately connected. Many so-called 'New Zealand' films are actually strongly anchored in Australian expertise. The *Lord of the Rings* trilogy (Jackson, 2001–03), for example, while often celebrated as a flagship for national identity, employed Australian cast and crew members and benefited greatly from expertise generated by Australian productions such as *The Matrix* (Andy Wachowski and Lana Wachowski, 1999). Similarly, films such as *The Piano* (Jane Campion, 1993), funded by Australian and French investors, directed by an Australian-trained New Zealander and featuring American and New Zealand actors, reflect the convergence of Australian and New Zealand film-making as well as representing a new paradigm of international art cinema (O'Regan 1996).

Australia and New Zealand are identified and brought together by the idea of the Antipodes, a term which traditionally refers to the places of the globe which are diametrically opposite to Europe. In cultural terms being Antipodean means to be other, displaced, a reflex of European metropolitan culture and yet part of it elsewhere (Beilharz 1997; Smith 1992). The Tasman Sea, often colloquially referred to as 'The Ditch', both links and separates Australia and Aotearoa (New Zealand). On the one hand, the two countries retain distinct political, social, economic and cultural characteristics, which are reflected in their different positioning in the global market. But they also participate in an economic system, trading relationship, and cultural economy that is progressively more integrated and characterized by the free exchange of both capital and labour.[1] The economic relations between the Trans-Tasman neighbours, however, have worked primarily in favour of Australia, and the dominant Australian business interests in New Zealand have often resulted in uneven financial and migratory flows.

Since the 1970s both countries' governments have supported the local film industries in an effort to foster a sense of national identity and counter Hollywood cultural hegemony. Today the film industry is regarded, particularly in New Zealand, as an important and growing economic sector. While Australian and New Zealand films have often competed at the global level for a share of the same markets,

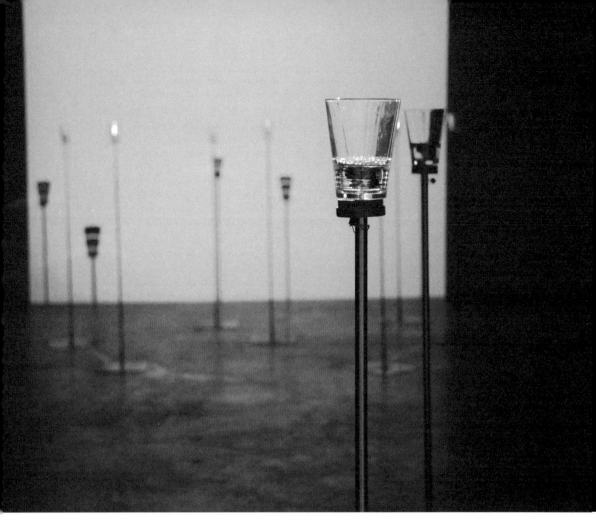

Re/Sense (Raewyn Turner, 2010),
Image courtesy of the artist.

the relationship between the two industries has been characterized by a significant exchange of creative talent. This exchange has often been fostered by the involvement of international investors (particularly American and European) in the Australian region. By focusing on the examination of selected producers' and directors' careers, this chapter will attempt to identify the different factors responsible for influencing the mobility of film-makers across the Tasman.[2]

The relationship between the Australian and New Zealand film industries has been shaped by close historical, linguistic and cultural ties. Significant interrelationships were already apparent even before the emergence of cinema technology. During the nineteenth century theatrical circuits linked the Australian East Coast with New Zealand cities (Thomson 1995: 404). Until the 1930s the work of successful vaudeville impresarios like the Fullers brothers, who had a strong presence in both Australia and New Zealand, favoured the Trans-Tasman exchange of creative personnel (West 1995: 238). Silent film-makers such as Raymond Longford and Franklyn Barrett started their careers in theatre touring towns on both sides of the Tasman before moving onto cinema. These exchanges continued during the period of early silent film-making: when Australian Raymond Longford started producing and directing films, for example, he decided to shoot *A Maori Maid's Love* (1916) in New Zealand (Rutledge 1979). Similarly, Beaumont Smith used Australian and New Zealand locations for *The Betrayer* (1921) and *The Adventures of Algie* (1925). English-born Franklyn Barrett pursued a successful theatrical and film-making career both in Australia and New Zealand. He joined the Melbourne office of Pathé Frères in 1908 and directed travelogues such as *The Sea Coasts of New Zealand* (1908) and *Across the Mountain Passes of New Zealand* (1910) which are some of the first films that offered New Zealand up to the gaze of European viewers (Leotta 2011). These early film-makers were also often responsible for the mobility of actors across the Tasman: Vera James, for example, started her career in New Zealand as a stage actress, but was eventually recruited by Barrett as the protagonist for two iconic Australian films, *A Girl of the Bush* and *Know Thy Child* (1921).[3]

After World War I, New Zealander Pat Hanna became renowned in Australia for his Digger travelling shows. One of his monologues *The Gospel According to Cricket* (1900) became a big seller both in Australia and New Zealand. The Digger shows' popularity led to Hanna making his first film *Diggers* (1931) as actor and writer for Efftee Studios led by Frank W Thring. *Diggers* has an important place in the history of Australian cinema as it was the country's second talking feature (Reade 1979: 91–92). After a series of disagreements with Thring, Hanna formed his own film production company where he produced, directed and starred in *Diggers in Blighty* and *Waltzing Matilda* (both 1933) that were poorly distributed and did not achieve the success he had hoped for (Reade 1979: 91–92).

New Zealanders continued to play a significant part in the development of Australian cinema even during the following decades. In some case these individuals simply followed the movements of their parents. Bert Bailey, for example, a particularly important figure in both Australian theatre and film into the 1940s, was born in Auckland from a New Zealand family. However he was already living in Sydney by the age of four (Australian Literature Resource 2010). In some other cases the move was the result of a deliberate choice. Cecil Holmes is a perfect case in point. Holmes started his career in New Zealand making a number of documentaries for the National Film Unit during the 1940s, but subsequently moved to Australia for political reasons.[4] In Australia Holmes directed a number of documentaries for the Commonwealth Film Unit and three feature films, including *Captain Thunderbolt* (1953) for fellow New Zealand expatriate and producer Colin Scrimgeour (Campbell 2010). Holmes also directed a series of ethnographic films for the Australian Institute of Aboriginal Studies and taught film-making to young Indigenous people (Campbell 2010). The Cecil Holmes Award given by the Australian Directors Guild is named after him.

Like Cecil Holmes, Roger Mirams is a key figure in the history of Australasian cinema. Mirams was one of the original partners in Pacific Films that he founded in 1948 with former National Film Unit staffer Alun Falconer. In 1952, with New Zealand film pioneer John O'Shea, he co-directed *Broken Barrier*, the first fictional feature film to be produced in New Zealand since 1940. Mirams moved to Australia in 1956 to work on the coverage of the Melbourne Olympic Games and decided to settle in Sydney following the Olympics. He first founded an Australian branch of Pacific Films and then his own film production company, Roger Mirams Productions, which produced a number of successful films and television shows (Shelton 2012).

The growing interconnections between the Australian and New Zealand industries became more apparent during the 1980s when shifts in cultural policy, and the creation of tax breaks aimed at film productions, stimulated the exchanges between the two industries. These interconnections often occurred within the context of the increased international involvement (both Hollywood and Europe) in the Australasian region.

One of the film-makers who embodies the significant interconnections between Australian and New Zealand cinema during this period is John Maynard. Maynard was born in Australia and was appointed foundation director of the Govett-Brewster Art Gallery in New Plymouth (New Zealand) in 1967 (Shelton 2012). In 1979 he turned his attention to film, producing his first feature, Geoff Steven's *Skin Deep*. Maynard's next feature was Vincent Ward's *Vigil* (1984) the first New Zealand film to be selected for competition at the Cannes Film Festival. After working on Australia/New Zealand co-production *The Navigator* (1988) he launched Jane Campion's career, producing her Australian-shot debut, *Sweetie* (1989) and in the process, becoming the only Australasian producer to get three consecutive pictures into competition for the Palme D'Or.

Maynard eventually returned to Australia (because of the bigger market and greater opportunities) where he produced a number of successful Australian features including *The Boys* (Rowan Woods, 1998), *The Bank* (Robert Connolly, 2001) and *Romulus, My Father* (Richard Roxburgh, 2007). Maynard has also been an active independent distributor in Australia and New Zealand for 25 years and his company Footprint Films has a reputation for creating innovative and cost effective marketing campaigns. Maynard married New Zealander Bridget Ikins, the producer of Campion's second film (*An Angel at My Table* [1990]) which was post-produced by Maynard in Sydney. Ikins, in turn, produced the Alison Maclean -directed New Zealand feature *Crush* (1992) before moving to Australia where she has produced several Australian films and TV shows (Shelton 2012).

New Zealand brothers David Hannay and Charles Hannah also played an important role in reinforcing the ties between Australian and New Zealand cinema. David Hannay was one of Australia's most experienced film and television producers, having been involved in the development, production and marketing of more than fifty film and television productions. He worked with thirteen directors on their first feature films both in Australia and New Zealand (IMDb 2012). In 1996 he received a Lifetime Achievement Award from the Producers and Directors Guild of Australia. He was also named Film Pioneer of the year by the Society of Australian Cinema Pioneers 'for outstanding service to the Motion Picture Industry'.

David's brother Charles entered the film industry in 1984 as Managing Director of David Hannay Productions after a successful career as an international corporate executive and restaurateur (IMDb 2012). Since 1984 Hannah has produced/executive produced and/or financed thirteen feature films including *Tasmania Monogatari* (Yasuo Furuhata) which when it was released in 1990 was in the top ten of all time Japanese hits, *Newcastle* (Dan Castle, 2008), a surf movie shot in Australia, and *The World's Fastest Indian* (2005), one of New Zealand's most successful films of all time, directed by Australian-born director Roger Donaldson.

In some cases successful New Zealand-born producers have moved to Australia for a career change. Roger Simpson is a perfect case in point as before moving to Australia during the 1970s and beginning a new career as film-writer and producer, he had practised law for several years in New Zealand (Australian Literature Resource 2012). The majority of New Zealand-born producers however, including Don Reynolds, Matt Reeder, Tim White, Caterina De Nave and Helen Bowden have moved to Australia looking for more work and opportunities after beginning their career in New Zealand. Helen Bowden, for example, produced her first short film in New Zealand but has been living in Sydney since the 1990s. Bowden is one of the five founding partners of Matchbox Pictures, a major Australian film and television production company and the lead producer on *The Slap*, an eight-part drama broadcast on Australian television. Her first feature *Soft Fruit*, screened in Critics' Week in Cannes in 2000, brought together a number of New Zealand female film-makers living and working in Australia. The film was directed by Christina Andreef who began her career writing scripts and working as assistant director for New Zealand film-makers such as Alison McLean and Jane

Campion. Jane Campion herself in turn participated in the making of *Soft Fruit* as executive producer.

As with film producers, the trans-Tasman expatriation of film directors has been largely an uneven phenomenon with more New Zealanders moving to Australia than the other way around. Tony Williams' career path, for example, illustrates this point. Williams was one of the directors who wanted to make a film in New Zealand during the 1970s before the time of the New Zealand Film Commission. He managed to do so by seeking and obtaining financial support from an Australian broadcaster. In 1977 he shot *Solo* which featured two Australian lead actors: Lisa Peers and Vincent Gill (Shelton 2005). One of the producers of *Solo* was the above-mentioned Australian-based New Zealander David Hannay. *Solo* was the first co-production between Australia and New Zealand and, along with *Sleeping Dogs*, contributed to the emergence of a new feature film industry in New Zealand. After *Solo* Williams moved to Sydney where he directed *Next of Kin* (1984); his career then led him to the top echelons of advertising in both Australia and New Zealand (Phillips 2012).

One of the most notable trans-Tasman film expats is Vincent Ward. In 1988 Ward directed *The Navigator*, the first official Australia/New Zealand co-production, and one which represented the unfulfilled promise of an integrated trans-Tasman market. Ward and his producer, Australian born John Maynard, could not find enough money to produce *The Navigator* in New Zealand. Ward left New Zealand for Sydney where he managed to find funding for the project, however the Australian producers pushed for a co-production agreement and this eventually led to the formulation of the 'Memorandum of Understanding Regarding the Coproduction of Films' signed by the Australian Film Commission and the New Zealand Film Commission. After *The Navigator* Ward continued his nomadic film-making career moving first to London to make *Map of the Human Heart* (an Australia/Canada/UK co-production directed in 1992), then to Los Angeles where he made one feature – *What Dreams May Come* (1998). Recently Ward has returned to New Zealand where he has made *Rain of the Children* (2008) and *River Queen* (2005), a film that was particularly successful among Australian audiences.

Ward's career path, which took him from New Zealand to Australia, Europe and the United States, is quite similar to that of Jane Campion, one of the most successful Australasian film-makers. Campion was born in Wellington, New Zealand, and currently lives in Sydney, Australia. Having graduated with a BA in Anthropology from Victoria University of Wellington in 1975, and a BA, with a painting major, at Sydney College of the Arts in 1979, she began film-making in the early 1980s, attending the Australian Film, Television and Radio School. Her first short film, *Peel* (1982) won the Palme D'Or at the Cannes Film Festival in 1986. Her first feature film *Sweetie* was produced by John Maynard, the Australian producer who played a crucial role in the development of New Zealand cinema during the 1980s and was responsible for launching the career of other talented directors such as Vincent Ward. *The Piano*, Palme D'Or winner in 1994, received a pre-production development grant from the Australian Film Commission. The film was produced by Australian Jane Chapman and is officially designated as an Australian film, even though everything on-screen was shot in New Zealand.

Jane Campion's Australian based work is sometimes claimed for New Zealand cinema. *Sweetie*, for example, was screened in Sydney as part of a festival of New Zealand cinema (O'Regan 1996). Campion's nationality has often been contested. She has lived in Australia for seventeen years, was trained at the AFTRS and has often used Australian film subsidy to develop her talent and film skills. At the same time she has often claimed how her work has been deeply influenced by the films of veteran New Zealand film-makers such as John O'Shea. Sometimes she describes herself as an Australian, but just as often she associates her work with her Kiwi identity, most recently shooting *Top of the Lake* (2013), a drama series for the US Sundance Channel, in the southern lakes of the South Island.

Roger Donaldson reversed the usual flow of film-makers moving from New Zealand to Australia. He started his career as a still photographer in Australia and came to New Zealand during the 1960s to avoid being drafted to fight in Vietnam. Under the banner of his production company, Aardvark Films, he directed a number of self-financed documentaries. His first feature film, *Sleeping Dogs* (1977) launched the career of Kiwi actor Sam Neill and became one of the most significant films in the history of New Zealand cinema. After directing *Smash Palace* (1982) which featured iconic New Zealand actor Bruno Lawrence, he moved to Los Angeles where he was enlisted by Dino DeLaurentiis to remake *The Bounty* (1984), which was partly shot in New Zealand and used Australian actors such as Mel Gibson. During the making of this film, Donaldson met Anthony Hopkins, who twenty years later would star in *The World's Fastest Indian* (2005) produced by New Zealand-born and Australian-based Charles Hannah.

The constant flow of expatriate film-makers across the Tasman has played a crucial role in the development of both Australian and New Zealand national cinemas. However, apart from some very rare exceptions, the significant exchanges between the two industries have not led to the formulation of shared cinematic narratives, nor strong audience loyalty. Despite the common history and culture very few films have dealt with stories that bring together Australian and New Zealand characters and locations. The very limited number of co-productions and shared narratives between the two countries is explained by the fact that since the 1980s the Australian and New Zealand industries have been very competitive with each other. The two industries have had a similar positioning in the global market and have been aiming at the same distributors and audiences. Policy makers and industry stakeholders have often chosen to ignore the exchanges between the two industries because of an anxiety about how the transnational context of film production affects the distinctiveness of national cinema. Similarly despite the significance of these interconnections the academic literature on Australian and New Zealand film (Verhoeven 1999; Mayer and Beattie 2007; Goldsmith and Lealand 2010; Bennet and Beirne 2011) has not yet engaged in a systematic investigation of the interconnections between the two national cinemas. Further research about the mobility of film-makers between Australia and New Zealand is needed to highlight obstacles and opportunities offered by the global dispersion of film production in the region.

Alfio Leotta and Tom O'Regan

References

Australian Literature Resource (2010) 'Bert Bailey', http://austlit.edu.au/run?ex=Show Agent&agentId=A%2C-G. Accessed 4 February 2013.

Australian Literature Resource (2012) 'Roger Simpson', http://www.austlit.edu.au/run?ex=ShowAgent&agentId=A%23}c. Accessed 4 February 2013.

Beilharz, Peter (1997) *Imagining the Antipodes: Culture, Theory, and the Visual in the Work of Bernard Smith*, Melbourne: Cambridge University Press.

Bennet, James and Beirne, Rebecca (2011) *Making Film and Television Histories: Australia and New Zealand*, London: Tauris.

Campbell, Russell (2010) 'Holmes, Cecil William – Biography', *Dictionary of New Zealand Biography. Te Ara – the Encyclopedia of New Zealand*, http://www.TeAra.govt.nz/en/biographies/5h32/1. Accessed 20 December 2012.

Conor, Brigid (2011) 'Problems in " Wellywood": Rethinking the Politics of Transnational Cultural', *LabourFlow TV*, 13 (7), 27 January, http://flowtv.org/2011/01/problems-in-wellywood/. Accessed 23 February 2012.

IMDb (2012) 'David Hannay', http://www.imdb.com/name/nm0360362/. Accessed 19 December 2012.

Goldsmith, Ben and Lealand, Geoff (eds) (2010) *The Directory of World Cinema: Australia and New Zealand*, Bristol: Intellect.

Leotta, Alfio (2011) *Touring the Screen: Tourism and New Zealand Film Geographies*, Bristol: Intellect.

Mayer, Geoff and Beattie, Keith (2007) *The Cinema of Australia and New Zealand*, London: Wallflower.

O'Regan, Tom (1996) *Australian National Cinema*, London: Routledge.

Phillips, Jock (2012), 'Advertising – Creative advertising', *Te Ara – the Encyclopedia of New Zealand*, http://www.TeAra.govt.nz/en/advertising/5. Accessed 21 December 2012.

Reade, Eric (1979) *History and Heartburn: The Saga of Australian Film 1896–1978*, Sydney: Harper and Row.

Rutledge, Martha (1979) 'Barrett, Walter Franklyn (1873–1964)', *Australian Dictionary of Biography*, National Centre of Biography, Australian National University, http://adb.anu.edu.au/biography/barrett-walter-franklyn-5145/text8615. Accessed 29 March 2013.

Shelton, Lindsay (2005) *The Selling of New Zealand Movies*, Wellington: Awa Press.

Shelton, Lindsay (2012) *Personal Interview*, Wellington.

Smith, Bernard (1992) *Imagining the Pacific: In the Wake of the Cook Voyages*, Melbourne: Melbourne University Press.

Thomson, John (1995) 'New Zealand Theatre in Australia', in P Parson and V Chance (eds), *Companion to Theatre in Australia*, Sydney: Currency Press, 404–05.

Verhoeven, Deb (1999) *Twin Peeks: Australian and New Zealand Feature Films*, Melbourne: Damned Publishing.

West, John (1995) 'Fullers', in P Parson and V Chance (eds), *Companion to Theatre in Australia*, Sydney: Currency Press: 238–39.

Notes

1. The 1973 Trans-Tasman Travel Arrangement has allowed for the free movement of citizens from one nation to the other, however, there has been free flow of people and labour between the two countries since the beginning of the twentieth century.

2. More research is needed to investigate the factors that affect the trans-Tasman mobility of screenwriters, actors and film crews.

3. Her father secured the New Zealand distribution rights for *A Girl of the Bush* directed by Franklyn Barret in 1921 (O'Regan 1996).

4. In 1948 Holmes was dismissed from the NFU because of his membership of the NZ Communist Party. Though he was later reinstated in employment, Holmes decided to shift permanently to Australia in November 1949 (Campbell 2010).

The Orator

O Le Tulafale

Country of Origin:

New Zealand/Samoa

Studio/Distributor:

Blueskin Films
New Zealand Film Commission

Director:

Tusi Tamasese

Producer:

Catherine Fitzgerald

Screenwriter:

Tusi Tamasese

Cinematographer:

Leon Narbey

Production Designer:

Robert Astley

Composer:

Tim Prebble

Synopsis

The first feature film in the Samoan language is also the first to be written and directed by a Samoan, Tusi Tamasese. Set entirely in rural Upolu in Samoa, the story centres on Saili, his wife, Vaaiga, and daughter, Litia. All three are challenged by different conflicts, and the film begins with Saili's, which is about the culturally appropriate burial of his parents, and claiming their land. This is linked with Saili's need to seek a chiefly title as an orator. His parents are inexplicably buried on a bush allotment, and when he tries to work the land around it he is harassed by others who challenge his right to do so. The scene of Saili uprooting freshly planted yams and taro, repeated rhythmically during the film, comes to stand for his lack of movement and failure to take up his responsibilities. There are considerable forces aligned against such progress though. Many others seek the title he believes to be his; a series of these aspirants approach the high chief, Tagaloa, but are shown to be unfit in various ways. This provides Tamasese with the opportunity to gently satirize the pretenders, especially the young man who has grown up overseas and cannot even sit cross-legged, as custom demands. Yet Saili hangs back. Part of his dilemma is that the role requires oratory. For a film about oratory, *The Orator* challenges its audience with minimal dialogue; Saili is especially silent. Instead he shows his respect for Tagaloa by leaving baskets of taro, while hesitating to pursue his claims. Saili's other challenge is his dwarfism. He is bullied both in the bush and in his other job

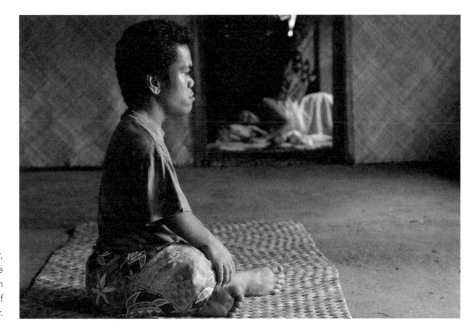

The Orator, 2011. Image reproduced with the permission of the director.

Editor:

Simon Price

Duration:

106 minutes

Genre:

Drama

Cast:

Fa'afiula Sagote
Tausili Pushparaj
Salamasina Mataia
Ioata Tanielu

Format:

35mm

Year:

2011

as night-watchman for a store. His size makes him vulnerable to physical attack, and also the object of scorn.

Vaaiga has been banished from her family and home village as a result of giving birth outside of marriage, but her brother, Poto, makes overtures to her to return, despite the fact that she has been gone for years, and her daughter is on the cusp of adulthood. He believes that his own sickness is a result of the family's cruel treatment of Vaaiga, yet he is equally cruel in attempting to get her away from Saili and her life in a different village. The revelation that Litia is having an affair with a married man prompts conflict between the family and other parts of the village, while Vaaiga sickens, ominously following her brother's visit.

As might be expected, the climax of the film is an oratory battle between Poto and Saili, a battle which is both compelling and dramatic. Saili's challenge, to take up his position fully in both family and village, is realized in an emotional yet restrained way, and the film resolves sadly but with hope.

Critique

For a first film, the direction of *The Orator* is remarkably assured. While the tone is generally sombre, and the pace measured, Tamasese's occasional use of humour reaches out to its audience, especially Samoans, with jokes about rugby and English accents. New Zealand screenings have attracted enthusiastic audiences from local Samoan communities. The film's *mise-en-scéne*, with its emphasis on lush vegetation and simple interiors, strongly evokes the materially simple lives lived by Saili and his family. The lack of non-diegetic music, unusual in feature film, leaves space for the sounds of plants, people, animals and weather conditions. This makes the natural world vibrantly present.

One of the film's great achievements is the way it lets customs and cultural practices speak for themselves. The depiction of *ifoga*, for example – ritualized public apology in order to receive forgiveness – is never explained, yet there is enough context to make it meaningful enough. There is no compulsion to explain here; story is everything, and such practices, though highly significant in the film, always serve the greater narrative. Customs are not challenged either, but the misuse of them is, especially when claims of wealth threaten to subvert them. Ultimately the film affirms traditional methods of restoring the peace, of bringing about reconciliation and resolving conflict. Similarly, the high chief is seen to be wise and considered in his methods of leadership, and resistant to foreign money, which seems to be a threat to right practice.

Given the paucity of representations of Samoans in film, casting a dwarf as chief protagonist can be seen as something of a challenge to other depictions. Instead of a Samoan mountain of a man, Tamasese rejects these stereotypes to tell the story of a small man whose dilemmas concern not so much his size as his place in his world. In doing so he avoids sentimental narrative resolutions in favour of a dignified and undemonstrative yet deeply moving film.

Mandy Treagus

Perfect Strangers

Country of Origin:

New Zealand

Studio/Distributor:

Gaylene Preston Productions
Huntaway Productions
Twentieth Century Fox

Director:

Gaylene Preston

Producers:

Robin Laing
Gaylene Preston

Screenwriter:

Gaylene Preston

Cinematographer:

Alun Bollinger

Production Designer:

Joe Bleakley

Composer:

Tim Prebble

Editor:

John Gilbert

Duration:

100 minutes

Genre:

Twisted fairy tale
Feminist genre bender
Gothic romance

Cast:

Sam Neill
Rachel Blake
Joel Tobeck
Robin Malcolm
Madeleine Sami

Format:

35mm

Year:

2003

Synopsis

In a provincial New Zealand town, Melanie and two co-workers from the fish and chips shop clean themselves up and hit the pub for their usual Saturday night of drinking while looking for an acceptable man to pick up. This time, instead of going home as usual with Bill, Melanie meets The Man and they go off to his boat, where a red rose and champagne await. But Melanie falls asleep before they get beyond talking. When she awakes, they are out to sea on their way to an uninhabited island. Despite anger at being whisked away into the unknown, Melanie is also attracted to this handsome stranger. When they land, he literally wines and dines her. But while she is ready for sexual advances, he wants her to love him as he says he already loves her. When they quarrel, his temper scares her and she knifes him. Once he is the victim, she tries to save him, but he dies, having promised never to leave her. She puts him in the freezer and continues to talk with him and otherwise feel his presence. She manages to fend for herself until Bill arrives, returning to what apparently has been his bach *or* holiday home all along. Unhappy to see him at first, Melanie eventually goes along with his plan to take her back to the mainland, giving The Man a burial at sea along the way and the film ends with a party for Melanie and Bill at the pub.

Critique

Although nothing in Gaylene Preston's previous documentaries and generally upbeat features had prepared New Zealand audiences for *Perfect Strangers*, Preston's words had repeatedly laid out the goal she set and achieved with this – her 'most personal' – film. Her first commercial success, a documentary, allowed her access to the international markets for selling distribution rights for feature films where she learned that the formula for success was to have a beautiful woman in distress be rescued by a strong man. Her first fiction feature, *Mr Wrong* (1985), was her deliberate attempt to make a gender-bender genre film.

As the work of a mature film artist, *Perfect Strangers* is a more advanced attempt to thwart almost all the conventional expectations of a thriller with a female protagonist and a romance component. Preston calls *Perfect Strangers* 'an interrogation of what story is, and how dangerous it is', especially when the particular story in question is about 'the dangerous deception of desire'.[1] 'In storytelling I'm particularly interested in what the audience might or might not want [...] [which] can get us into enormous trouble as the audience.'[2] For example, we sympathize with Melanie's attack on The Man (Sam Neill) because of his behaviour toward her, but his death is not necessarily best for Melanie (Rachel Blake), since it leaves her stranded on the island.

This approach to audience expectations led New Zealand critics and viewers unwilling to accept her use of a well-known genre to question audience assumptions about that genre to spurn *Perfect Strangers*. Outside New Zealand the film's reception has been

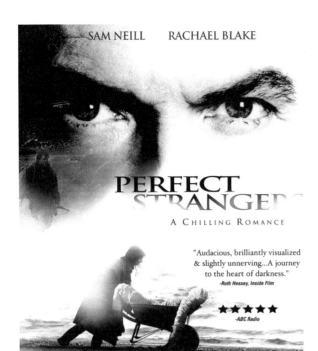

SAM NEILL   RACHAEL BLAKE

PERFECT STRANGERS

A Chilling Romance

"Audacious, brilliantly visualized
& slightly unnerving...A journey
to the heart of darkness."
-Ruth Hessey, Inside Film

★★★★★
-ABC Radio

FIRSTLOOK
HOME ENTERTAINMENT

Perfect Strangers, 2003.
Image reproduced with the
permission of the director.

warm. It is an exceptionally feminist version of the Gothic, largely
because Preston 'wanted to take this film into gothic and out of
gothic and all over the place'. She also 'wanted to make a film that
would reflect the unconscious as well as the conscious'.

Although Preston emphasizes that '*none* of this film is
autobiographical', it does link to some family history. While making
War Stories Our Mothers Never Told Us (1995) Preston learned
that her mother had had an affair while her husband was overseas
during World War II. The affair ended when her father returned,
but Gaylene can remember times when her mother seemed to be
somewhere else, a theme further explored in her 2010 film *Home
By Christmas*. When Melanie seems lost inside her head, in another
world, especially at the end of *Perfect Strangers*, it is easy to think
that Preston may be using observations she made of her own
mother.

Perfect Strangers takes advantage of naturally dramatic scenery,
filmed as it was primarily around Greymouth, on the West Coast
of the South Island, where Preston was born. Weta Digital assisted
with the creation of a storm at sea. As usual, Alun Bollinger
is Preston's cinematographer; under Preston's direction, he
unobtrusively shoots one-shot scenes with two or more actors or,
through his own experience and innate timing, matches his moving
camera exactly with an actor's movement through a scene. The
actors are perfectly cast, and the two leads (Blake and Neill) are
exceptionally well paired. Yet one of *Perfect Strangers*'s strongest
components is its sound design, by Tim Prebble, and its music, for
which Plan 9 (David Donaldson, Stephen Roche and Janet Roddick)

are responsible. Preston herself, though, came up with the idea of starting the film with sounds before any image, and of making those sounds deceptive. What might have been sounds from a horror film turn out merely to be slowed down noises of a knife chopping onions, and Melanie's groans as she chops. Elsewhere, motivation for an otherwise unmotivated glance off-screen by Melanie comes from inserting the sound of a fantail (a native bird) above her head.

Retrospective looks at Preston's oeuvre tend to acknowledge *Perfect Strangers*'s high calibre, but in a country accustomed to 'man alone' stories, this 'woman alone' tale has not received its due recognition for what its talented film-makers achieved.

Harriet Margolis

Notes

1. Personal communication with author, Wellington, 2 August 2012.
2. In her commentary on the DVD.

Pictures

Country of Origin:
New Zealand
Production Company:
Pacific Films
Director:
Michael Black
Producer:
John O'Shea
Screenwriters:
Robert Lord
John O'Shea (from an idea by Michael Black)
Cinematographer:
Rory O'Shea
Production Designer:
Russell Collins
Composer:
Jan Preston
Editor:
John Kiley
Duration:
87 minutes

Synopsis

During the final years of the New Zealand Wars (1845–72), photographer Walter Burton is attached to a Colonial Office Railways surveying expedition and seizes the opportunity to record the experiences of Maori prisoners of war at the hands of the colonial troops. Having been denied permission to exhibit his photographs, Walter is reduced to studio portraiture; a practice that whilst lucrative stifles his desire to reveal the truth of the Colonial endeavour. Joined by his brother Alfred, also a successful photographer, Walter takes to drink while Alfred enjoys success for the quality of his picturesque colonial landscapes and his willingness to avoid the kinds of events that Walter seeks to portray. As Alfred's journeys into the New Zealand hinterland continue, accompanying the womanizing and racist surveyor Roachfort, he comes to realize some of what his brother was seeking to expose and, after saving the life of Roachfort who had fallen foul of a Maori tribe for his attempts to seduce their young women, Alfred himself grows contemptuous of the Colonial Office and their mission in New Zealand. Walter finally attempts to exhibit his photographs and, after his photographic plates are destroyed, commits suicide. A postscript notes that Alfred abandons photography to become an elocution teacher.

Critique

As Nick Roddick succinctly notes, 'The reassessment of history is never an easy task, especially a history as clouded with noble self-deception as that of the colonization of New Zealand.'

Pictures attempts to explore those processes of self-deception and, while not entirely successful, is an important film for the ways

Genre:

Drama

Cast:

Kevin J Wilson
Peter Vere-Jones
Helen Moulder
Elizabeth Coulter
Terence Bayler
Matiu Mareikura

Format:

35mm

Year:

1981

in which it conducts its examination of the role of representation in the construction and distribution of ideas of the colony, both for the colony itself and in order to attract continued support from the British Empire. Yet the film cannot avoid falling prey to those same issues, meaning that the film occupies a fraught position of ambivalence with regards the material it is seeking to explore.

As befits a fictionalized biography, the characters are written with broad brushstrokes in order to support the larger allegorical purpose. Walter (Peter Vere-Jones) functions as the flawed protagonist, effectively silenced by the Colonial Office in the film's opening moments and occupying a position of self-loathing throughout the remainder of the film. His long-suffering wife Helen (Elizabeth Coulter) is the gentle and understanding counterpoint to Alfred's (Kevin J Wilson) unhappy immigrant wife Lydia (Helen Moulder), while the surveyor Roachfort (Terence Bayler) is portrayed as an unscrupulous cad not above using the Burton's wardrobe props as devices to seduce a series of young Maori women. But what is most fascinating about *Pictures*, and which reveals the tension and ambivalence inherent in its exploration of these events, is the manner with which it represents the Maori themselves. Roachfort, throughout the film, employs a Maori guide Ngatai (Matiu Mareikura) and it is Ngatai who functions as our only bilingual exposure to a Maori perspective. Later, as Alfred questions Ngatai about his enterprise as a guide, Ngatai comments that he does alright with the money Roachfort and Albert provide but that it is no substitute for the land lost to the colonial enterprise noting that he has "Plenty of money. But no home". No further hint is given as to Ngatai's past and, later, he is jailed for being a troublemaker, thereby being removed entirely from the narrative. Both of the Burtons have a number of encounters with Maori but these are never subtitled and while this does reproduce the experience of the colonial surveyors, it leaves the audience none the wiser as to any sense Maori might have had regarding the events occurring around them, about which they were rarely consulted.

In a similar vein, *Pictures* offers a criticism about the representation of the landscape within the larger colonial project, with Walter's 'actualities' standing in stark counterpoint to Alfred's tamer and, for the Colonial Office, far more agreeable picturesque scenes. Given the current climate of large-scale film-making in New Zealand, this remains an important notion and yet *Pictures* cannot help but fall prey to the same demands that Walter is at pains to critique. As a consequence *Pictures* is full of actually quite lovely landscapes, excellently rendered by the cinematographer Rory O'Shea. Again, this serves to demonstrate how deeply embedded ideas about the relationship between landscape and representation are and how difficult it is to criticize or explore these ideas from within them. One could argue that such difficulties are one of the things that marks out producer and co-screenwriter John O'Shea's earlier films and that, far from being a failing of the films, is in fact, a necessary precondition for those films that seek to explore the bi-cultural history of New Zealand.

Enormous care was taken with the filming of *Pictures*, with five years being spent gathering props and materials for the project, including the Burton's own cameras and some five hundred costumes. The film itself formally mirrors the period it represents and has been criticized for being slow and stilted in the way it seeks to echo the strictly controlled artifice of Victorian society. Nevertheless, *Pictures* offers an intriguing exploration of Colonial New Zealand and, uniquely, of the role the making of images themselves played in that process.

Scott Wilson

References
Roddick, Nick (1982), 'Pictures', *Monthly Film Bulletin*, October.

The Price of Milk

Country of Origin:
New Zealand
Studio/Distributor:
John Swimmer Productions
Director:
Harry Sinclair
Producer:
Fiona Copland
Screenwriter:
Harry Sinclair
Cinematographer:
Leon Narbey
Production Designer:
Kirsty Cameron
Editor:
Cushla Dillon
Duration:
87 minutes
Genre:
Drama
Cast:
Danielle Cormack
Karl Urban
Willa O'Neill
Michael Lawrence
Rangi Motu

Synopsis

On a small picturesque farm, Rob and Lucinda lead an idyllic existence, secure and comfortable in their relationship and with their herd of cows. Beneath the surface, however, Lucinda begins to question Rob's commitment to her and, at the urging of her friend Drosophila, seeks to invoke Rob's ire as a way of reigniting the spark in their relationship. When their quilt is stolen in the night by a mysterious group of Maori, Rob's indifference leads Lucinda to exchange his cows for the quilt, an act that literally renders Rob speechless and which leads to him moving out of their home. Unexplained events continue to plague both Rob and Lucinda, all of which seem linked to the Jacksons, a mythical collection of fairy-like creatures who may or may not be the same Maori who stole the quilt in the first place. Finally, as Lucinda exchanges a necklace with Mrs Jackson, matriarch of the Jackson family, Rob mistakenly weds Drosophila, quickly learning that it was she who motivated Lucinda's actions to begin with. As Rob returns to Lucinda to apologize, Mrs Jackson returns the quilt to him commenting that Lucinda can keep it 'for as long as she wants but, maybe later, I might want it back'.

Critique

The opening moments of *The Price of Milk*, comprising a series of shots of the luscious green pastureland Rob (Karl Urban) grazes his cows on, which then fade into a close-up of the couple asleep beneath their quilt, quickly make it clear that we are to understand the quilt, and the film itself, as an allegory. Around this is woven Rob and Lucinda's (Danielle Cormack) relationship and, through all of this, is threaded the presence of the Jacksons who steal the quilt, an action that incites the film's major conflict, and who then return it which allows the film to resolve peacefully. Thus the quilt both stands for the land and for ownership or possession, and the struggle over the quilt represents a particular exploration of land issues, settlement and Indigeneity, all of which is punctuated by Sinclair's particular brand of visual humour: Rob's dog Nigel

Format:

35mm

Year:

2000

is agoraphobic and spends much of the film scuttling across the landscape safely inside a cardboard box; Lucinda, at one point, sits sadly outside in a bathtub filled with her tears.

However, unlike other films that have tackled, directly or indirectly, New Zealand's bi-cultural experience with land, *The Price of Milk* speaks to a particularly Pakeha (European New Zealander) set of concerns with sensitivity and humour, with the film's allegorical position allowing it to maintain some distance from these other, deeper issues. Thus while superficially *The Price of Milk* is a charming, magic-realist exploration of love, a fact that has been much commented upon in local and international reviews, it also explores Pakeha anxiety about land ownership and the kinds of relationship Maori have with the land which are often, to non-Maori, unfathomable.

The Jacksons who are, with Drosophila (Willa O'Neill), the film's antagonists, are not explained by the narrative in the way that Drosophila is. Their intentions remain mysterious throughout and their relationship to contemporary (Pakeha) New Zealand is unclear. The many Jackson nephews are all gang members, but their gang-patched jackets reveal that they are affiliated with nothing more dangerous than a golf club; the necklace Lucinda exchanges in return for the quilt is a worthless glass bauble but it is this which the nephews exchange – viewing it as an enormous diamond – for a huge power station whose sole purpose is to keep Mrs Jackson (Rangi Motu) warm. Finally, the quilt is returned to Rob by Mrs Jackson who encourages him to keep it for as long as he wants but notes that she might also want it back at some point in the future. The Jacksons' ability to appear mysteriously in Rob and Lucinda's bedroom at night demonstrates that they have the power to go anywhere, but despite the film's framing of them as menacing dark figures at the foot of Rob and Lucinda's bed, their actions are never threatening. So *The Price of Milk* asks, at one level at least, 'what do Maori want' and concludes that beyond wanting some kind of reciprocal relationship with the land, they remain unknowable.

Drosophila, by comparison, is a far more familiar narrative figure and, as her name indicates (a drosophila is a fruit fly), she is the more obvious source of concern for the love story, playing Rob and Lucinda off against each other in order to marry Rob and provide her own fairy-tale story to match theirs. Despite this, she remains mostly harmless and is forgiven by the film, if not by Rob and Lucinda, as the story concludes. Finally, *The Price of Milk* offers a shift towards multicultural representation with the local storekeepers – the Bhanas – playing a central role in the narrative and leading towards one of the film's most memorable scenes where Lucinda, clad in a bright red sari, trails a long train of fabric behind her as she runs across the beautifully green landscape. This action places New Zealand's Indian population as firmly in the landscape as the film's Maori and European characters and helps cement the film's gentle interrogation of place and belonging.

Scott Wilson

The Strength of Water

Country of Origin:

New Zealand

Studio/Distributor:

Filmwork and Pandora Film
Filmstifung North Rhine
Westphalia

Director:

Armagan Ballantyne

Producer:

Fiona Copland

Screenwriter:

Briar Grace-Smith

Cinematographer:

Bogumil Godfrejow

Production Designer:

Rick Kofoed

Composers:

Peter Golub
Warren Maxwell

Editor:

Elizabeth King

Duration:

86min

Genre:

Drama

Cast:

Hato Paparoa
Melanie Mayall-Nahi
Jim Moriarty
Nancy Brunning
Isaac Barber

Format:

35mm

Year:

2009

Synopsis

A mysterious young male stranger arrives in an isolated Maori community in a coastal town in New Zealand and disrupts the lives of 10-year-old twin brother and sister Kimi and Melody. The arrival of the stranger (Tai), precipitates a tragic accident which forces the twins apart, with Kimi having to find the strength to let go of what he loves most. Tai is punished but Kimi finds a way of reuniting with his sister, in a way which becomes his source of salvation.

Critique.

Pakeha (European New Zealander) director Armagan Ballantyne's 2009 debut feature film *The Strength of Water,* with a screenplay by Maori playwright Briar Grace-Smith, who is of Nga Puhi and Ngati Wai descent, is set among a small Maori community who live in a coastal town in the Hokianga region in the far north of New Zealand. Workshopped with Briar-Smith and Ballantyne at the Sundance Directors' and Screenwriters' Labs in Utah in 2006, and developed at the Binger Institute in Amsterdam, it was a German/New Zealand co-production, made mostly with a cast of amateurs, and premiered at the Berlin Film Festival, where it gained considerable praise.

It focuses on two 10-year-old twins, Kimi and Melody, who deliver eggs around the local community from a hand cart, and their fatal encounter with Tai, a drifter seeking refuge in his grandfather's house, which is considered 'tapu'. Set in what Craig Mathieson (2009) described as 'a landscape where the elements waste everything away', including its inhabitants, it mobilizes a strong sense of the force of the land, which extends into aspects of 'Gothic magic realism', as displayed in Grace-Smith's earlier plays and writing for the Maori Television series *Mataku* (various creators, Maori Television, 2002–2005) and *Kaitangata Twitch* (created by Margaret Mahey, Maori Television, 2010–11) (see Maufort 2007: 248). Frequently compared to the more commercially successful *Whale Rider* (Niki Caro, 2002), 'endlessly and pointlessly' as *Dominion Post* reviewer Graeme Tuckett noted (2009), *The Strength of Water* is a low-key, subtle and gentle study of an isolated Maori community in which, as Jake Wilson commented in *The Age*, '[t]he damp green hills and choppy seas play a role as important as any of the characters'.

Traditional Maori elements are strong in *The Strength of Water,* as Ann Hardy has pointed out, along with more hybrid elements:

> It incorporates traditional mourning rituals at a *tangi* [funeral] for the female twin, sees another character as linked to the mythical beings known as *patupaiarehe* [spirit beings who live in deep forests], employs the practices [...] of hanging photographs of the dead in the *wharenui* [meeting house] as an indication of the male twin's distress and recovery, and uses a device familiar from international films [...] of having a ghostly character support a process of psychological healing for the surviving protagonist. [...] The shots of landscape

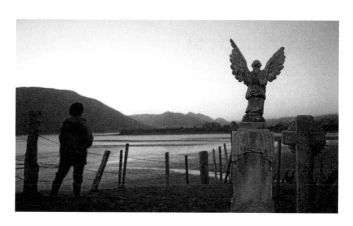

The Strength of Water, 2009. Image reproduced with the permission of the director.

and animals composed by Polish cinematographer Bogumil Godfrejow embody the concepts of *wairua* [(general, enduring life force] and *mauri* [personal, temporary life force] but are also reminiscent of similar shots from films by Tarkovsky or Ozu situated in Christian and Buddhist aesthetic systems, respectively. (Hardy 2012: 18)

Yet despite being located in a specific region of New Zealand among an Indigenous community hanging on to traditions, the film presents, as Peter Calder noted, 'a story that is richly and intensely of this land but whose concerns are so universal that it could, with small adjustments, be set in Iceland or Japan' (2009). It is a powerful film, full of *Maoritanga*, which deserves as much as the more commercially successful *Whale Rider*, despite its significant differences from the latter film.

Tony Mitchell

References

Calder, Peter (2009) '*The Strength of Water*' [Review], *NZ Herald*, 27 August, http://www.nzherald.co.nz/entertainment/news/article. cfm?c_id=1501119&objectid=10593311. Accessed 10 February 2013.

Hardy, Ann (2012) 'Hidden gods – Religion, spirituality, and recent New Zealand cinema', *Studies in Australasian Cinema*, 6: 1, pp. 11–27.

Mathieson, Craig (2009) 'A mystical play on grief in an imposing landscape', *SBS*, 2 December, http://www.sbs.com.au/films/ movie/5702/The-Strength-of-Water . Accessed 10 February 2013.

Maufort, Marc (2007) 'Recapturing Maori Spirituality: Briar Grace-Smith's Magic Realist Stage Aesthetic', in Marc Maufort and David O'Donnell (eds), *Performing Aotearoa: New Zealand Theatre and Drama in Aotearoa*, Brussells and New York: P.I.E. Peter Lang, pp. 247–67.

Tuckett, Graeme (2009) 'The Strength of Water' [Review], Dominion Post, 4 September, http://www.stuff.co.nz/entertainment/film/film-reviews/2835137/The-Strength-of-Water.

Wilson, Jake (2009) 'The Strength of Water' [Review], The Age, 3 December, http://www.theage.com.au/news/entertainment/film/film-reviews/the-strength-of-water/2009/12/02/1259429403364.html. Accessed 10 February 2013.

Woodenhead

Country of Origin:

New Zealand

Studio/Distributor:

Pictures for Anna

Director:

Florian Habicht

Producer:

Florian Habicht

Screenwriter:

Florian Habicht

Cinematographer:

Christopher Pryor

Production Designer:

Teresa Peters

Composer:

Marc Chesterman

Editors:

Florian Habicht
Christopher Pryor

Duration:

90 minutes

Genre:

Drama

Cast:

Nicholas Butler
Teresa Peters
Tony Bishop
Matthew Sunderland
Warwick Broadhead
David Hornblow

Format:

35mm, black and white

Year:

2003

Synopsis

In the remote town of Woodland, gentle simpleton Gert works at the local dump under the cruel tutelage of Hugo, despite being generally adored for his role in keeping Woodland clean. Hugo asks Gert to safely deliver his cherished daughter Plum to the neighbouring town of Maidenwood, a task that other suitors have unsuccessfully attempted in the past. As the couple set out, Hugo sends his henchman Goerdel out to trail the pair and ensure no harm comes to Plum. After Goerdel disables their car, Gert and Plum continue on foot and, later, on donkey, until night falls, forcing them to shelter in a mysteriously empty, yet fully stocked house. Their passions inflamed by food and drink, the couple make love – an act expressly forbidden by Hugo – and continue their journey the following day. Hugo, having learnt of Gert's betrayal, orders Goerdel to kill him and retrieve his daughter. Further misadventures include Plum's abduction by an escaped circus strongman, Gert's torture at the hands of Goerdel, and Plum's eventual marriage to Goerdel, an act she agrees to in order to save Gert's life. Finally, as Hugo succumbs to the industrial waste of the dump, he grants Gert control and the film ends with Gert returned to his original position, happy with his lot.

Critique

Woodenhead is a unique film, not least of which because of the manner of its creation. Habicht suggests that his process of recording the dialogue before the images came to him in a dream in which disgraced lip-synchers Milli Vanilli appear as angels, advising him to follow their example. Regardless, what emerged is a darkly comic fairy tale, entirely in the spirit of the Brothers Grimm, wherein sex and violence inhabit the same landscape as pure motives and gentle innocence. The dream-like quality of the film, delivered in a crisp black and white by Pryor's cinematography, is further enhanced by the fact that the majority of on-screen actors did not provide their own dialogue and that, for the most part, conversations occur while the actors' mouths are closed, suggesting both a series of interior monologues and telepathic connections. These disjunctions, which would ordinarily be expected to disrupt the audience's experience, work to generate a quite arresting – if occasionally oblique – narrative, all of which renders Gert's (Nicholas Butler) return to the quiet of Woodland after the death of Hugo (Warwick Broadhead) something of a relief.

The landscape is vitally important to *Woodenhead* and, as is so often the case with fantasy films, it is emptied of almost all other inhabitants, rendering it both curiously familiar (the black sand beaches of the film's climax locate it specifically on the North Island's West Coast) and conveniently generic. When lost, Gert and Plum (Teresa Peters) wander through a pine forest, not an older and more iconic native forest. By drawing on a specifically European set of story conventions, Habicht is freed from having to either account for or include notions of Indigeneity and the film's use of landscapes means that whilst it could only have been filmed in New Zealand, it equally looks like it belongs in the fantasy landscape it constructs.

Habicht's attention to landscape reaches its surreal heights towards the film's conclusion as Gert, beaten, bruised and forlorn, listlessly wanders an empty black-sand beach. In an exchange that may or may not be a dream, he encounters a carnival ringmaster who is accompanied by a cluster of grotesques and who offers Gert a permanent role with his group. Instead, as Gert turns and walks slowly back to Woodland, the legs of three unannounced dancers rise up from the sand in front of him. This choreography, which initially eroticizes the landscape and, as it gently proceeds, becomes less erotic than it is melancholic, offers a sense of the landscape as an active participant in the story that has unfolded. This is entirely in keeping with the Grimm's own construction of the folk-tale landscape as a place that is actively aware of the narratives that occur within and upon it but which is, ultimately not concerned with the lesser actions of we flawed mortals.

To that end, the isolated communities of Woodland (which we briefly see a little of) and Maidenhead (which is never shown) appear more like outposts or enclaves than towns and the film carries the same kind of post-apocalyptic feeling that is so palpable in films that also draw on medieval (or earlier) narrative types; thus, like Bergman's *The Seventh Seal* (1957), Vincent Ward's *The Navigator: A Medieval Odyssey* (1988) or the Coen brothers' *O Brother, Where Art Thou?* (2000), *Woodenhead* generates the sense that it could equally be happening in some distant future as much as a parallel present.

Woodenhead was well received both nationally and internationally; its screenings during the 2003 New Zealand International Film Festival were extended to cope with its success and Habicht's decision to film on a digital format, and then treat the footage in post-production in order to generate a sense of celluloid, clearly demonstrates the manner with which cheaper modes of production (*Woodenhead*'s budget was NZ$30,000) can give rise to startling and arresting works of art. Habicht continues to explore the freedom made available by digital film-making, with his *Kaikohe Demolition* (2004) and *Love Story* (2011) both utilizing the techniques developed and at play in *Woodenhead* to great effect and critical acclaim.

Scott Wilson

DIRECTORS:
WOMEN DIRECTORS OF FEATURE FILMS IN NEW ZEALAND

Whenever women directors are grouped together in an international context, New Zealand's Jane Campion is always among the first mentioned. Niki Caro, Christine Jeffs and Alison Maclean are often included too. This global reputation is remarkable when New Zealand's population is only 4.4 million. Within New Zealand, Gaylene Preston is prominent as well, with a career that outstrips that of any director of her generation. These women's collective presence is so strong that until very recently it was generally believed that New Zealand had no woman director 'problem'. But the low numbers of feature films directed by – and about – women are similar to those in many other countries. In the ten years to December 2012, women wrote and directed 12 per cent of feature films made in New Zealand by New Zealanders, men wrote and directed 72 per cent and the balance had mixed gender writer/director teams. Five per cent of feature films had women as writers and directors *and* a female central protagonist and a further 5 per cent that men wrote and directed also told stories about women.

The New Zealand Film Commission (NZFC), the state funding body, has no gender equity policy and, unlike Screen Australia, it does not generate gender data. Recent research, however, shows that it consistently invests far less in women-directed narrative feature films than in men's. It also invests much less in women's projects on the pathways to feature film-making (short films, feature development funding and talent investment programmes). The research also shows that women directors tend to be represented in NZFC investments in the proportion that they (or their producers) apply to the various programmes, with occasional exceptions. For example, although women were attached as directors to 27 percent of the successful NZFC Fresh Shorts programme in 2012 and this roughly reflected their representation in applications, in 2011 when the applications were at the same level, half the successful projects had women directors attached. Outside NZFC-funded projects, women directors tend to be better represented in telemovies funded by NZ On Air (NZOA) than in NZFC-funded features. Many women direct documentaries, some of them with a global perspective, but there are no documentary-specific statistics. (In 2013 the NZFC and NZOA established new documentary funds so it will soon be possible to track those). New Zealand women directors are also profoundly under-represented in 'self-funded' feature film-making, undertaken with an un(der)paid cast and crew and dependent on in-kind support of equipment and other resources from individuals, institutions and crowd-funding. In a recent list of New Zealand feature films made over the past decade, of all the features written and directed by women, just one was self-funded, Athina Tsoulis's *Jinx Sister* (2008), 6 per cent, while of the films written and directed by men the proportion was 36 per cent. Two more, Astrid Glitter's *John* (2005), and Rosemary Riddell's *The Insatiable Moon* (2010) were written by men. Andrea Bosshard co-directed two, *Taking the Waewae Express* (2007) and *Hook, Line & Sinker* (2011). Alyx Duncan's *The Red House* won the Sorta Unofficial New Zealand Film Awards (the MOAs) Best Self-Funded Film Award in 2012, but was partially funded under the Screen Innovation Production Fund – a now defunct Creative New Zealand programme – by Asia New Zealand and by the NZFC for post-production. There is to date only one New Zealand webseries written or directed by a woman, Roseanne Liang's *Flat 3* (2012). Women directors are a tiny minority in the local 48 Hours competition; and in a recent major Make My Movie competition organized by people also involved in 48 Hours, women directors' representation in the twelve finalists was limited to one co-director.

It is not possible to identify definitively the factors that affect women's participation as feature film directors in New Zealand. The starting point is always that a film director's life is very demanding for anyone, woman or man. Gaylene Preston has speculated that there are few women directors in the 48 Hours competition because women participate strongly in 'director' roles alongside men right up to the moment that shooting starts, but at that point they tend to take one step back and the men take one step forward. She suggests that this stepping forward/stepping back could be negotiated so that more women get directing experience and take responsibility for what appears in the frame. If this 'stepping back' exists in 48 Hours, perhaps its presence supports the view that it is pervasive on all the pathways to feature film-making, because many women are less 'competitive' and less 'obsessive' than men. It may also help explain why many more women are producers than directors and why many women prefer to produce projects by and about men.

But there are external factors too, both general and specific. In general, women have less time and less access to resources, as measured by Statistics New Zealand/Tatauranga Aotearoa's *Time Use Survey* (2011) and Creative New Zealand's *Portrait of the Artist* (2003). More specifically, in the NZFC feature development process from 2006–09 the proportion of women-directed projects declined as they moved through the system towards production. This may have been because women-directed projects were less able to access the necessary extra funding and distribution agreements from sources beyond the NZFC, or because there was bias within the NZFC, conscious or unconscious.

Global influences may also affect contemporary women's feature film-making in New Zealand. These include the rise of less expensive digital film-making which in theory places feature film-making within the reach of all; media convergence; and the shift towards multiple small screens. In this context, feature film directors choose to work in television and commercials for economic or other reasons. For instance, Alison Maclean defines herself as a New Zealander, a New Yorker and a film-maker. She is currently developing a New Zealand project, an adaptation of Eleanor Catton's *The Rehearsal* (2008). But although Alison Maclean cannot make her self-written features as often as she would like, she enjoys the challenges of all that she does – film, television and commercials. She enjoys directing commercials – the images and the storytelling, the directors of photography and crews – they are compressed, short and fast compared with features. Television, in contrast, is very competitive and hard and she has decided to redirect her energies to commercials and films only, though she made two episodes of Bob Martin and Matt Watts' *Michael: Tuesdays and Thursdays*, a Canadian television series (CBC 2011) and loved it. She is also finishing a short, *The Professor*, about a woman who dreams of marrying a cowboy, and preparing *The Other Side*, a low-budget feature (personal communication, 2012).

Although the factors that affect the scope of New Zealand women directors' current participation in feature film-making are complex and affected by global influences, because New Zealand is small it is possible to isolate some New Zealand-specific current issues – re documentary and hybridity; Maori women directors; diasporas; producers; scriptwriting; and motherhood.

Documentary and hybridity

Globally, women film directors are more strongly represented as makers of documentaries than of narrative features. It is no different in New Zealand. Gaylene Preston continues to make documentaries as well as narrative features. Other established documentary film-makers include Pietra Brettkelly, Annie Goldson and Leanne Pooley whose *Topp Twins: Untouchable Girls* (2009) was particularly popular and had theatrical screenings in the United States.

After funding documentary post-production for some time, the NZFC has recently begun to fund development of documentary features, established Te Whai Ao for emerging and experimental documentary film-makers and created the Joint Documentary Fund with NZOA. It has not to date, however, funded development and production of documentaries by New Zealand directors that are set outside New Zealand, like Pietra Brettkelly's *The Art Star & the Sudanese Twins* (2008) and *Flickering Time Bomb*, which in 2013 she is shooting in Afghanistan, or Annie Goldson's series of documentaries about New Zealanders caught up in political events in Asia and the Pacific: *Punitive Damage* (1999), *An Island Calling* (2008) and *Brother Number One* (2011).

A recent New Zealand trend towards hybrid features that incorporate re-enactments, or mix elements of fiction and fact is led by women directors – Gaylene Preston's *Home by Christmas* (2010), Alyx Duncan's *The Red House* (2012) and Leanne Pooley's *Beyond the Edge* (2013), about Sir Edmund Hillary's ascent of Everest. Furthermore, as media converge, and with (for example) Jane Campion's six-part television mini-series *Top of the Lake* being shown at the 2013 Sundance Film Festival and at the Berlinale, Gaylene Preston has taken this hybridization further, into television, with her *Hope & Wire* (TV3, 2014), a fictional series based on stories from the Christchurch earthquakes. This is very different to a docudrama.

Maori directors

About 15 per cent of New Zealand's population identify as Maori and given the robust participation of Maori men in feature directing, including telemovies, the low representation of Maori women as directors of feature films is a mystery. The last feature film a Maori woman wrote and directed was Merata Mita's *Mauri* (1988), although actor, television and stage director Katie Wolfe directed telemovie *Kawa* (2011), written by Kate McDermott, following the success of her short films *This Is Her* (2008) and *Redemption* (2010) which she also co-wrote and self-defines as her 'first Maori film'. Briar Grace-Smith, also a playwright and television writer, has now written three features: *The Strength of Water* (Armagan Ballantyne, 2009) winner of Best Script at the Writers Guild-run Script Writers Awards New Zealand (SWANZ) 2010; *Billy* (telemovie, Peter Burger, 2011); and *Fresh Meat* (Danny Mulheron, 2012). She also wrote and directed the short *Nine of Hearts* (2012).

There is no lack of experienced Maori women directors who could make features. Awanui Simich-Pene directed Riwia Brown's *Irirangi Bay* (2012) in Maori Television's Atamira series of plays. Television documentary director Paula Whetu Jones attended the Canadian Women in the Directors Chair programme in 2009 with a feature script. Others are successful short film directors, for example actor and stage director Rachel House, who studied at the Prague Film School, and was awarded Best Director there for her first short film *Bravo* (2008) and the Best Film Audience Award for her second short *New Skirt* (2008). She also directed short film *The Winter Boy* (2010), a short, written by Kylie Meehan and funded by the NZFC, which appeared in many festivals. Playwright and documentary maker Renae Maihi wrote and directed *Purerehua*, an NZFC-funded short in 2011. Actor Nancy Brunning directed *Journey to Ihipa* (2008), written by Vicki-Anne Heikell. Reina Webster, a graduate of the prestigious Tisch School of the Arts, has directed music videos, commercials, documentaries and episodic television and wrote and directed the short *Little Things* (2004). Whetu Fala has directed two short films: *Mokopuna* (1992) and *The Hibiscus* (1995), written by Makerita Urale. Jillian White's *Moko* (2000) was shown at Sundance. Riwia Brown, writer of *Once Were Warriors* (1994), is the writer and director of a forthcoming NZFC-funded short animation *In the Rubbish Tin*. Libby Hakaraia wrote and directed a short, *The Lawnmower Men of Kapu* (2011), which won the People's Choice Award at the 2012 Wairoa Maori Film Festival. Catherine Bisley has written, directed, and co-produced two self-funded short films, *the fish will swim* (2009) and *Alwyn Motel* (2012), has a third, *Wide Eyed*, in production and funded through Premiere Shorts, and two feature films in development.

Diasporas

Virginia Woolf wrote, 'As a woman I have no country. As a woman I want no country. As a woman, my country is the whole world.' Internationally, thanks to virtual communities on the interwebs, many women directors now participate in the daily diasporas, or 'scattering' of visual and spoken languages, of ideas and of cultures. This often incorporates aspects of intersectionality and makes Virginia Woolf's concept of women's global citizenship a reality. New Zealand women directors also participate in, have participated in, or have been affected by diverse short- and long-term physical diasporas into and out of New Zealand – not always by choice and not always as adults. The influences of these diasporas complement individual directors' engagements (if any) with virtual communities and enrich our pool of films by and about women, whether or not these films are made within New Zealand.

Jane Campion and Alison Maclean have been settled outside New Zealand for a long time but in 2012 Jane Campion returned to New Zealand to make *Top of the Lake*, her first New Zealand-based work since *The Piano* (1993). As noted, Alison Maclean is preparing to return to make an adaptation of Eleanor Catton's multi-award-winning novel, *The Rehearsal*, with novelist Emily Perkins as a co-writer.

Based in New Zealand, Christine Jeffs and Niki Caro travel overseas to direct. Christine Jeffs's most recent feature, United States-made *Sunshine Cleaning* (2008) will be followed by romantic comedy *Wonderful Tonight*, also being made in the United States, which in late 2012 was in pre-production. Niki Caro's Disney sports drama, *McFarland*, is also in pre-production. In the next generation, there is Miro Bilbrough based in Sydney (*Venice*, 2012).

Women who were born outside New Zealand, or whose parents immigrated here, are strongly represented within the small group of New Zealand women who have made features here over the last decade. They include Sima Urale, Samoa's first woman director, whose short *O Tamaiti* (1996) won the Silver Bear at Venice, and who directed the feature *Apron Strings* (2008), written by Indian-born Shuchi Kothari (*Firaaq*

[2008]) and Dianne Taylor. Sima now heads the New Zealand Film & Television School. Roseanne Liang (*My Wedding & Other Secrets* [2011], based on her documentary *Banana in a Nutshell* [2005]) is the child of immigrant parents. Leanne Pooley emigrated from Canada. There are others making successful short films, including Zia Mandviwalla whose *Night Shift* with a Pacific Island protagonist was accepted in competition in Cannes in 2012 and Sapna Sanant, an Indian director whose *Kimbap* (2013) is about a Korean family in Auckland.

Dana Rotberg, the Mexican director, settled in New Zealand a few years ago and her *Tuakiri Huna/White Lies|Tuakiri Huna* (2013) is based on a Witi Ihimaera novella, *Medicine Woman* (2007). She defines the film as Mexican as well as New Zealand and in doing so illustrates the potential of various New Zealand diasporas:

> I am a Mexican woman. And yes it is a Mexican film definitely because my soul is there. But at the same time it's a New Zealand film because it happens in this country, this story of colonization is not the same as it happened between the pre-Hispanic and the Spanish people of my country. And of course the story comes from you [Witi Ihimaera] and Ruatahuna and the Ringatu people, and so the blood of it is Maori. It is a film that holds all those sources of identity and I think that is one of the reasons why it is such a powerful film (South Pacific Pictures, 2013).

A small, highly specific, short-term and potentially influential diaspora to and from New Zealand is facilitated by the very popular annual Killer Films (New York) internship for emerging film-makers. Four of the five participants selected for this initiative have been women writers and directors: Michelle Savill, Catherine Bisley, Dianna Fuemana, Sally Tran. Another influential diaspora in and out is associated with the work of Peter Jackson and Fran Walsh. Two women directors from this diaspora are Nathalie Boltt and Clare Burgess whose short *The Silk* (2012), an adaptation of New Zealand writer Joy Cowley's story of the same name (1985), has won a group of awards on the film festival circuit.

Producers

The role of producers is crucial. South Pacific Pictures (SPP), led by John Barnett, is exceptional for its contribution to films (and television) by and about women. Internationally, SPP is probably best known for Niki Caro's *Whale Rider* (2002), but for more than decade women have created and written at least half of SPP's feature film and television output, which often features interesting women as central characters. Furthermore, it has been a training ground for women directors. For example, credits for first season of the award-winning and Emmy-nominated SPP series *Being Eve* (Katherine Fry, 2001) included Vanessa Alexander (who wrote and directed the feature *Magik and Rose* [2001]) as producer, Niki Caro (*Whale Rider, North Country, A Heavenly Vintage*) and Briar Grace-Smith (*The Strength of Water, Fresh Meat*) as writers and Armagan Ballantyne (*The Strength of Water*) as a director. Most recently, SPP has produced *My Wedding and Other Secrets*, a romantic comedy co-written by Roseanne Liang and Angeline Loo and directed by Roseanne Liang, and Dana Rotberg's *White Lies|Tuakiri Huna*. Jo Johnson, the SPP Development Executive has written about SPP's record in these terms:

> This is not 'good business sense', but because the women involved are the best creative talent available and the stories depict a mix of characters from the real world. We have never found gender to be an issue with respect to employing creative personnel, be they writers, directors, production designers, editors, composers, etc (Evans, 2011a).

Given SPP's commercial successes, however, it is arguable that their choices to employ, and to continue to employ, women have in fact been made on business grounds. The culture that SPP has developed also attracts women. When it advertised for applicants to its Emerging Writers Lab in 2011, half the applicants were women, *and* half of those accepted were women. Somehow, women screenwriters felt welcome and wanted to participate, in a way that they might not in NZFC programmes or in 48 Hours.

Other producers have been less embracing of women's contributions and many women producers – much more strongly represented than directors in any analysis of women's participation in the industry – appear to prefer to produce projects with male directors. For example, *West of Memphis* (Amy Berg, 2012), a documentary made in the United States, is the first feature produced by Peter Jackson and Fran Walsh that an (American) woman has directed. On the other hand, Fran Walsh has for many years produced and co-written Peter Jackson's films, often with Philippa Boyens.

Some New Zealand women write and produce but do not direct, a useful way to achieve autonomy. Within the diasporas Emily Corcoran, based in London, wrote and produced *Sisterhood* (2008), filmed in London and New Zealand and wrote and is producing *Stolen*, to be shot in New Zealand in 2013. Donna Malane and Paula Boock's Lippy Pictures is a highly successful, award-winning partnership which works to date only with male directors. It has produced two telemovies *Until Proven Innocent* (Peter Burger, 2010) and *Tangiwai: A Love Story* (Charlie Haskell, 2011) and written a third, *Bloodlines* (Peter Burger, 2010). In 2013 their *Pirates of the Airwaves* (Charlie Haskell), a docudrama about Radio Hauraki, a pirate radio station established in 1966, is in post-production. Another telemovie, *Field Punishment no. 1* (Peter Burger), has also received funding. Lippy Pictures is crossing over to film, with one feature film in NZFC-funded development, *The 10pm Question* (no director yet attached), adapted from Kate di Goldi's novel of the same name (2008) and another, *Hungry Ghost* (Elio Quiroga), adapted from Ian Wedde's novel *Chinese Opera* (2008), for which they are seeking international investment.

Scriptwriting

There is no shortage of talented women screenwriters in New Zealand. Women participate strongly at New Zealand's only MA scriptwriting programme, at the International Institute of Modern Letters at Victoria University of Wellington where they consistently represent about half of each year's class and have won seven of the eleven annual awards for Best Portfolio. At SWANZ 2012, Juliet Bergh and Jessica Charlton won both the Best Feature Film Script and the Best New Writer Award for their script for *Existence*, which Juliet directed. Women wrote seven out of ten final scripts for the inaugural Best Unproduced Feature Script, won by Linda Niccol, who wrote three of those seven scripts; Casey Whelan wrote two of them and was highly commended. Martha Hardy-Ward (who also writes for television and theatre) wrote Michelle Savill's *Ellen is Leaving* (2012), which won Best Short Narrative at SXSW in 2103. As already noted, Briar Grace-Smith has written three produced features. Two of her plays were included in the six-part Atamira Maori Television series in 2012, alongside Riwia Brown's *Irirangi Bay*.

In conjunction with the SPP Emerging Writers Lab statistics, and the presence of consistently award-winning writers for television (including telemovies) and for theatre, like Fiona Samuel, Paula Boock, Donna Malane, Madeline Sami and Rachel Lang, these facts seem to indicate that the 'problem' is not related to lack of writing talent.

But it is problematic that women writers of feature-length work do not necessarily write about women and have contributed few – if any – complex women protagonists to New Zealand film. In a recent Radio New Zealand interview about her second crime novel with a woman protagonist, *My Brother's Keeper* (2013), Donna Malane reflected on the lack of women protagonists in Lippy Pictures projects:

> To be honest, I'm not used to writing female protagonists in my screenwriting. For some reason, Paula Boock [and I] end up telling stories that are primarily about men. And it's quite bizarre really, because there aren't many writer/producers around and Paula and I formed Lippy Pictures and then we've gone on making male-dominated stories and it's a bit of a joke actually […] the film we're working on at the moment has I think forty-five male characters and one female […] It's just embarrassing because we would love to write stories for and about women but […] somehow these ones we develop just seem to be about men (Freeman, 2013).

Donna added that she and Paula would like her crime novels to go to screen.

Motherhood

Some women delay having children until they have made their first feature. Others do not want to spend at least two years on developing and directing a single film because they believe that this would damage their relationships, especially if they are mothers. There is now, however, a strong tradition in New Zealand of women directors who are also mothers of young children, usually very well supported by an extended 'family'. Gaylene Preston and Niki Caro provide cross-generational models for directors like Kirstin Marcon (*The Most Fun You Can Have Dying* [2012]), Simone Horrocks (*After The Waterfall* [2010]) and Roseanne Liang.

Simone's experience on-set affected her decision to become a director:

> The film industry is not a family friendly industry, for men or for women. It's tough the way we work, it makes it hard to maintain relationships. When my daughter started school, I really felt the need to be around when she came home. I hadn't always been there for her while she was a baby, and I have some very real regrets about that. So I took a year off and did a screenwriting course. When people asked me why I gave up camera to become a director, I'd say I looked around on set, and the only people who were allowed to have a family (or at least had enough power that if they needed to bring the kid and a nanny with them to work, they could) were the director, the producer and the stars. I'm not good with money, and I can't act, so I joked that if I wanted to stay in the business, my only option was to direct (Evans, 2010).

Rosanne wrote:

> I felt really supported and lucky being able to make my film and raise a young baby at the same time. The filmmaking time was really intense and took a lot of hours, but it was also finite, so all I needed to do was make sure I was supported during those crazy weeks of production. I had the help of my husband, my family, and also wonderful childcare people, including someone sourced through production. I talked to female directors who had done it before and got solid, practical advice, as well as pointers about how my emotions might go haywire during the process! I made sure I got to see baby every day, even if it was only for 30 minutes. I tried to make sure that work was work, and time with him was

time with him. It was really hard, absolutely, but I felt so supported throughout the whole process, like there was a big crowd of people who were there for me. I'm so humbled, and I think back on that production time with immense gratitude and fondness (Evans, 2011).

Kirstin Marcon's experience was a little different:

> I personally didn't put having children on hold. My son was three-ish when I first read the novel, and he's eleven now as we approach the release. He's thoroughly sick of this film by the way! The year of actually making the film was tough on him, I was away for five months, and during the shoot I was barely available. I am very lucky in having an extremely supportive partner. I wanted to make the film badly, and I've been willing to make sacrifices to do it. The biggest sacrifices would be time spent with family and friends, time to myself, and literally years of income (Evans, 2012).

Other mothers, like Rosemary Riddell (*The Insatiable Moon* [2010]), come to directing once their children are grown.

The future

New Zealand has plenty of women with on-screen stories to tell and the skills to tell them. Women who want to direct have models of successful New Zealand women directors who work around the world and of women who combine feature film-making with motherhood. New Zealand's state funding for feature films and the state-funded pathways to feature film-making are not however accompanied by institutional measurement of investment by gender nor a gender equity policy and the culture of its vibrant 48 Hours film competition appears not to be inviting for women directors. It is arguable that until these institutions acknowledge and address gender issues within their cultures women directors will continue to be under-represented in New Zealand feature film-making.

Marian Evans

References

Creative New Zealand (2003) *Portrait of the Artist*, http://www.creativenz.govt.nz/en/arts-development-and-resources/research-and-arts-sector-resources/portrait-of-the-artist. Accessed 23 May 2013.

Evans, Marian (2012) '48 Hours Podcast', *Wellywood Woman*, 4 April, http://wellywoodwoman.blogspot.co.nz/2012/04/v48-hours-women.html. Accessed 23 May 2013.

Evans, Marian (2010) 'After The Waterfall', *Wellywood Woman*, 28 June, http://wellywoodwoman.blogspot.co.nz/2010/06/after-waterfall.html. Accessed 23 May 2013.

Evans, Marian (2010) *DEVELOPMENT: Opening space for New Zealand women's participation in scriptwriting for feature films?*, Ph.D. thesis, Wellington: Victoria University of Wellington

Evans, Marian (2009–13) 'Gender Issues for New Zealand Women Filmmakers', *Wellywood Woman*, http://wellywoodwoman.blogspot.co.nz/p/gender-and-new-zealand-industry.html. Accessed 23 May 2013.

Evans, Marian (2012) 'Kirstin Marcon & *The Most Fun You Can Have Dying*', *Wellywood Woman*, 15 April, http://wellywoodwoman.blogspot.co.nz/2012/04/kirstin-marcon-most-fun-you-can-have.html. Accessed 23 May 2013.

Evans, Marian (2011) '*My Wedding and Other Secrets*', *Wellywood Woman*, 3 March, http://wellywoodwoman.blogspot.co.nz/2011/03/my-wedding-and-other-secrets.html. Accessed 23 May 2013.

Evans, Marian (2011a) '*ORIENTAL BAY – WINTER 2011 – NIGHT*', 3 August, http://wellywoodwoman.blogspot.co.nz/2011/08/night-time-in-oriental-bay-winter-2011.html Accessed 23 May 2013.

Freeman, Lynn (2013) 'Writer Donna Malane', *Arts on Sunday*, 10 February, http://www.radionz.co.nz/national/programmes/artsonsunday/20130210. Accessed 23 May 2013.

New Zealand Onscreen (n.d.) 'Katie Wolfe Biography', *People*, http://www.nzonscreen.com/person/katie-wolfe/biography. Accessed 23 May 2013.

South Pacific Pictures (2013) 'Witi Ihimaera in Conversation with Dana Rotberg; An Edited Transcript of a Video Interview', *White Lies/Tuakiri Huna Press Kit*, Auckland. pp. 19–24.

Statistics New Zealand/Tatauranga Aotearoa (2011) *Time Use Survey 2009–10*, http://www.stats.govt.nz/browse_for_stats/people_and_communities/time_use.aspx. Accessed 23 May 2013.

ANNIE GOLDSON, FILM-MAKER

Annie Goldson of Auckland has been making films, and helping others to make them, since the early 1990s. She has taken many roles in production, writing, script supervision and teaching; she has also published several essays reflecting on her own film-making practice. This article focuses on the films she has directed.

In an early work, *Wake* (1994) – not listed, curiously, in her IMDb filmography – she brings several concerns into dynamic interrelationship: family history and memory; cinematic self-reflexivity; feminism, and the involvement of early feminist film theory and practice with speaking and viewing positions. In her own film education, Annie Goldson clearly absorbed the path-breaking work of Claire Johnston, Laura Mulvey and others in journals like *Screen* and *Framework*, and the crucial feminist claim that the personal domain is, irretrievably, a political one as well.

Wake has been well received in the special, privileged circuits of conferences and university classrooms but it could be better known. Strategies which were termed 'experimental' in the film work of the later twentieth century became influential, then easily accepted in mainstream cinema, so that Goldson's use of home-movie footage, shot on 16 mm in the early 1960s, now seems a perfectly coherent representation of memory. The blurry, uneven segments were filmed by her father; they offer distant impressions of an English immigrant family's initial voyage out, and evoke both the strangeness of the experience for the children who were very young at the time, and also the sense of distance in time, the sense that retrieval can only be fragmentary. A few very old images from watercolour paintings with interspersed views of Auckland and of Lyttleton Harbour in the South Island.

The viewer makes the connections with reminiscent anecdotes from three other English-born speakers, a middle-class white woman whose husband left her for a Maori girl soon after their arrival; a working-class gay man who hoped to find easy acceptance in New Zealand society; and a young woman, who thinks New Zealand offers opportunities she might not have had in England. The interviewer's questions are elided; we get only the responses, so that the focus is held on the subjects. Their evidence yields a complex picture. The two women say they have had little or no contact with Maori; the man says he gets on easily with the Maori he has known. The film is in a sense an essay on a settler society; and here 'essay' means enquiry or exploration. The film-maker, and her subjects, are finding out where they are.

Goldson followed that film with an essay in political and cultural history, *Seeing Red* (1995). This called back, for a younger generation, an incident from New Zealand's entanglement in the global Cold War. In 1949 Cecil Holmes (b.1921–d.1994) was a young documentary maker working for the National Film Unit, and at that time an active Communist (he left the party in 1957). While he was drinking in a hotel with friends, his briefcase was stolen from a car, most likely by a security agent. Papers inside it revealed information about a stop-work meeting, being planned in protest against the government's economic policies. The issues were hardly revolutionary, but the information was given to the press, and Holmes was sacked from the Film Unit. He won the ensuing legal case, and his name was cleared; but he left New Zealand for good, to pursue a long career in Australia (making many documentaries, particularly on Aboriginal life and struggles, and trying under extreme difficulties to make features). Goldson uses a mix of strategies – archival film, interview, re-enactment – not simply to tell the story of the 'satchel snatch' and its aftermath, but also to reflect on documentary practice per se, questioning its political value. If this film is her least successful, in the sense that the mix is somewhat discordant, it is also of considerable importance in its work on the Griersonian documentary tradition. Cecil Holmes's films belong in that tradition; Goldson's own work both benefits and moves on from it.

In a lecture based on the experience of making *Wake*, she speaks of the way after that film she 'retreated back to exploring other people's lives and traumas, rather than her own'. Looking at her later films, particularly at the strong and challenging essays of recent years (*An Island Calling* 2009; *Brother Number One*, 2011) it is hard to see how they constitute any kind of retreat. Each film, too, is very strongly centred on a chosen subject, and makes its particular claims; for that reason, I cannot see them as marking stages in a narrative of a director's development. She says that *Wake* is her 'most personal film', in the sense that its content is linked to her own life; but all her films draw their vitality from the personal domain – a mother's in *Punitive Damage* (1999), a brother's in *An Island Calling*, and again a brother's in *Brother Number One* (where the tyrant's title is mocked and doubled in the story). The lighter film-essays *Georgie Girl* (2001) and *Sheilas* (2004) have strong personal centres, the first as a warm, spirited portrait of the transexual politician Georgina Beyer, the second as a recollection of several women's lives as marked by second-wave feminism since the 1970s.

In *Elgar's Enigma* (2006), the presentation of the composer's late cello concerto is linked to a thread in his biography. Nothing could be harder than making a film about a piece of music, since music in cinema is generally supposed to subtend imagery, performance or documentary exploration. We are told, often very firmly, that music cannot be illustrated, that Disney's *Fantasia* (1940) should be erased from the memory (impossible, of course); that music should be taken on strictly in terms of sound and aural form. *Elgar's Enigma* flies freely over all those edicts, picking up that composer's marvellous cello concerto, probing it and drawing it into relationship with a story of love and loss in Elgar's life. Here is documentary in the service of music, helped by the reflections of the musicologist Brian Trowell and of Ken Russell (who made his own film on Elgar in 1962). The film brings out the special drama of the concerto with its four movements – adagio, allegro, adagio, allegro – presented in relation to Elgar's responses to the carnage of World War 1. In this account, he was particularly affected by the death in action in France of a young man called Kenneth Munro, the son of a woman to whom he had once been engaged. She had broken the engagement and immigrated to New Zealand; Elgar never forgot her. The story is powerful enough, but with the master-cellist Lynn Harrell, the music wins.

An Island Calling is a haunting and haunted work, the meditation of Owen Scott on the murder of his brother John and of John's partner, Greg. Having made a life together in Fiji, where the Scott family had lived for generations, and the place to which John had been drawn back after years away, the two were brutally killed by Apete Kaisu, a family friend who had become obsessed by Old Testament edicts against homosexuality. Relations between men were part of life, of indigenous Fijian masculine life especially; but their practices were not on parade. John and Greg, with their flamboyant parties, were too much in the public view.

Through old photographs and reminiscent narration, the film brings back the story and the place; we meet Owen on his return to Fiji after years away, and track his emotional reconnection; both because of the murder and in spite of it, the place becomes once again his home. The film catches in its tropical beauty, its apparent peacefulness; there are the church gatherings, sonorous hymn singing, images from John's funeral, and the commentary given by Apete's proud, benign but uncomprehending mother, a splendid, imperial Fijian. Suva appears as it was before independence in 1970 – 'it was a white place', Owen remembers, for 'white mischief days'; a colonial town ruled by English society, regaled by the young Queen's visit in 1954. They lived in spacious bungalows; beyond the verandas and the Royal Suva Yacht Club, the Indians and indigenous Fijians led other kinds of lives. Annie Goldson and her cinematographer Wayne Vinten respond to their faces and presences. The film's various strands offer a short history of Fiji from the 1950s on, to George Speight's coup of 1998 and then Bainimarama's in 2006: now a vibrant, struggling multi-cultural south Pacific state, waiting painfully for another chance at democracy.

Goldson followed that film with another centred on a quest. *Brother Number One* is the most rigorous and widest-ranging of her films; it takes the audience back into the years through which Cambodia became a prison camp under the murderous regime of the Khmer Rouge, of Pol Pot (*Brother Number One*) and his brutal armies. By sheer unfortunate chance, in August 1978 Kerry Hamill, a carefree young sailor at large in tropical seas, strayed off course into Cambodian waters. Along with his English travelling companion, John Dewhirst, he was taken into custody; the two were held and tortured over months in the worst of the Khmer Rouge prisons, 'S21', and then executed on the strength of a forced and fictional 'confession'.

They were two of millions. More than thirty years later, Hamill's younger brother Rob learns of the impending trial of a leading Khmer Rouge prison chief, 'Comrade Duch'. He travels to Cambodia and engages in the process as a civil party, the representative of one of the victims. Rob is a former Olympian rower; he raises the question of how grief and loss can be linked to hard, concentrated physical effort. In a conversation with his wife Rachel, filmed before he leaves, he also asks what good the trial, and his part in it can do; she believes that making the effort to retrieve the past is of great importance, that people cannot simply 'move on'. The film tracks Rob through the gruelling process in the court, when he and Comrade Duch face each other; it also follows him into the prison and the archives of the Khmer Rouge period.

One thing becomes clear: Kerry went down fighting. His 'confession' is littered with satire. We see the words keep emerging from an ancient typewriter, with references to 'Major Ruse' and 'Colonel Sanders', to the way, as he assures his interrogators, yes, the CIA certainly had offices in small towns all over New Zealand; intrepid, mocking messages to anyone of his own tribe who might come upon the document. Meanwhile Duch has converted to Christianity and worked for World Vision; this does him no good. His sentence, at first reduced from 35 to 19 years, is revised upwards to life imprisonment. Meanwhile Rob Hamill says in the court that after wanting Duch to experience what he inflicted on others – 'to be shackled, starved, whipped and clubbed' – he can now let the story go.

For him and his family, this is a point of arrival; if healing is possible, the experience has clearly taken them some way towards it. It is otherwise for the audience. It is open to the viewer to see the recurrent shots of beautiful small children, in both Phnom Penh and provincial New Zealand, as figures of hope and renewal. There are other ways to see them; that sunny normality pays the penalties of ignorance. The film keeps on showing us that we have reached only the edges of the story, showing the horrific interiors of S21; aged survivors with their memories, and their unanswerable questions on what happened to spouses, parents, friends; other survivors who want to believe that Pol Pot actually had some good ideas, which were ruined, in their view, by 'infiltrators'.

What is clear, however, is the value of the trial. It is better to know than not to know; it is better that the truth comes out and that justice is served. In their differing frameworks, Annie Goldson's films keep a consistent grip on that purpose. For her services to the film industry, she was awarded the ONZM (Officer of the Order of New Zealand) in the Queen's Birthday honours list of 2007; she has her special place in a national film culture marked by great vitality in documentary, an area where women are major contributors.

Sylvia Lawson

Acknowledgements

I thank Annie Goldson for her generous help with this article, and for supplying DVD copies of the films discussed above.

THE FILM PORTRAIT OF A NEW ZEALAND STORYTELLER:

GAYLENE PRESTON'S *HOME BY CHRISTMAS* (2010)

Experience which is passed on from mouth to mouth is the source from which all storytellers have drawn. And among those who have written down the tales, it is the great ones whose written version differs least from the speech of the many nameless storytellers. [...] In every case the storyteller is a [wo]man who has counsel for [her] his readers. But if today 'having counsel' is beginning to have an old-fashioned ring, this is because the communicability of experience is decreasing.

Walter Benjamin, 'The Storyteller'

Gaylene Preston's *Home by Christmas* (2010) commences with the voice of the director, which situates the opening images of the film. The image of an approaching steam engine full of boisterous, carefree passengers, puffing clouds of grey smoke, is followed by a cut to the film-maker seated across from her father in a quiet garden at her home. A tape recorder sits between them. The film-maker's voice-over exposition that follows allows us to understand the context of the interview, introducing Ed Preston (played by Tony Barry) as the reluctant participant who has at last agreed to humour his daughter and talk about his experiences during World War II. The story he tells is framed as a flashback, commencing in 1940 in the West Coast town of Greymouth on the South Island. Young and impulsive, Ed Preston (played by Martin Henderson) joins his mates who all enlist in the New Zealand Army on their way home from rugby practice. When he returns home to tell his wife Tui (played by the director's daughter Chelsie Preston-Crayford) who is pregnant with their first child, she is understandably distressed. Ed cavalierly dismisses her concerns, envisaging a short stint as an enlisted man and 'a free holiday'. With the lure of an army rehabilitation loan firmly in his sights, he reassures Tui that he will be 'home by Christmas'. The film that follows serves as a memoir, which chronicles the evolution of Preston and his family from a vantage point that the film-maker characterises that 'secret place that nobody talked about, during the war'.

First, let us look at the storyteller, the source of flashback narrations in *Home by Christmas*. His role is largely drawn from the portrait film, a practice that film historian Paul Arthur defines as, 'present-tense studies of individuals [...] made by autonomous filmmakers or small collaborative units' (Arthur 2003: 94).[1] In its characterization of Ed Preston, *Home by Christmas* uses basic formal elements and motifs of portraiture. In the interview, Preston relies primarily on frontal medium-shot compositions in which her father's face and hands remain in focus and serve as his means of expression (Arthur 2003: 95). As in portraiture where subjects are commonly filmed in vernacular surroundings rather than overtly symbolic or stylized environments, in *Home by*

Christmas the storyteller is interviewed in the film-maker's private home on HD, which she maintains, 'gives it a kind of digital 80s feel; it's flatter; it's beige; it lacks mood, but it feels authentic' (Wiles 2010). Longer takes and a reasonably stationary camera during the filmed interview again fall within the stylistic parameters of the portrait form. In his discussion that focuses on American documentary and avant-garde films of the 1960s, Arthur traces the lineage of the portrait form to the Italian neo-realist film movement and the writings of realist theorist André Bazin, who lauded 'the reconstituted reportage' of quotidian events in the films of Roberto Rossellini and Vittorio De Sica (Bazin 1971: 20). As Arthur (2003: 97) observes, neo-realism prided itself on the portrayal of 'everyday protagonists' as opposed to the presentation of glamorized, heroic action in Hollywood films. Bearing the traces of the neo-realist movement, the American film portrait of the period similarly defined itself in opposition to Hollywood's aesthetic and ideological formations, serving as 'a democratic forum for the display of alternative lifestyles and social diversity, a utopian gesture toward a future in which everyone really could be famous for fifteen minutes' (Arthur 2003: 98).[2] *Home by Christmas* reworks the portrait film genre to present the storyteller's vision of the past within the social and political context of New Zealand.

Not unlike subjects of film portraiture, the storyteller in *Home by Christmas* is a character in an 'extant fiction', which has been developed from nonfiction practices (Arthur 2003: 97). Film-maker Preston creates the persona of the storyteller Ed Preston from fifteen hours of recorded interviews with her father in which he recounts his memories of the war. In a bravura performance, Australian actor Tony Barry in the central role of Ed retells the latter's story before Alun Bollinger's camera that meticulously records the most subtle nuances of facial expression and gesture. Periodic close-ups recall moments from Carl Dreyer's silent protoportrait, *The Passion of Joan of Arc* (1928), in which the unadorned face of actress Renée Jeanne Falconetti serves as a mirror to the soul of the martyred Christian warrior. Whereas Falconetti's subtitled script in Dreyer's film reproduces the transcripts of the actual Rouen trial word-for-word, the voice-over recitation and exchanges between Barry and Preston in *Home by Christmas* rely on both improvisation and recollection. Preston recalls:

> We both improvised, but it's a strange kind of improvisation because you're not allowed to make it up; you have to improvise using what you've heard. I wouldn't let him [Barry] learn the words. It's a very interesting medium; once you take an interview out of a tape into a transcript, then edit the transcript and then go back to editing the original sound tape, it's amazing how much you've edited out from the sound tape – just in little wee ways of saying, 'the' instead of 'a' or you know just changing things slightly. It was very interesting going back and doing a new sound edit and those sound edited tapes were what were used for Tony. […] Fortunately he was really busy, and he didn't learn any lines. I had told him not to learn them. But actors will always want to learn the lines because that's what actors do. They learn the words. (Wiles 2010)

The taped interview that provides the substance of the film's story is transformed into a written transcript, an historical document of sorts, which is then edited, and altered once more during the filmed performances of both the interviewer and the interviewee. Unsurprisingly, Barry's uncanny capacity to capture the essence of aging war veteran Ed Preston was acknowledged by the Qantas New Zealand Film Awards in 2010. Yet the film does not insist upon the verisimilitude of the storyteller's performance as would a narrative fiction film that trades on the flashback image as manifest truth. As the interview unfolds, the participants' creative interpolation is placed in evidence. The 'visibility of the discursive present', which film historian Lynn A Higgins maintains was dramatized in New Novels and New Wave films, here shows remembered experience 'to be of the same substance as fabulation' (1996: 23). Higgins states, 'What distinguishes contemporary works is that they are told not only *from* the present but self-consciously *through* the act of narration, which thus becomes their origin' (23). A practice that evolved in tandem with the New Wave film movement, American film portraiture similarly placed stress on the '*performance* of piquant stories' in such films as *Lonely Boy* (Roman Kroiter and Wolf Koenig, 1961), a portrait of pop idol Paul Anka, *Happy Mother's Day* (Richard Leacock, 1963), the documentary portrait of Mary Ann Fischer, mother of the Fischer quints, and *Portrait of Jason* (Shirley Clarke, 1967), a study of male prostitute Jason Holiday (Arthur 2003: 96). In Preston's film, the recitation of the storyteller cannot be viewed simply as the progressive unpacking of biographical material but as a self-conscious staging of the 'drama of remembering and forgetting' (Higgins 1996: 23).

Home by Christmas reinvents the portrait genre to suit its own topical agenda however, in its inclusion of elements commonly associated with biography, especially flashbacks that incorporate still photographs and archive footage. The storyteller's wartime recollections are mostly framed in flashbacks, which unfold in New Zealand and across successive continents. The first such flashback in the film is Ed Preston's recollection of his enlistment in the armed forces. A black-and-white photograph of the family pickup truck labelled 'Preston's Greymouth Fish Merchants' appears, showing the young Ed (played by Martin Henderson) in the driver's seat. This slightly canted snapshot would merit a place of privilege among others within the family photo album, but here it comes to life when the sound of an engine turning over and the appearance of forward movement give it narrative momentum. This family photo stands at the interface of document and fiction, history and memory; a record of the past that through the addition of sound and motion, and also the photo-shopped appearance of a fictional character, becomes part of the fictive world of the flashback narration. The image serves a similar function to that of 'the flash memory image', which film historian Maureen Turim describes as 'a brief flashback that leads to a more expansive recall' (1989: 208). Turim explains how the flash image of memory in modernist films such as *Hiroshima, mon amour* (Alain Resnais, 1959) serves to encode the fictional character's involuntary recall breaking through repressive forces. Here, however, the single photographic image cannot be read simply as a memory fragment, as it mixes fiction with documentary codes to introduce elements of defamiliarisation in the voice-over description and images of the past.

Photography itself forms a motif within the film. Black-and-white period photographs that document the successive stages of Ed's cross-continental trajectory within his flashback narration of the war (soldiers waving goodbye from a train station, gaunt faces peering out from behind the wire fence of an Italian prison camp, the austere spectacle of the Swiss Alps) serve as authentic records of the scenes they show. Photographs are invoked as the incontestable evidence that the places and people recalled in flashback narrations, indeed, existed; each one anchors the storyteller's subjective memory to collective history. The periodic appearance of documentary war photographs alternates with that of fabricated family portraits of fictional characters, which mark important moments of transition within the lives of Ed and his wife at home. The first exchange of family photographs marks the couple's mutual joy at the birth of their son. Yet the inverted, intrusive image of the handsome, young photographer setting up to take the photo of Tui and her newborn baby ironically foreshadows the topsy-turvy future of the family; the image figuratively replaces the previous one, which shows the dark silhouette of an anonymous soldier at sea closed off from family intimacies as the porthole slams shut. Family photographs are at first accompanied by heartfelt exchanges in letters read aloud, seeming to surmount the obstacles of time and space; however, as the years pass, photographs increasingly testify to the emotional and geographical distance that separates Ed and Tui. The portrait of Ed in uniform that initially serves as the sole, tangible connection between himself and his young family later appears among others in the newspaper that lists local men missing in action. This image of Ed reappears once more transformed into a fantastic hallucinatory vision that Tui experiences while picnicking with their son. To escape from her solitude, Tui commences work at the studio of the photographer who has faithfully chronicled the development of her son in photo shoots. A pair of black-and-white photographs of remote mountain vistas hanging in frames on the wall directly behind her desk at work mirror those that appear within Ed's flashback recollection of his risky escape into Switzerland; the two distinctive dimensions of the photos in separate flashback structures within which they appear provide a visible indication of the inconceivable distance between Tui's own insular world in wartime New Zealand and that of her husband en route through the Alps.

Whereas photographs appear in profilmic reality as iconic emblems of the past, flashbacks shot in 16 mm and in heightened colour on split focus lenses, according to Preston, give filmic expression to the way in which memory works. She explains,

> Split focus lenses work on a mirror system which means as you're moving the camera or even if you're not moving the camera, you can move the focus in the frame. Similar to how your memory works, you have a frame, and you can move the focus in it. (Wiles 2010)

One such flashback occurs as Ed remembers his sojourns to the New Zealand club in Cairo. The voice-over recollection begins as period newsreel footage locates the club within the hustle and bustle of cosmopolitan Cairo. A montage sequence then shows a city teeming with street merchants, sex shop signage, belly dancers and brothels. When queried about whether the men stationed there pursued 'holiday romances', Ed cannily responds that he and the boys were more interested in the beer than in the brothels. He then redirects the discussion to the more sinister dimensions of his time there, such as an eerie late night journey through the City of the Dead, an infamous hideout for thieves and murderers. In contrast with these remembered experiences of the city and its environs shown in hand-tinted archive footage, the flashback that follows continues in colour 16 mm film. The camera's focus quietly shifts from Ed and his mates playing cards and drinking beer in the golden glow of late afternoon to the black-and-white snapshots before them on the table of Tui (represented in the photo by Chelsie Preston-Crayford) and her newborn son, Edward Junior. The family photos precipitate another embedded flashback of Ed back at home lying in bed by Tui's side wrapped within the play of shadows cast by the pale blue-moon light. A return to the snapshots marks the close of the recollection.

These multiple and embedded flashback narrations are mediated by the voice-over and visible presence of the storyteller, enabling the spectator to retroactively read individuated memory fragments as more complete, complex memories. The multiple flashbacks unfold in the manner of a Chinese box, commencing with a cryptic exposition of life abroad encoded as a documentary travelogue, followed by a revelatory recollection framed to allow the shift to its focal point – the family photos – which in turn, precipitate another more intimate memory of home encoded as a lyrical daydream. Sound and music complement the voice-over narration, facilitating this progressive intensification of focus. In the initial flashback, Ed's voice-over account of Cairo nightlife is mixed with ambient street sounds and a rousing choral refrain of men's voices singing, 'I love you in the evening.' In the subsequent flashback, voice-over, music and sound drop out, allowing the audience to focus on young Ed's on-camera repartee with his mates that turns to the family photos. Non-diegetic theme music composed by Jan Preston naturalizes the subsequent transition into the daydream flashback at home with Tui. Composer Preston acknowledges that the function of music in this film composed of such diverse elements was precisely to 'bind these elements together' (*Homebychristmas.com* 2010). Yet the dynamic contrasts of documentary reportage and fictional re-enactment, tinted newsreel footage, and heightened colour film, photographic and cinematic representation, self-consciously force the spectator to attend to the means of filmic narration. During this series of flashbacks, the spectator must simultaneously assume two vantage points, one that remembers the formal elements of narrative and one that forgets these mechanisms due to the naturalizing work of sound and music within the film (Turim 1989: 16–17). In flashback films, as Turim observes, the balance struck between knowledge and forgetfulness that is operative in all filmic fictions to a greater or lesser degree 'often tilts towards a knowledge of structure, an awareness of the process of telling stories about the past' (16–17). The mosaic composition of flashbacks in *Home by Christmas* encourages the spectator to assume an intellectual distance from the remembered events being shown, while the resonance of the voice-over narration enhanced by background sound and theme music ensures the spectator's emotional engagement with the fictive world of the film.

Film-maker Preston describes *Home by Christmas* as 'a collage, a patchwork quilt of a film' (Wiles 2010). A multicoloured patchwork bedspread thrown across the bed in the sunroom where Tui sits with her newborn son listening to the radio provides an emblematic segue from the previous flashback series. An authoritative male voice-of-God narration sourced in the radio broadcast to which Tui listens resonates with patriotic and nationalist zeal. Its orchestrated rationale presents a sharp contrast to the understated tenor of Preston's voice-over recollection, introducing newsreel footage of New Zealand infantrymen trudging across the desert sands with an inflated wartime rhetoric that elevates the everyday man to the rank of idealized hero winning 'fame and honor across the ocean'. In stark contradiction to the broadcaster's spiel, the young Preston is shown to be a sweet-natured, hard-working Kiwi bloke who, like many others, becomes trapped within a mindless war machine. Subsequent flashback memories of the explicit circumstances of the Desert Campaign framed within Preston's subjective point of view mark a radical departure from the officious, faceless propaganda recounted on the radio. A startling, hallucinatory image of an army jacket falling from the sky punctuates Preston's recollection of desert battle and shows the flip side of romanticized heroism. The jarring juxtaposition of male voice-over narrators in the desert war segment sharpens the distinction between personal memory and public rhetoric, while drawing attention to the ideological and formal operations involved in the construction of the conventional war adventure story.

Providing a seamless segue, the *mise-en-scène* of Tui and the baby is clearly designed to replicate the snapshots that were the focal point of attention within the previous flashback series; however, this sunroom scene cannot be considered a flashback recollection from Ed Preston's perspective. Indeed, the unfolding story of the Preston family at home in Greymouth is largely informed from this point onwards by the voice of Tui Preston whose own flashback recollection of the war years is documented in *War Stories My Mother Never Told Me* (1995). Tui's previously untold story of a secret love affair that she reveals for the first time in *War Stories* not only testifies to the loneliness and separation she faced in her husband's absence, but to the lure of a sexual freedom hitherto unavailable to women. Film-maker Preston describes the discrepancy between the voices of her parents:

> 'Tui – she's a completely different kind of storyteller to my father anyway. I couldn't have chosen two more different storytellers really. [...] One [Tui] very elliptical storytelling full of internal disharmony and indecision, and one [Ed] terribly matter-of-fact about awfully big things. (Wiles 2010)

The interweaving of these disparate voices within the film narration forms what the film-maker calls, 'a story net'; an oral history that extends beyond the borders of the Preston family to the wider community of New Zealand and beyond. *Home by Christmas* draws on the intrinsic tension in film portraiture between realist and modernist aesthetic tendencies to present the story of an 'everyday protagonist' during the war years (Arthur 2003: 94–95, 114). Biographical flashback narrations, which introduce archival image sequences of the past as well as subjective memory images, reflect a modernist impulse in their exposition of material contradictions.[3] Yet the inscription of filmic modernism through the flashback in *Home by Christmas* is finally subordinated to those realist principles that inform portraiture, which include social observation, the nonfiction character, the quotidian event and the natural setting (Arthur 2003: 114, 94–95). Prioritizing her own roots in documentary practice, the film-maker assumes the role of recorder and reproducer, which recalls that of the African *griotte*:

> In the oral tradition, the griot[te] is endowed with multiple functions, as musician dancer, and storyteller; [s]he is the storehouse of oral tradition. The peripatetic nature of his [her] performance enables him [her] to recount to listeners the history of the entire community. His [her] audience can in turn pass such knowledge on to others who are not present, in an endless transmission – passing from mother to sons and daughters, generation to generation. (Ukadike 1994: 204)

In *Home by Christmas*, Preston takes on the role of *griotte* to preserve an unheralded account of the past that has been either denied or erased. Outside the circle of the Preston family, the spectator is nonetheless compelled to participate in the transmission of the tale.

Mary M Wiles

References

Arthur, Paul (2003) 'No Longer Absolute: Portraiture in American Avant-Garde and Documentary Films of the Sixties', in Ivone Margulies (ed.), *Rites of Realism: Essays on Corporeal Cinema*, Durham: Duke University Press, p. 94–98, 113–114.

Bazin, André (1971) 'An Aesthetic of Reality: Neorealism', in Hugh Gray (ed. and trans.), *What Is Cinema?*, Vol. 2, Berkeley: University of California Press, p. 20.

Benjamin, Walter (1968) 'The Storyteller: Reflections on the Works of Nikolai Leskov', in Hannah Arendt (ed.) *Illuminations*, New York: Schocken Books, p. 84, 86.

Higgins, Lynn A (1996), *New Novel, New Wave, New Politics: Fiction and the Representation of History in Postwar France*, Lincoln: University of Nebraska Press, p. 23.

Preston, Jan (2010) 'Behind the Scenes: Part Seven Soundtrack', http://www.homebychristmas.com/home/behind-the-scenes/.

Turim, Maureen (1989) *Flashbacks in Film: Memory and History*, New York: Routledge Press, p. 16–17, 208.

Ukadike, Nwachukwu Frank (1994) *Black African Cinema*, Berkeley: University of California Press, p. 204.

Wiles, Mary M (2010) '"A Gentle Voice in a Noisy Room": An Interview with New Zealand Filmmaker Gaylene Preston', *Senses of Cinema*, 56, http://www.sensesofcinema.com/2010/feature-articles/%E2%80%9Ca-gentle-voice-in-a-noisy-room%E2%80%9D-an-interview-with-new-zealand-filmmaker-gaylene-preston/.

Notes

1. I am indebted to Arthur's excellent discussion of portraiture in American films from the 1960s, which has provided the source of inspiration for this essay.
2. Arthur does point out that despite their common roots in realist principles, neo-realism and portraiture do 'diverge significantly in their aesthetic and philosophical assumptions' (2003: 97).
3. In *Flashbacks in Film*, Maureen Turim discusses how World War II, and the holocaust in particular, has been a crucial reference point for modernist flashbacks (1989: 231–42).

DIRECTOR STUDIES

COSTA BOTES
A JAZZ APPROACH TO FILM

Working as an independent film-maker in a small country such as New Zealand is not for the faint hearted, but it is a career Costa Botes has pursued single-mindedly, with occasional financial respite as a director-for-hire, since 1982. His credits include director, writer, camera, editor and producer, with his contribution to most productions including credits in more than one role. He has won several awards for his work both at home and abroad and many of his films have screened in festivals around the world. In 2005 he established his company Lone Pine Film and TV Productions Limited. Alongside his work as a hands-on film-maker, Botes teaches and writes about film and mentors emerging film-makers.

Botes's interest in film was sparked early. As a child he loved the regular family trips to the movies and, having been introduced to the joys of 16 mm Bolex home movies by a school friend, bought a second-hand camera so he could pursue his interest. He studied for a Diploma of Fine Arts at Ilam in Christchurch and as a student film-maker his abilities were recognized, and his passion confirmed, when his work was screened by the New Zealand Federation of Film Societies and the New Zealand International Film Festival.

While he is perhaps most widely known for his collaboration with Peter Jackson on the much-loved mockumentary *Forgotten Silver* (1995), Botes's considerable output includes a number of shorts (e.g. *Stalin's Sickle* [1986], *Mislaid* [2005]), a feature-length drama (*Saving Grace* [1997]), music videos (e.g. *She Drives* [2004], *Bed Monkey* [2007]), several music and concert films (e.g. *Kathmandu Blues* [2010], *Struggle No More* [2006]), television documentaries (e.g. *Catching the Tide: Sam Hunt's Cook Strait* [1987]) and television dramas (e.g. *The Tribe* [1999–2003, TV4]) and a growing body of impressive feature-length documentaries which are gaining local and international attention as first-class examples of the craft.

Peter Jackson was an important early influence. Botes says, 'I was always inspired by him and feel he added hugely to my growth as a film-maker' (personal communication, 6 August 2012). After they met in the 1980s, the pair worked together on a number of projects which did not get off the ground, before their first successful collaboration, the short comedy *Valley of the Stereos* (1992). Starting with Botes's story idea, they workshopped the scripts with George Port, who directed the film and undertook much of the production work. Jackson's WingNut Films is the credited production company.

Botes describes his next collaboration with Jackson, *Forgotten Silver*, as 'possibly the most challenging yet satisfying film experience I have had to date' (personal communication, 6 August 2012). Produced by WingNut Films and taglined 'The incredible true story of the world's greatest unknown film-maker' (*CostaBotes.com* n.d.). *Forgotten Silver* had the country in a spin when it first screened on television one Sunday night in 1995. Viewers asked, why have we never heard of this brilliant Colin McKenzie, a New Zealand film maker to rival DW Griffith and Cecil B de Mille, whose ground-breaking shooting and screening innovations spanned four decades? After that first screening, stories of academics, inventors and other less learned folk claiming to have known of McKenzie and his work were legion, dying down only when it was revealed the whole thing was a brilliant hoax.

The initial idea for *Forgotten Silver* came from Botes, as did many of the story ideas, and his credits on the film are co-writer and co-director (with Jackson). It was a fruitful collaboration.

> It was Peter's idea to put ourselves into the story as modern day film archeologists, a genius stroke that enabled me to weave in all the other parts of a challenging narrative. Peter's love of silent movie comedies and his technical grasp of how to achieve the same effects made him a natural choice to direct most of the fake McKenzie film clips. I was more behind the overall story and tone and style of the film. An especially challenging aspect was the vast number of faked still photographs required. I think photographer Chris Coad and I have been comparatively unsung in this respect. The editing, started by Eric de Beus and completed by Mike Horton, was quite an odyssey too. (Costa Botes, personal communication, 7 August 2012)

The film now has cult status, continues to screen in festivals around the world and is used in classrooms as a pioneering example and outstanding exemplar of the mockumentary genre.[1]

Botes's last engagement with Jackson, also extremely challenging, stretched from 1999 to 2004. Initially, he was hired to write a synopsis of JRR Tolkien's *The Lord of the Rings* (1955). Seeing an opportunity, he suggested to Jackson that he could also document the production process of the film trilogy and was hired by New Line Cinema for this purpose. Botes found his brush with Hollywood very bruising. Disagreement with the company over how his footage was to be used led him to producing his own version in the form of three feature-length documentaries, rich in fascinating detail and describing in a free flowing style every aspect of each film's production. In total, the documentaries contain some 200 self-contained stories and vignettes. While using Botes's material for their own Extended Edition DVDs, the company eventually also released his documentaries.[2] On the positive side, the experience taught him much about film-making using the new technologies – handheld digital cameras and cheap editing equipment far superior to what had formerly been available.

> I taught myself to edit on Avid, and then Final Cut pro. I began to really enjoy the process of just going out alone and 'finding' a movie. It felt more like making music, or writing, both activities I enjoy and which come easily to me. (Costa Botes, personal communication, 7 August 2012)

Love of music, especially roots music, is a key aspect informing Botes's film-making practice. A musician himself, he often films performances, enjoying the seat-of-the-pants work of shooting in challenging venues with one camera and then editing the *vérité* footage to look seamless, a process he happily describes as 'courting disaster' (personal communication, 17 July 2012).

Something Botes aims for in his work is to convey to the viewer the feeling of being part of the filmed experience. He has become very skilled at shooting one-off musical events quickly and cheaply, using minimal resources, rounding them out in the edit with archival footage, interviews and observational sequences. These skills can be seen in such films as *Songs for a Bigger Island* (2010), a documentary in which Cook Islands singer Willy Crummer makes his first recording in many years; in the performance piece *Yes That's Me: Dave Murphy Plays the Blues* (2008) and in *Kathmandu Blues* (2009), where footage of a blues festival in Nepal is augmented by gorgeous images of landscapes and street life. Differing from those films in that there is a narrative strand, *Struggle No More* (2006), is an absorbing account of the varying fortunes of the highly talented and largely unknown Wellington band The Windy City Strugglers.

When Botes became aware that 'the best bits of my films seemed to occur when unexpected things occur and I seize the moment' he 'decided to embrace chaos, chance and change instead of trying to control them' (*Target Audience Magazine* 2012) honing his approach to film-making to echo his experiences as a musician.

> Long before I start editing, the movie is already taking shape in the fundamental choices I have already made [...] in an ideal situation the feeling I commonly have now is that the movie is 'making itself' [...] Consciously (and subconsciously) I have been grasping at a process that is musical. It's just like when one improvises in a band – the chords and the scales are all so familiar, one ceases to think about them. You're just listening to the music. The fingers go hopefully to the right places and something coherent happens. It's a jazz approach to film-making, and I'm much more excited about that than the 'kitset' or 'sheet music' approach used in the traditional industry. (Costa Botes, personal communication, 17 July 2012)

Determined to retain the artistic freedom to tell a story that deserves telling, rather than cater to the tastes of the more conventional commercial market, Botes is inspired by individualistic film-makers Les Blank, the Maysles brothers and Werner Herzog. Alongside his deep interest in music, most recently he has been attracted to 'found' stories involving compelling individuals, often people on the fringes of the mainstream, driven by a deep and all-consuming passion. While focusing sharply on his protagonists, Botes has an eye for detail and a sense of rhythm that ensure these documentaries are both cinematic and dynamic. Archival footage from a wide variety of sources and a carefully modulated score are also trademark features of these documentaries.

Botes's contribution to *Lost in Wonderland* (2009) as producer, cinematographer and editor came about through his meeting independent film-maker Zoe McIntosh, who had an idea for a film she wanted to research and direct. The result of this collaboration documents the life and achievements of a gutsy public figure, lawyer Dr Bob Moodie, whose colourful cross-dressing and steely defence of the underdog have kept him in the media spotlight in New Zealand for many years. Alongside coverage of his brilliant career, Moodie's fortunes as a victim of chaotic social welfare practices highlight the historical iniquities of the system and the lasting damage they cause. Awards for *Lost in Wonderland* came in the form of Best Cinematography and Best Popular Documentary at the 2010 New Zealand Film and TV Awards.

On his next single-person focused documentary *Candyman: The David Klein Story* (2010), Botes was producer, director, cinematographer and editor. The film chronicles the journey of a man who went from obscurity, to fame, then back to obscurity in the space of a few short years. David Klein revolutionized the US candy industry when he came up with the idea for a gourmet jelly bean to be produced in a vast range of wild new flavours and dazzling colours. While Jelly Bellies quickly became the candy of choice for everyone from the 1970s disco crowds to President Ronald Reagan, giving Klein his moment in the sun as high-profile, jovial Mr Jelly Belly, in a moment of weakness he signed away his share of the business to the Goelitz family who manufactured the product. The tragedy of this triumph of Goliath over David is made more poignant when Klein's son Bert confronts his father in bitter accusations reminiscent of Biff Loman facing up to his deluded father Willy in Arthur Miller's *Death of a Salesman* (1949). In addition to appearing in a number of festivals, *Candyman* won Director's Choice Best Feature Documentary at Rincón, Puerto Rico in 2010.

Daytime Tiger (2011) resulted from an invitation from prolific short-story writer and poet Michael Morrissey, author of the original *Stalin's Sickle* story (1981), who invited Botes into his home to document how, through will-power, he was able to use the tempests of his bipolar illness to creative advantage. In the resultant film, which Botes produced, directed, shot and edited, Morrissey raves – at Botes and his handheld camera, at his long-suffering wife Anne – extolling his own brilliance ('we are the ultimate geniuses, Jimi Hendrix and I') while resorting to physical violence with a machete when words are not enough. Later, astonished at what he saw of himself in Botes's riveting film, Morrissey finally agreed he needed the calming influence of medication. While not an easy watch, *Daytime Tiger* holds up a fascinating and very sobering mirror to the destructiveness of untreated bipolar disorder, while at the same time offering a glimpse into how hard-won positive change can greatly increase a person's potential for happiness.

The Last Dogs of Winter (2011) is a visually gorgeous film, again produced, directed, shot and edited by Botes. The compelling narrative documents the efforts of intrepid local Brian Ladoon, another of Botes's passionate fringe-dwelling characters, to save the Qimmiq breed of Canadian Eskimo Dog from extinction. The glorious frozen landscape of the Northern Manitoba appears as an eloquent character in all its seasonal moods, as do the wandering polar bears. A New Zealand flavour is added by the presence of Caleb Ross, an actor Botes met when working on *The Tribe*, who works alongside Ladoon caring for the dogs. Ross also contributed production and camera support.

Working as an independent film-maker in New Zealand is nothing if not challenging, not the least of the challenges being to fund your projects. While Botes receives some minor funding from bodies like the New Zealand Film Commission and Creative New Zealand and some sponsorship from companies such as Park Road Post, most of his projects are made from money provided by private individuals, not the least of these being Botes himself. But he remains unfazed, keeping his focus firmly fixed on making films from ideas that excite him, intent always on doing his best work.

Helen Martin

References

Target Audience Magazine (2012) 'New Zealand Filmmaker with a Knack for Making the Unusual Compelling', 28 January, http://targetaudiencemagazine.com/2012/01/new-zealand-filmaker-with-a-knack-for-making-unusual-compelling/.

CostaBotes.com (n.d.) 'Forgotten Silver', http://costabotes.com/forgotten-silver/.

Notes

1. See Botes's discussion of *Forgotten Silver* at http://www.nzonscreen.com/title/forgotten-silver-1995/background#critique_0).
2. For more on the 'Making of *Lord of the Rings*', see http://costabotes.com/making-of-lord-of-the-rings/.

YVONNE MACKAY,
NEW ZEALAND DIRECTOR

Yvonne Mackay's first love is directing feature films and her career exemplifies the creative determination necessary to make feature films in a small country like New Zealand. She began making television programmes in the mid-1970s and has participated in key moments of change within the New Zealand film and television industry, including significant struggles by women to be recognized as craft equals. Yvonne, with her adaptation of Joy Cowley's *The Silent One*, (1984), was the first woman to direct a drama feature in New Zealand. She has won numerous international awards for her direction of feature film, telemovies and drama series for the discriminating audience of children, young people and their families. These productions can be said to form critical landmarks in a distinguished directing career in New Zealand which has seen her turn her hand successfully to a wide range of television genres.

Her original career choice was opera but in the mid-1970s, whilst studying in London, she decided to switch from training as a coloratura opera singer to learning film-making. As she puts it

> I looked at what I would be doing. I would be singing in Germany, being a maid or a countess in a Mozart opera and I was never coming home, so I wrote two letters to teachers and said I was going to the London Film School (Yvonne Mackay interview, 15 November 2012) .

Practicalities presented by the 20-minute film audition prevented that happening but she returned to Wellington determined to study film, which she did through a pioneering Victoria University extension film school course. Her film project, the 25-minute film *Old Man's Story* (1977), which Dave Gibson, a fellow student on the Victoria University course, produced, became part of a series of six short films. Roger Donaldson and Ian Mune had already produced and directed five of the series, based on short stories by Frank Sargeson and Janet Frame. *Old Man's Story* by Sargeson fell neatly into the collection, which was later sold at Cannes. Yvonne Mackay remains true to her vision of telling stories about the South Pacific since that first film production. She is not a scriptwriter but describes herself as a director who realizes a film from a script, and has demonstrated an exceptional ability to find, commission and closely collaborate with a range of acclaimed New Zealand storytellers.

During the mid-1970s Yvonne Mackay worked in the first dedicated television production hub, Avalon Studios, outside Wellington. She attributes her directorial opportunities to a guild system, the Television Producers Guild which, at the time, was positively discriminating to encourage women and Maori creatives into the television creative sector. She became the first female floor manager at Avalon, during the same period that Pamela Meekings-Stewart was breaking new ground as a producer of studio magazine shows. When she first arrived at Avalon she recalls being asked 'what do you want to be a director for?' She had directed previously in radio drama and is clear about the thrill that television direction gave her.

> In radio all I had was a bunch of actors, a different play every week and one technician. Suddenly I am thrown from being the first floor manager to being a director of the soap opera drama *Close to Home*. I loved it up in the control room watching five cameras whizzing around and two great boom swingers and eight sets and actors. It was almost like going live (Yvonne Mackay interview, 15 November 2012).

She knew then that she did not want to be a producer. She wanted to direct and be acknowledged for those skills. She forced the issue from within the guild by demanding that directors should get the same salary increments as producers. On another occasion she made a special episode of the long-running farming programme *Country Calendar* (NZBC/TVOne, 1966 – present) that included dramatic re-enactment of an outbreak of foot-and-mouth disease in New Zealand. This was scheduled to play while she was away in Cannes, France supporting her film *Old Man's Story*. She asked the guild to arbitrate whether she as the director should be allowed to decide the final cut to put to air, or whether the producer could pull rank and play it to suit the schedule. She won.

The founding of the independent production house Gibson Films with Dave Gibson and David Compton enabled her to step into direction of independent productions. Dave Gibson and she had met on the Victoria University Extension Film Course, and, as she puts it, whereas David Gibson was happy with television, she hankered for feature films. Later the company became the Gibson Group, to reflect a strategy designed to enable different niches of production. This was owned 50 per cent by Gibson and Mackay. This company went on to carve out an important place in the growing local television business, with Dave Gibson producing and Yvonne Mackay directing projects. In 2006 Yvonne Mackay started her own production company, ProductionShed.TV.

In the early years of the company Dave Gibson and Yvonne Mackay aimed to fill a gap in young people's and family provision. This was not just a business decision. It reflected her belief in the power of stories for children, and young people, which was based on her own seminal childhood experiences. 'Story and nursery rhyme were there (for me) at the age of three years,' she says, recollecting the legacy of nursery rhymes and stories she learnt from her dying grandmother, and she recalls as an older girl the joy of bossing around school mates in her own school plays 'when everyone was stonkered and naughty in the late afternoon' (Yvonne Mackay interview, 20 January 2013).

Many of her script ideas were, and continue to be, drawn from the rich seam of New Zealand children's literature and she sees her role as that of realizing the film from the written form. This respect for the author and story remains the signature approach of Yvonne Mackay as director. She has worked and become friends with many of her New Zealand storytellers. In the early years she explored the many editions of the New Zealand School Journal, where she found authors like Joy Cowley and Margaret Mahy, children's writers later to receive international acclaim. She also commissioned promising writers from scratch for personal projects. As she puts it, 'I was forever reading children's novels and thinking 'will this make a film?'. John Banas, who went on to win awards for adult content (*Seige* (2012)) wrote one of Yvonne's early children's films, *Nearly No Christmas* (1983); Burton Silver wrote *The Monsters Christmas* (1981); and Jack Lazenby wrote the story for her first film, *Black Hearted Barney Blackfoot* (1980), for which Ian Mune did the screenplay. This caused some consternation when entered into television awards because it had no dialogue as such, instead featuring wonderful sounds devised by Mune, Mackay, and composer Jack Body.

The Silent One

The making of the feature film *The Silent One* in 1984 was a significant and audacious first feature film project. Not only was it the first feature film that Yvonne Mackay directed but it was also the first dramatic feature to be directed by a woman in New Zealand, as previously stated. It was also Dave Gibson's first production feature. As Yvonne Mackay observes, so many people were learning on the job, including Lee Tamahori as first assistant director, 'We took 80 cast and crew from New Zealand and plonked them amongst 2,000 Cook Maori people and tried to do this most difficult logistically and ambitious film. Most of us were doing it for the first time' (Yvonne Mackay interview, 15 August 2012).

The idea of purchasing the film rights for Joy Cowley's book, *The Silent One*, was suggested to Yvonne Mackay by Burton Silver, the scriptwriter on the infamous *Country Calendar* spoofs she was directing at the time at Avalon. He thought it would make a fantastic children's film. It is a story of good and evil set on a Pacific island. *The Silent One* is a mythological children's story about the spiritual relationship between a deaf mute boy and a rare white turtle. The boy's 'difference' creates suspicion and blame when the village suffers drought, followed by a devastating storm. When the turtle befriends the boy they are hunted and ostracized.

The author, Joy Cowley, had yet to publish the manuscript when Yvonne Mackay read it, loved it and won rights to the story. At the time she did not take heed of the old axiom of not working with children or animals. Only later would she learn that the child actor could only free dive for 2 minutes and that turtles spend minutes on the surface and hours in the deep.

It was important to Yvonne Mackay that she remained truthful to Joy Cowley's spiritual story, whilst at the same time adapting the story to acting and budget constraints, which saw the story shift from Fiji to the Cook Islands. She worked with the feature film screenplay writer Ian Mune and Joy Cowley on the script, treatment and locations on Aitutaki and became immersed in the culture.

The Silent One, in which Pakeha (European New Zealander) Pat Everson and Maori George Henare both starred as Cook Island Maori, is of its time (the early 1980s). For example it would not be acceptable for Pat Everson to play the Cook Island Maori mother today, but at the time she gamely agreed to being painted brown each day and endured dark contact lenses and wig in 40-degree heat. The divide between good and evil is also perhaps too firmly etched for current tastes. There is occasional crude stereotyping, for example in scenes of the 'witch doctor' who influences 'the tribe' against the 'good chief', but it remains an archetypal story of redemption where a spiritual white turtle, and a boy outsider who comes from nowhere, saves a village.

The production faced unpleasant and unforeseen surprises. The team discovered that the supposedly idyllic lagoons on Aitutaki had been dynamited for fish and the coral was white and dead so a hasty decision was made to shoot underwater coral reefs on the Australian coast off Heron Island. The shoot itself presented challenges for a director who admits that she cannot swim. Yvonne Mackay describes sitting on a barge under a black blanket in tropical heat watching the monitor attached to the underwater camera. The camera operator had to swim up to her to communicate. The turtle had to be a 100-year-old kitchen table sized turtle for the scenes of the boy riding it to look right. The child actor was a free diver but could spend only 2 minutes at the very most under water with the turtle which could sit down on the bottom for two hours, and did on occasion.

Finding funding was a further challenge. The project was pitched to American investors who were interested in a child/animal relationship film, preferably starring a horse or dog. The turtle was a surmountable hurdle. But the setting on a remote Pacific

Island was a difficulty for American investors, who wanted a white child to star. Some money was put into the project but it was not a happy relationship. The company had rights to open the film in the United States but went bankrupt before this happened. It released the film on television instead, thus ruining the US release.

Whilst in the Cook Islands filming she was asked by a Hollywood reporter if the film was 'the beginning of her going to LA'. As she recalls, she responded, 'Why should I have to go to LA? Why can't I stay in my own country and tell my own stories which can be relevant around the world?'(Yvonne Mackay, 15 August 2012). She is proud of how exotic the film looked overseas, while at the same time managing to tell a universally appealing human story. The popular and critical acclaim for *The Silent One* internationally, for her, vindicates her stand advocating the power of local, truthful storytelling. The film went on to win awards at Italian, German, Portuguese, French and Russian film festivals. It eventually won fifteen awards.

She muses in 2012 that

> To be honest, looking back, when I did *The Silent One*, I thought it was the beginning of a film career but I had to go back and serve the company I owned 50 per cent of and keep on directing those television programmes (Yvonne Mackay interview, 15 August 2012).

The decision to stay in New Zealand necessitated a business plan that included work in television in a range of genres. Over the following decades Yvonne Mackay directed many well-received television series (*Duggan*, 1997 - 1999), television dramas (*Clare* (2000), *The Insider's Guide to Happiness* (2004) and *The Insider's Guide to Love* (2005) and *Typhon's People* (1997), which was cut into a feature film by Jamie Selkirk and sold to France) and documentaries (*Aspiring* (2006) and *Leo's Pride* (2006)). But, despite critical success in television, Yvonne Mackay continued to hanker for film, even though she knew she had a great company making money from television. As she puts it

> [O]ver here was me wanting to be Jane Campion or Lee Tamahori or one of these feature film people who can devote every day of their life thinking passionately about their next feature film […] but I would have to go back in and roll my sleeves up and do the television drama instead (Yvonne Mackay interview, 20 January 2013).

Early in her career she set up First Sun, a company designed to develop feature films but, according to Mackay, one by one feature film scripts ended up being used in different ways, for example as telemovies like *Clare*, which dramatized the Cervical Cancer enquiry at National Women's Hospital and which she had first envisaged as a 6-million dollar film. But feature films continued to be on her horizon.

Sometimes feature film opportunities seemed tantalizingly close but were blocked by funding decisions, some of which she believes were tangentially related to her being a female director. She mourns the loss of one feature film project in particular and believes, to this day, that it was the best script (written by Julian Dickon) to ever come across her desk. She lined up a formidable cast, Denholm Elliott, John Hurt and a young Liam Neeson, a requirement before any proposal could be pitched for public money. She, as director, and Dave Gibson, as producer, pitched *A Hard Road*, a story about conscientious objection during World War I, to the New Zealand Film Commission. As Yvonne Mackay relates it, one of the board members asked her what would happen when the first fight occurred between director and producer. 'What is going to come first, your marriage or your feature?' She believes that 'No one would have the nerve to ask a man that'. Another board member asked how a woman could direct a film about

World War I. She responded that it was a buddy film about a man who has convictions and another man who does not want to fight for an English king. She was finally asked where the roles for women were. The loss of this project was a personal heartbreak for her and she believes 'you could not get away with such "cheeky" questions in the wake of pioneering female commissioners like Ruth Harley and Catherina de Nave' (Yvonne Mackay interview, 20 January 2013).

Kaitangata Twitch

Yvonne Mackay lived as a child in Woodend in Canterbury, near the Maori settlement of Tuahiwi and later on the Banks Peninsula, and *Kaitangata Twitch* (2010) draws on her childhood experiences of the South Island.

Yvonne Mackay had already drawn extensively on Margaret Mahy's storytelling genius, firstly in *Cuckoo Land* (1986) which incorporated an early use of music clips and effects and was awarded a gold medal at the 1986 New York Film Festival. A kidult drama series, *The Haunting of Barney Palmer* (1986) followed. Later she directed *A Tall Long Faced Tale* (2008), in which Mahy (awarded the prestigious Hans Christian Andersen for children's literature in 2006) is interviewed by her own characters and Elizabeth Knox.

Kaitangata Twitch adapts a slim novel by Margaret Mahy and is set around Christchurch and the Banks Peninsula on the edge of an ancient harbour caldera where Margaret Mahy herself lived. It explores the familiar Mahy leakage between dreams and the present world. In essence it is a story about a young Maori girl discovering her roots, and the secrets and richness hidden deeply in local Indigenous traditions. The challenge as Mahy puts it is to

> look at what people do to the land. Clear it, bruise it, burn it. They smash it around, smooth it all out just to please themselves. Maybe there are a few pieces of land that want to stay the way they are. Maybe get their own back even, maybe Kaitangata is one of those pieces of land

> (http://www.kaitangatatwitch.co.nz/. Accessed 24 January 2013).

Twelve-year-old Meredith, with the help of a mysterious old Maori mentor, must reach into the myths and legends of the past to calm the angry and dangerous spirit of an ancient chief who possesses Kaitangata Island and its recurrent twitches. Whether or not she likes it, Meredith has been chosen to be the island's keeper. She must watch over Kaitangata and its rumblings. Whereas the local Maori tribe knew to leave it alone, rapacious modern land developers are disturbing its peace. So now Kaitangata is twitching again in a terrifying way after 50 years of stillness when a girl disappeared without a trace, apparently swallowed up by the island. There is powerful resonance in the fact that the film was shot the year before devastating earthquakes hit the Canterbury area in which it was filmed.

Yvonne Mackay was now working as a producer, as well as director, within her own new company, ProductionShed.TV. It was difficult to find funding to enable traction for the project. It helped that Margaret Mahy, now a celebrated children's author, provided the international name on which the project could begin to build. Seasoned scriptwriters Gavin Strawhan, Briar Grace-Smith (Nga Puhi and Ngati Wai) and Michael Bennett (Te Arawa) added creative heft. The 'bible' for the series, which could be used to pitch for more international money, was put together with help from NZ On Air, the free-to-air funding agency, Te Mangai Paho, the Maori language television funding agency and Maori Television (where it later became a top programme, out-rating primetime news).

After a fraught period of pitching the idea locally and overseas, Yvonne Mackay raised sufficient funding with Dorothy Pinfold to be able to hand over production to Christopher Hampson so that she could concentrate on directing ProductionShed.TV's first large children's project, a television series of thirteen episodes. CGI effects were created by Ian Taylor at Animation Research Limited (Ngati Kahungunu, Nga Puhi).

Kaitangata Twitch has sold around the world to Australia, Canada and Nordic and Eastern European countries and garnered awards: New Zealand Qantas Film and Television Awards, the Houston Worldfest Award and the Sir Julius Vogel Award. It also reached the finals of the prestigious Le Prix Jeunesse, the premier award for children's film. Dr Maya Goetz (judge on both Prix Jeunesse and the children/youth Emmy Awards) asserts that winning a Prix Jeunesse is more difficult than winning an Emmy because it requires outstanding quality and innovation (Maya Goetz, personal communication, 28 February 2013).

Funds for stories with resonance for children and families have always been very tight in New Zealand where there is now no public service broadcaster with the remit to innovate and take risks on big drama projects. Yvonne Mackay describes the frustration of not having the budget for pre-production and post-production gloss, or to be able to market it appropriately to reach wider audiences. She views festival invitations and awards as a critical strategy to be exploited by film-makers in small nations like New Zealand because publicity enables feature films to reach audiences cost-effectively. Such events also provide networking opportunities.

Despite the difficulties of creating feature films for children and young people, Yvonne Mackay continues to work on new projects. As she says

> Children don't vote and cannot choose what they watch, so making high-quality drama for them is more important than adult drama as far as I am concerned. It is where they get inspired to think about themselves. It's important that they know who they are and where they come from, so that they have the confidence to take their place in the world (Yvonne Mackay, 20 January 2013).

The ongoing challenges presented by feature film production in New Zealand is yet again illustrated by the re-versioning of a recent film project. In 2002, before she parted ways with the Gibson Group and started ProductionShed.TV, Yvonne was to direct an ambitious 18-million dollar feature about the Larnach family of Larnach's Castle in Dunedin. However the film was scrapped when, on the first day of principal photography the international funding did not arrive in the account. Yvonne, never one to give up on her dreams of bringing our stories to our screens, is now adapting the feature film script into a six-part television drama; a 'Downton Abbey Downunder' with former colleague John Banas.

Ruth Zanker

MERATA MITA

Director, screenwriter, actor and producer Merata Mita (b.1942–d.2010, Ngati Pikiao and Ngati Te Rangi) died suddenly on 31 May 2010 outside the studios of Maori Television in Auckland, months after she had been appointed a Companion of the New Zealand Order of Merit for services to the film industry. She had been working as co-producer on Taika Waititi's highly successful film *Boy* (2010) at the time. She was the first woman, and remains the first Maori woman, to single-handedly direct a feature film in Aotearoa (New Zealand), *Mauri/Life Force* in 1988. A fierce advocate of *mana wahine Maori* (the power of Maori women), she acquired considerable *mana* as a film-maker, and as an inspiration for Indigeneous film-makers around the world. Beginning as an intern in documentary film in 1977, as production liaison person and interviewer on an New Zealand/German co-production of a documentary about the Treaty of Waitangi, in 1979 she directed and co-produced *Karanga Hokianga/A Welcome to the Hokianga*, about a papal delegation's visit to a northern community to celebrate the Catholic Church in the Pacific, which 'concentrated on the profound aspects of [Maori] spirituality before the Europeans arrived, [and] was made on money raised by the Maori community up there' (in Mitchell 1985, 7). In 1980 she was researcher, reporter and presenter for the Maori current affairs television programme *Koha* (Gift), which screened on Television New Zealand.

> We were naïve enough to believe that these were programmes by Maori, about Maori, for Maori, since we would occupy less than 1 per cent of the total hours programmed by the two channels. I remember the shock I, and others of the team, felt when the Pakeha head of General and Special Interest Programmes told us we were in fact making programmes by Maori, about Maori, for the 'majority viewing audience', a favourite TV term for white New Zealand. [...] We had made it through the sacred portals of TV but our status was no better than that of honorary whites. (Mita 1996: 46)

Her role as presenter in the programme also created conflict with some Maori men, who saw her presence as akin to *whai korero* [formal speech making] on the *marae* [sacred communal space], a male preserve (Peters 2007: 105).

Nevertheless, she persevered independently, and even managed to get her 26-minute documentary *Bastion Point: Day 507* (1980) co-directed with her then partner Gerd Pohlmann and cinematographer Leon Narbey, about the 18-month land occupation in Auckland by Ngati Whatua o Orakei, screened on national television, after it won a prize at the Oberhausen Short Film Festival. Also made independently with the same team was her celebrated documentary about the 1981 Springbok tour of New Zealand, *Patu!/Strike* (1983), in which she developed what she stated was a combination of Maori philosophy and film technique: 'I can unite the technical complexity of film with a traditional Maori philosophy which gives me a sense of certainty, an unfragmented view of society, and an orientation toward people rather than institutions' (quoted in Jesson and Mita 1983). This translated in *Patu!* into what Geraldene Peters has identified as

> observational-style handheld camera, expressively textured soundtracks, ironic or associative juxtapositions in editing (sound against image/image against

image) borrowed and resurrected (reversal, or negative) film stock, sequences of photographic montage, inclusion of broadcast radio commentary, and the occasional use of Merata's voice-over narration. (Peters 2007: 107)

This was sometimes at the expense of clear expositional narrative and contextualization. *Patu!* was also, incidentally, the first feature-length documentary made in New Zealand by a woman, and Mita had to hide footage from the police and complained of police harassment during the editing. Local cinemas refused to screen the film because of its controversial and contentious nature, but it was shown at international film festivals, 'in *marae*, art galleries and country halls, school halls, as well as breaking attendance records in the Academy theatre in Auckland, Wellington and Christchurch. I didn't give a damn about making a film for overseas' (quoted in Mitchell 1985: 7). It received a standing ovation at the 1983 Wellington Film Festival, was highly regarded at the London Film Festival, and was listed on the New Zealand register for the UNESCO Memory of the World project. Mita considered her approach to film-making to be a communal one, as well as a Maori one, which was practised by including a training program for Maori film-makers as part of her work, and augmented by her close collaboration with Pakeha (European New Zealander) editor Annie Collins.

In 1983, she also played the role of Matu in Geoff Murphy's historical film based on Te Kooti's war in the 1870s, *Utu*, on which she also did production liaison. Murphy subsequently became her partner.

Mita made a number of documentaries before embarking on *Mauri*, which she wrote, directed and produced, and which was set in the 1950s in Te Mata, a fictional Maori community on the east coast of the North Island. She described it as a 'parable about the schizophrenic existence of so many Maori in Pakeha society' (1996: 49). As Helen Martin (1989) stated in her review of *Mauri*:

> Shot by a largely Maori film crew and employing many non-professional Maori actors, the film presents the complex web of relationships in an isolated North Island west coast settlement. Against a backdrop of seasonal changes the rhythms of birth, life and death are unified in the holistic primitiveness of the elements. Air, fire and water feature strongly, but it is the earth that is the centre and the source of the cycle's rhythms. Land and life force, or *mauri*, are inextricably linked – visually in Graeme Cowley's breathtaking cinematography and dramatically in the relationship of the characters to the land.

The opening scene confronts the spectator with the birth of a Maori baby, as a Pakeha doctor stands by redundantly, and *kuia* (female elder) Kara (played by Maori land-rights activist Eva Rickard) severs the umbilical cord with a *paua* shell, and then buries the placenta in the earth. As Mita explained:

> When a child was born it was normal practise for the afterbirth to be buried in a special family plot. Every family has such a place and the afterbirths of countless generations were returned to the earth in a ritual thousands of years old. This illustrates the bond between the people and the land and is called *whenua ki to whenua*, *whenua* being the same word in Maori for afterbirth and land. ('Mauri', New Zealand Film Archive)

The film's focus on seasonal Maori rituals is interwoven with what Harding (2011: 219–20) describes as three

> linked movements: the guardianship of Kara (which she passes broadly to her *mokopuna* [grandchild], Awatea); the ethnic inter-marriage between a Pakeha farmer

(Steve Semmens) and Maori woman (Ramiri) which also reclaims the *mana* of stolen land; and the belated redemption of the criminal Paki (who could not honourably marry Ramiri as he had violated the *tapu* of her dead relative and infringed the *mauri* of Ramiri's tribal group). These intense personal bonds are interlinked to demonstrate to a non-Maori audience how the sustaining concept of *mauri ora* [well-being] works as a vivifying and renewing principle of individual and collective identity within Maoridom.

Paki, played by Maori trade unionist Anzac Wallace, who also played the protagonist of *Utu*, is revealed to have been a gang member and jail escapee involved in a bungled robbery in the city, and to have impersonated Rewi, a local-born hitch-hiker he picked up on his way back to his village, who was killed when the car crashed, and is a relative of Kara. At the end of the film, the police close in on Paki, who seeks penance for his violation of *tapu* from Kara, while the recurring symbol of the flight of the *kotuku* (white heron) combines with Awatea's vision of Kara's soul flying to the ancestral home of Hawaiki and the birth of Ramiri and Rewi's child. There is a high proportion of untranslated *te reo Maori* (Maori language) in the film, which clearly indicates it was made primarily for Maori audiences.

Mita subsequently made a number of important documentaries, including *Mana Waka* (1990), a reconstruction of a documentary originally commissioned by the Tainui Princess Te Puea Herangi for the 1940 centennial of the Treaty of Waitangi. The archival footage dealt with the war canoe fleet Ngatokimatawharua, Takitimu and Aotea, but was unfinished due to lack of government funding. Working with Annie Collins as image and sound editor, Mita was commissioned to re-edit the film for the 1990 sesquicentennial of the Treaty. She stated:

> The film has a wairua [spirit, soul] of its own. The film's mana is inherent in its subject matter. My job as a director was to make sure that that mana manifested itself in the final cut. The film was mute, made without sound, so I designed a soundtrack which would endorse the hard physical work that was done, that would evoke past memory, culture and identity, and enhance the film's spirituality. (1996)

The soundtrack contains wood chipping and native birdsong evoking the bush (New Zealand forest), and the film was edited at the Turangawaewae *marae* in Ngaruawahia, near where it was originally conceived.

In 1996 she made *Te Pahu: The Maori Drum*, about the absence of the drum among traditional Maori musical instruments. This includes an interview with the pioneer of the revival of *taonga puoro*, or pre-European Maori musical instruments, Hirini Melbourne (Ngai Tuhoe and Ngati Kahungunu, b.1949–d.2003), also a composer, singer, university lecturer and poet, who had been the music director of *Mauri*. *The Dread* (1996) told the story of a group of Maori woodcarvers in Ruatoria, a remote east coast town in the North Island, who follow the principles of both Marcus Garvey, the prophet of Jamaican Rastafarianism, and Te Kooti, the Maori guerrilla warrior who founded the Ringatu religion, calling themselves Ngati Dread. A television documentary about her, *Merata Mita: Making Waves*, screened in 1998, directed by Hinewehi Mohi (Ngati Kahungunu and Ngai Tuhoe), a singer-songwriter – former member of the Maori group Oceania – and television producer. Mita's documentary *Hotere*, about the prominent Te Aupouri *iwi* artist, based in Port Chalmers on the Otago Peninsula, renowned for his reclusive silence, and political and ecological themes in his work, was completed in 2001. *taonga puoro* (Hirini Melbourne was again musical director) are mixed with improvised jazz and poetry for the film was provided by Hotere's former wife, the poet Cilla McQueen.

The documentary ends with Hotere, in an archival recording, relating his *whakapapa* (lineage). Hotere was awarded an Order of New Zealand in 2012 and died in 2013.

A mentor for the Sundance Film Festival's Native Film Initiative, and the National Geographic All Roads Indigenous Film Festival, Mita also taught Indigenous screenwriting, aesthetics and production at the University of Hawai'i, and was executive producer on *The Land Has Eyes* (2004), the first feature film directed by a native Fijian, Vilsoni Hereniko. Her final documentary, *Saving Grace*, went to air in 2011. She described it as one of her most important, dealing with ways in which Maori can prevent violence against children. Her project for a feature film based on the 1992 novel *Cousins* by Patricia Grace (Ngati Toa, Ngati Raukawa and Te Ati Awa), about the vastly different upbringings of three young Maori women, remains uncompleted.

Tony Mitchell

References

Harding, Bruce (2011) '"The Donations of History": *Mauri* and the Transfigured "Maori Gaze": Towards a Bi-national Cinema in Aotearoa', in Alistair Fox, Hilary Radner and Barry Keith Grant (eds), *New Zealand Cinema: Interpreting the Past*, Bristol: Intellect, pp. 218–37.

Jesson, Bruce with Merata Mita (1983) 'Film and the making of Politics', *The Republican*, February, p. 15.

Martin, Helen (1989) '*Mauri*' [Review], *NZ Listener*, 9 September.

'Mauri'. http://www.filmarchive.org.nz/feature-project/pages/Mauri.php. Acccessed 11 October 2013.

Mita, Merata (1996) 'The Soul and the Image', in Jonathan Dennis and Jan Bieringa (eds), *Film in Aotearoa New Zealand*, second edition, Wellington: Victoria University Press, pp. 36–54.

Mitchell, Tony (1985) 'A Dangerous Independent: An Interview with Merata Mita', *Filmviews Quarterly*, 124, pp. 6–7.

Peters, Geraldene (2007) 'Lives of Their Own: Films by Merata Mita', in Stuart Murray and Ian Conrich (eds), *New Zealand Filmmakers*, Detroit: Wayne State University Press, 2007, pp. 103–20.

BARRY BARCLAY

Barry Barclay (b.1944–d.2008, Ngati Apa descent) will be remembered as the first Maori, and the first Indigenous film-maker anywhere in the world, to direct a feature film. After rejecting a vocation in an Australian Roman Catholic order, he returned to Masterton in New Zealand, and got into television via radio, making a number of trade films and advertisements. In 1970 he joined Pacific Films and began working with renowned producer-director John O'Shea. One of his early films was *The Town That Lost a Miracle* (1972) a half-hour remembrance of the visit of 'Opo the crazy dolphin', who some Maori believed was a *taniwha* (supernatural creature), to Opononi on the Hokianga harbour in the summer of 1955–56. Produced by John O'Shea, and made with the writer James McNeish, it showed no footage of the dolphin, but concentrated equally on different people's remembrance of the event, an approach that would come to distinguish Barclay's approach to documentary film in general. Celebrated writer Michael King described it as 'hauntingly disturbing', commenting in *The Listener*,

> As the documentary showed graphically, the coming of Opo released contradictory forces that are perhaps latent in all New Zealand communities but rarely seen so nakedly: loyalty and envy; gentleness and viciousness; trust and scepticism; generosity and avarice. At its most fundamental level, *The Town that Lost a Miracle* was about the citizens of Opononi, not their dolphin […] The emphasis was on the importance of what was said rather than who said it. (King 1972)

Barclay would go on to work with King, who subsequently won a National Television Award as writer on the acclaimed (and also highly criticized) 1974 series *Tangata Whenua/People of the Land*, a ground-breaking six-part documentary about Maori life and culture screened on Television New Zealand. Outside of Pacific Films, Barclay concealed his membership of the radical Maori activist group Nga Tamatoa (Young Warriors) at the time, as did Merata Mita, but his radical *marae* [communal] approach to film-making and storytelling, which allowed everyone to have equal status, had a strong effect on the series. Barclay introduced members of the Nga Tamatoa in the fifth part of the series, where they provided a focus on the necessity of maintaining Maori linguistic and cultural traditions and agency in the 1970s. As Stuart Murray states in his book *Images of Dignity: Barry Barclay and Fourth Cinema*:

> The *Tangata Whenua* series was a milestone in the history of New Zealand television, bringing images of Maori communities and practices to a national audience that was, up to that point, largely ignorant that such worlds existed. […] Barclay's central concerns of respect and reciprocity for the community giving the images to the film-maker were first given real shape in the series, and the consequences of this were not just a formal approach to the demands of documentary film-making but also a political stance on what these images might mean and how they should be used. (Murray 2008: 35)

The emphasis is on conversations rather than voice-over, which simply supplies basic information such as translations, with fixed, often long-lens camera shots.

His next project was the impressionistic short *Ashes* (1975), based on TS Eliot's poem 'Ash Wednesday' (1930), featuring an early performance by Sam Neill as a conflicted priest confronted by three women, typical of the adventurous approach taken by Pacific Films at the time. In 1977 he made *Aku Mahi Whatu Maori/My Art of Maori Weaving*, which documented one of the last examples of old-style cloak weaving in New Zealand, confounding his Art Council funders, who wanted a glossy 35 mm product to show in overseas embassies, by making a low-key 16 mm film. He then went overseas, beginning work on his first feature-length documentary, *The Neglected Miracle* (1985), a multiple-financed film about the threat to biodiversity in plants, many of which have a Third World origin, by genetic manipulation in Europe or the United States. The result is that many farmers in poor regions where foods have their natural origins are often forced to pay for modified versions of crops developed in the West. Filmed in Peru, Nicaragua, Costa Rica, the Netherlands, Italy, France, Australia and New Zealand, it took seven years to complete, and involved 56 hours of interviews. As Stuart Murray (2008: 8) commented:

> In *The Neglected Miracle* the left-wing liberational politics of a global Marxism meet the details of Fourth World indigenous claim. It is arguably the one film by Barclay which fits the criteria of Third Cinema, though even here it promotes a certain difference, being unusual in its lack of a didactic commentary.

Returning to New Zealand, Barclay completed his first feature film, *Ngati/Tribe* (1987), working from a script by actor, writer and human rights activist Tama Poata (Ngati Porou, b.1936–d.2005), who won Best Original Screenplay in the 1988 *New Zealand Listener* Film and Television Awards. Barclay won Best Film, and veteran actor Wi Kuki Kaa won Best Actor. The film also won Best Film at the Taormina Film Festival and screened in Critics' Week at the Cannes Festival. The soundtrack, by musician Dalvanius, which mixed 1980s bass and synthesizer with some traditional Maori *waiata* (song), won a New Zealand Music Award. As Barclay stated:

> It's about being Maori – and that is political […] political in the way it was made, a serious attempt to have Maori attitudes control the film. Political in having as many Maori as possible on it or being trained on it. Political in physically distributing the film or speaking about it and showing the film in our own way. (Quoted in Lomas 1987)

Set in and around the fictional town of Kapua on the east coast of the North Island in 1948,

> (and Barclay has stressed that *Ngati* has a primal relationship with the Ngati Porou tribe of the film's North Island east coast setting, and then with other tribal communities), the figuring of children and elders, of the land and sea, of the day-to-day activities of social life, constitute an aesthetic and politics of image that stresses the contemporaneity of *iwi* [tribal] culture. (Murray 2008: 58)

The film opens with the Kapua community gathered around the bedside of the dying Ropata, whose leukaemia is being treated by both Maori and Pakeha (European New Zealander) medicine. A brash young doctor, Greg, arrives in the community from Australia, and gradually discovers that he was born in Kapua, and is in fact Maori, which changes his attitude to one of humility and reverence. On a broader scale, the local freezing works are threatened with closure, because some Maori farmers are sending their livestock to other abattoirs. Eventually Ropata's father Iwi (Wi Kuki Kaa) takes over management of the local livestock station, ensuring a constant supply of stock to the freezing works. There is a good deal of *te reo Maori* (Maori language) in the film, not all of it subtitled. In 1990 Barclay published a book, *Our Own Image*, which discussed his experiences making *Ngati*, as well as issues such as film as a *hui*, or 'gathering', and the idea of 'talking in', or film as a *marae*-style meeting of equals, aided by the use of long zoom lenses.

In 2002 Barclay delivered a speech at the University of Auckland's Centre for Film, TV and Media, presenting a manifesto of sorts on Fourth Cinema, which he equated with Indigenous cinema (with a capital 'I'), then in its relative infancy. This included *Mauri*, *Once Were Warriors*, the Maori *Merchant of Venice* (Don Selwyn, 2002), *Ngati* and Barclay's subsequent feature film *Te Rua/The Store House* (1991), along with films by Australian Aboriginal directors Tracey Moffat and Ivan Sen, Fijian director Vilsoni Hereniko, Cheyenne/Arapaho director Chris Eyre, Inuit director Zacharias Kunuk and Saami director Nils Gaup. Of course the volume of films in Fourth Cinema has since grown exponentially, but Barclay stressed the importance of 'interior' aspects as well as exterior features such as 'the rituals, the language, the posturing, the décor, the use of elders, the presence of children, attitudes to land, the rituals of a spirit world' (2003: 7). He also talked of the importance of Indigenous systems of distribution of Fourth Cinema film. The following year Barclay published a letter in the New Zealand trade journal *Onfilm*, replying to John Barnett, the production executive behind Pakeha director Niki Caro's 2002 feature *Whale Rider*, emphatically not part of Fourth Cinema, who had spoken about the film's fidelity to both Ngati Porou cultural narratives and an 'international story'. Barclay stated:

> Don't badger us that this is the glorious path we must all go along, head to tail; don't put us down when we raise our concerns about how non-Indigenous artists handle this type of material; and don't go hyper-promoting, in any triumphalist way, 'universal story' to the detriment of genuine Indigenous efforts. Above all, don't tell us that we, as Maori, must like this film. (Quoted in Murray 2007: 88)

Barclay's second feature film, *Te Rua* was partly financed by German sources, and dealt with spiritual guardianship (as opposed to material ownership). It concerned an attempt by Maori from the fictional Uritoto *hapu* (sub-tribe) to retrieve three carvings sold to a German in the late nineteenth century and housed in the basement of a Berlin museum. The film alternates between scenes in Berlin and stylized *marae* scenes filmed with characters talking direct to camera, as well as scenes shot at Cape Palliser on the Wairarapa Coast, the site of the original theft of the paintings by a member of the Uritoto. A Maori performance poet on tour in Berlin becomes involved in the campaign to retrieve the carvings, along with his uncle Rewi (Wi Kuki Kaa), a lawyer based in Europe. Their attempt fails, but instead they take three busts from the museum as 'hostage', but Peter is shot, and they are arrested by German police. After they refuse an offer by the museum to return the carvings quietly, the ensuing public uproar causes the museum's head to sign a document returning the spiritual guardianship of the carvings to the Uritoto. Sometimes a difficult film to follow, Murray suggests that 'there is no doubt that some of the feeling of a disjointed narrative produced by *Te Rua* is due to Barclay's refusal to engage with the orthodoxies of narrative film-making' (2008: 76).

Barclay returned to documentary with *The Feathers of Peace* (2000), although it is a fictionalized documentary about the enslavement and displacement of the Moriori people of Rekohu/'Misty Skies', or the Chatham Islands, by the Taranaki tribes Ngati Tama and Ngati Tutumu in the 1860s. Based on a book by Michael King, *Moriori: A People Rediscovered* (1989), and a documentary by Bill Saunders made in 1980, it dealt with a highly contentious issue compounded by a Native Land Court which awarded the Maori invaders virtually all of the islands in 1870, despite the fact that many of them had returned to Taranaki in the 1860s. The similarities to the colonial acquisition of New Zealand by force did not, of course, escape notice. Barclay's approach to the subject was experimental, using news-style reportage, in which all parties are interviewed, and as Murray comments, the film 'offers its own cinematic narrative as a counter-history, a space for Moriori in particular to articulate their version of events, and to lay a claim for an idea of justice' (2008: 78).

Barclay was appointed one of the nation's Artist Laureates in 2004 in recognition of his contributions to cinema over four decades, and made one more film in 2005, *The Kaipara Affair*, as well as publishing a book about Maori guardianship, *Mana Tuturu: Maori Treasures and Intellectual Property Rights*. The former was a documentary in many senses about the concerns of the latter; dealing with legal aspects of fishing rights in the Kaipara Harbour. Murray describes it as

> his most sophisticated engagement yet with the wider national context of government or bicultural relations. It is also his most poetic, particularly in the complexity of its structure and the methods through which it delivers its narrative. Finally, it is, in the way it marshals its activism and suggests ideas of community, the film that most exemplifies Barclay's emerging definition of "Fourth Cinema"'. (2007: 150)

A 133-minute version of the film was shown on the New Zealand-Film festival circuit, but it was cut down to 70 minutes for television screening in New Zealand by TVNZ, who funded the film, a process that Barclay objected to strongly. Barclay subsequently made DVD copies of the full-length feature available to communities involved in similar struggles to those presented in *The Kaipara Affair*.

Barclay was made a Member of the Order of New Zealand in 2007, and died suddenly of a stroke in 2008. Graeme Tuckett's documentary *Barry Barclay - The Camera on the Shore* was shown at the Auckland International Film Festival in 2009. His legacy of Fourth Cinema has spread globally.

Tony Mitchell

References

Barclay, Barry (1992) 'Amongst Landscapes', in Jonathan Dennis and Jan Bieringa (eds), *Film in Aotearoa New Zealand*, Wellington: Victoria University Press, pp. 116–29.

Barclay, Barry (2003) 'Celebrating Fourth Cinema', *Illusions*, 35, pp. 7–11.

Lomas, Rongotai (1987) 'A First for the Maori Ngati', *Illusions*, 5.

King, Michael (1972) '*The Town that Lost a Miracle*' [Review], *NZ Listener*, 3 July.

Murray, Stuart (2008) *Images of Dignity: Barry Barclay and Fourth Cinema*, Wellington: Huia Publishers.

Murray, Stuart (2007) 'Activism, community and governance: Barry Barclay's *The Kaipara Affair*' (2005), *Studies in Australasian Cinema*, 1: 2, pp. 147–59.

Murray, Stuart (2007) 'Images of Dignity: The Films of Barry Barclay', in Ian Condrich and Stuart Murray (eds), *New Zealand Filmmakers*, Detroit: Wayne State University Press, pp. 88–102.

CHRISTINE JEFFS:
SURVIVING IN TRANSNATIONAL SEAS

Even within as small an entity as 'the national cinema of New Zealand' there is time for discernible epochs and space for alternative histories, or, as a recent comprehensive review of New Zealand film history put it, there are always 'currents in the mainstream' (Pivac, Stark and McDonald 2011). Recently, the most visible of those currents have something of a masculine character, whether it be the industry resources devoted to supporting Peter Jackson's global blockbusters, *The Lord of the Rings* (2001–03) and *The Hobbit: An Unexpected Journey* (2012); the true-life drama of a man devoted to speed (*The World's Fastest Indian* (Roger Donaldson, 2005); or the comedies produced from the experience of New Zealand male writers, such as *Boy* (Taika Waititi, 2010), *Sione's Wedding* (Chris Graham, 2006) , *Sione's 2: Unfinished Business* (Simon Bennett, 2012) *Fresh Meat* (Danny Mulheron, 2012) and *Mt Zion* (Te Arepa Kahi, 2013).

This, however, has not always been the case. The two decades from the mid-1980s to the early 2000s in particular were notable for the achievements of New Zealand women film-makers with Merata Mita, Yvonne McKay, Gaylene Preston, Alison Maclean, Jane Campion, Niki Caro and Christine Jeffs all operating at a high level of visibility and bringing to the New Zealand industry some of its greatest critical successes. They included the recognition given at Cannes and numerous other festivals to McLean's, Caro's and Jeffs's short films (*Kitchen Sink* [1992], *Sure to Rise* [1994] and *Stroke* [1994], respectively), and to the features *Rain* (Christine Jeffs, 2001) and *Whale Rider* (Niki Caro, 2002).

With the exception of Merata Mita, who died in 2010, these film-makers are still working, but with public profiles that are now more subdued, at least in New Zealand. There are a number of possible reasons for the diminution of the presence of women as directors in our national cinema, some of which may be related to gender and age but others of which are related to the flows of people, technology, funding and projects that characterize the contemporary audio-visual industries. This chapter focuses on a case study of the director Christine Jeffs as emblematic of a contemporary set of currents that hides some film-makers from local view at the same time as they are working assiduously in other contexts and formats.

The forces that promote transnationalism, bringing people together to work on projects for global markets, are capable of providing a sustainable 'portfolio' career for female, as for male, directors but they also make it very difficult to maintain a visible cohort of mature directors associated with a national cinema framework, especially if they prefer to work on 'serious' drama, rather than in 'quirky' or high-concept modes.[1]

Jeff's first feature *Rain*, a psychodrama based on the eponymous novella by Kirsty Gunn (1994), is one of the key texts of New Zealand national cinema. The story of a family destroyed through the interactions of boredom, self-absorption, curiosity and desire, the film is set at a beachside holiday house one summer in the 1980s. Located in an era where beach houses were not yet the preserve of the rich , and steeped in the amber tones of popular 1980s design, *Rain* has been described by one critic as 'raw Kiwiana – processed through a clear and deliberate arthouse aesthetic' (Matthews 2001). Featuring competition between a narcissistic mother and her pubescent daughter for the sexual attention of a stranger the film ends in tragedy when their joint neglect results in the death by drowning of their very young son and brother,

Jim. With its themes of an unhappy marital relationship arising from a spiritual vacancy in the adults and the mortal dangers involved in acting on desire or moving beyond childhood, *Rain* is also very 'Kiwi' in its alignment with the pessimistic, fatalistic, variety of Antipodean film-making identified by Sam Neill and Judy Rymer as 'the cinema of unease' (1995) or with what Mita called 'white, neurotic, cinema' (1992).

Easy to parody in retrospect for their piquant mix of measured solemnity and operatic emotionalism (Jane Campion's 1993 film *The Piano* being the paradigmatic example of the form, albeit largely funded by the Australians and French), such melodramas have in fact embodied and negotiated a series of important accommodations between European and Pacific cultures and between both those cultures and the increasing capabilities of modern women. Decreasing encouragement for this kind of cinema (which usually takes the form of small-scale naturalistic dramas in domestic settings) by the Film Commission's funding policies from the mid-2000s as it sought to diversify into 'feel-good' movies and internationally marketable genre films, such as horror and co-productions, is one of the factors that has made it difficult for most women directors to extend their body of work in the New Zealand environment.

Nonetheless, at the time that *Rain* was launched: screened at the Director's Fortnight at Cannes, shown at the Toronto and Sundance festivals and on release in New Zealand cinemas for an extraordinary 6-month run (Jeffs 2013), the praise for Jeffs's direction made it seem likely she would have a productive career in New Zealand film.

> It could seem trite and obvious […] to name Christine Jeffs as the latest in a line that runs from Jane Campion to Alison Maclean to Niki Caro, and the film itself as something like a Kiwi *Ice Storm*, but there is that kind of sensitivity here and that kind of confidence. Call it a high-water mark. (Matthews 2001)

Rain was in fact Jeffs's second big success; the first had been the short film *Stroke*, which had featured in the *Un Certain Regard* section at Cannes in 1994. A wordless 8 minutes in duration *Stroke* depicts a gendered confrontation stripped down to basics then built up again into art through the use of symbolic graphic elements, bravura cinematography and a precise, inventive soundtrack which gives an epic dimension to an essentially small event. A rounded woman, Dorothy, wearing a swimsuit and petalled cap in soft shades of blue floats on her back in a circular space sketched out by her limbs. But this state of peace lasts just a few moments as a series of identical male bodies (clad in vertical black-and-white stripes) line up and launch themselves into the pool to the sound of shattering glass. Like a military force they surge into Dorothy's space, clearly not caring if they leave her broken in their wake. Her situation seems dire but she subverts it by swimming under this phalanx of men and making her way to the side. However, merely escaping does not satisfy her. She plods to the diving board and launches herself into the air over the astonished stares of the finally-halted swimmers, landing with such force that the whole pool resounds with the radiating circles of her energy.

Despite the cartoon-like simplicity of this narrative it contains a number of motifs that will reappear in Jeffs's later, more complicated works and provide evidence of an authorial presence, even in projects that are not primarily of her own devising. Dorothy's bliss in solitude reminds one of the importance accorded by Virginia Woolf to the necessity for women of having '[a] room of one's own' (1929) and all of the female protagonists in films directed by Jeffs --Janey in *Rain*, Sylvia Plath in the biographical film *Sylvia* (2003), and Rose and Norah in *Sunshine Cleaning*, (2008) – struggle to establish a zone (a literal or mental space) in which they can have control over their own circumstances. The achievement of that space is threatened by both the actions of others and by personal vulnerability, and it is often achieved in a situation where something else important is lost (Jim and the artless innocence he represents in *Rain*, eventually in *Sylvia*, Sylvia's own life). Once the women achieve self-determination however, it is not enough for them to rest and dream, as Dorothy is doing at the beginning *Stroke*: they go on to be creative and productive in their own terms. For Sylvia Plath, that productivity is, of course, in her renowned poetry, while for the working-class character Rose in *Sunshine Cleaning* it is the ability to run an excellent cleaning company in order to provide for her family. Even for 13-year-old Janey, who has to bear the guilt of her brother's death, there is also a gain: when she is in the woods with the older male photographer Cody, we see her taking his camera and turning it back on him, giving him orders on how to pose. She may, in the future one sometimes imagines for the characters beyond the film, be haunted but it is also possible to see her as becoming an artist in her own right.

The high standard of Jeff's handling of both visual imagery and the planning of soundtracks are also evident in this early work, giving rise later to the 'arthouse aesthetic' that Matthews (2001) commented on in relation to *Rain*. This skill in producing beautiful images, linked in finely judged sequences that provide narrative, thematic and emotional information simultaneously, rests on several sources in Jeffs's own background. After graduating from Massey University in 1983 with a BA in sociology and geography she began working in the film industry in Wellington doing post-production sound. It was by virtue of a connection made with Neil Finn of Crowded House when she directed a music video of the Finn Brothers (Neil and Tim) *Angel's Heap* that Christine could later call on him to contribute music tracks for *Rain*.

Moving from sound post-production into general editing Jeffs worked as an assistant on some of the most significant films in the first wave of feminist film-making including Melanie Reid's *Send a Gorilla* (1984), Gaylene Preston's *Ruby and Rata* (1990) and Alison Maclean's *Crush* (1992). Wanting to progress beyond the assistant role she attended the Australian Film, Television and Radio School in Sydney, graduating in 1990 with a diploma in editing, which gave her access to work on both films and commercials on her return to New Zealand. Because the film industry in New Zealand was small in the early 1990s, several directors improved both their skills and their incomes by working across the film and advertising industries. Jeffs proved very good at the condensed, impactful storytelling which advertising of an international standard requires and from 1995 to 2000 won several awards for her commercial direction for clients such as the Land Transport Authority and Xenical, including an Axis Award and an award at Cannes, and in 1999 came top of the Admedia Poll for Best New Zealand Director.

In the same year she set up her own production company (originally called 'The Girl', now Exile Films) with producer Ian Gibbons: an enterprise that continues until today. Since, in contrast to feature film-making, the director is effaced from public view in advertising, one strand of Jeffs's work has always been invisible almost from the start of her career. Nevertheless, working in advertising is an opportunity she says 'to make things, to put film through the camera, to use different lenses, to keep on trying new things' (Jeffs 2013) in an environment where opportunities to make features are infrequent.

As well as a directing style informed by years spent in editing, sound post-production and the well-resourced activity of commercial filming, plus a set of thematic concerns influenced at a formative time by feminism, the other major creative resource in Jeffs's working life has been her professional and personal partnership with John Toon. Toon is a New Zealand-born cinematographer and director who has collaborated with Jeffs ever since the production of *Stroke* and has been the cinematographer on all three of her features. The benefit of working together consistently, Jeffs says, is that 'John gives me space to work on performances. His lighting style is natural and not too obtrusive and together we create a warm atmosphere on the set that is good for the actors' (Jeffs 2013). Normally, Toon is accompanied by people he is used to working with in the gaffer and best-boy positions especially, so together the group of them constitute a small mobile unit in the 'ethnoscape' of global flows (Appadurai 1990) in the transnational film industry.

A success at Cannes attracts international attention and in the period following the release of *Rain,* Jeffs was sent many scripts for possible projects, primarily from agents based in the United States, but few of them 'spoke to her heart' (Jeffs 2013). Instead, it was contacts made during filming commercials in Europe that brought her to the attention of a British/American co-production and the actress, Gwyneth Paltrow, who was attached to its forthcoming project on Sylvia Plath. Christine was invited to direct the film at a late stage in its development, becoming what she describes as a 'director for hire' with limited scope to influence a rather conventional 'biopic' script. She did however try to connect with elements of the story and in particular, to work with the performances. Taking part in the rest of the casting, she remembers that it was a struggle to have Daniel Craig as 'a powerful and intense actor' (Jeffs 2013), less known then but now a celebrity actor in his subsequent role as James Bond, confirmed as Plath's husband, the poet Ted Hughes.

*Sylvi*a was filmed largely in England, including at Shepperton Studios in Surrey. But, in one of the twists made possible when production teams comprise people from around the world, Jeffs was able to have scenes supposedly set in east coast America during the summertime and planned to be shot in South Africa, diverted to locations around Dunedin in the South Island of New Zealand. The post-production of the film also stayed in New Zealand, with an editing suite set up in the small North Island town of Warkworth near Jeffs and Toon's country home. Compared to *Rain*, says Jeffs, there was less creative freedom for her on the project, in that were many more 'voices' contributing their opinions on the piece from both England and America. The result is a film that has credible characterizations, some compelling moments of emotional drama and generally looks attractive and convincing but which is lacking in the sophisticated, impressionistic use of cinematic language that was a feature of both *Stroke* and *Rain*. The somewhat literal quality of the film is underlined by the soundtrack which features directly expressive orchestral music rather than the tangential encounters of music, character and landscape that Jeffs had organized for *Rain*.

The launch of *Sylvia* was followed by another period of directing commercials, both in New Zealand and overseas, while generating proposals for original projects. These included scripts based on the works of American writers Richard Ford and Jane Smiley. An adaptation of Smiley's *Horse Heaven* (2003) is a project that has appealed to Jeffs for several years: she has owned several horses herself and competes in show-jumping and dressage. This project has come close to going into production with some notable actors attached to it, but needs an ensemble cast and therefore lacks the 'star' actor at its centre, which is required nowadays for large-budget productions to attract funding.

An intriguing niche in the death industry – post-mortem clean-ups – produced the material for Jeffs's next film project, *Sunshine Cleaning*, this time produced under the classification of independent American cinema, backed by the same producers responsible for the 2006 success *Little Miss Sunshine* (Jonathan Dayton and Valerie Faris). The script was by Megan Holley, who wrote it after meeting two male post-mortem cleaners working in Albuquerque and translating their situation roles for four main roles, including a pair of sisters. While, once again, technically a director for hire Jeffs came onto the project with enough leeway to put her own stamp on most aspects of the production, including de-emphasizing the roles of the other characters in favour of the sisters: hard-working, conventional Rose and her moody, misfit sibling Norah. Although it was a low-budget production, the script attracted some fine actors including Amy Adams and Emily Blunt in the main roles, with Alan Arkin as their self-employed and increasingly unsuccessful father, Joe.

By this stage in Jeffs's career it may seem that *Sunshine Cleaning*, based on American material, shot and funded in the United States with American and British actors, has no significant connection with New Zealand. That is true, in the literal, regulatory sense of definitions of the constitution of national cinema. However, the point is that Jeffs, like other directors at work transnationally, brings important personal preferences and aspects of her creative formation in New Zealand with her, as well as the aesthetic filter that her constant collaborator, John Toon, adds to the look of the film.

Viewed schematically, the narrative and emotional preoccupations of *Sunshine Cleaning* are transpositions of those also present in *Rain*: for instance, the tension between siblings insufficiently supported by self-absorbed parents (the absent mother in the film, absent because of suicide, is an extrapolation of the mother who wants to escape in *Rain* and of the path chosen by Sylvia Plath, if she were viewed from her children's perspective). Adulterous heterosexual relationships also feature in all three films, but in none of them are these relationships a solution to the protagonists' dilemmas. Instead, as was pointed out earlier, in a film directed by Christine Jeffs, the key dynamic will be about women coming to understand their own situation and choices. Those dilemmas will be rendered vivid and engaging through committed and subtle performances by the actors, most memorably the female actors.

> I am aware of my focus being on performances and relationships. [...] I stay involved in a scene with the actors, it's an intuitive thing, knowing when to stay with it, when you have got the performance, knowing when to cut. It's also about creating responses through the juxtaposition of images and sounds with just a little dialogue on top. (Jeffs 2013)

Wanting a film to be received in a certain way by audiences does not guarantee that it will be, but the evidence of reviews shows that Jeffs's emphasis on performance was in fact picked up by critics evaluating the film.

> Christine Jeff's production treats its protagonists like people, not caricatures, and that makes all the difference when it comes to identifying with these individuals. Perhaps the most compelling reason to see *Sunshine Cleaning* is the pairing of two of the best and most charismatic young actresses today. The movie is in part about sisterhood, and they play beautifully off one another. One could easily envision the movie being less interesting and the characters less compelling in the hands of lesser talents. So much of what makes Rose and Norah intriguing results from what we read in the eyes and the expressions of the performers. (Berardinelli 2009)

> New Zealand's Christine Jeffs, who directed Gwyneth Paltrow in *Sylvia*, shapes the script, by newcomer Megan Holly, into something with its own scrappy integrity. Rose and Norah are damaged goods, scarred by their mother's suicide, though they rarely speak of it. This funny and touching movie depends on two can-do actresses to scrub past the biohazard of noxious clichés that threaten to intrude. Adams and Blunt get the job done. They come highly recommended. (Travers 2009)

Working on lower-budget productions overseas has its constraints in that there is less scope for a visiting director to make the community connections that result in some of the innovative solutions to technical and artistic problems that are available when one lives and works in the same country: however the film crews are comparably professional in both New Zealand and the United States according to Jeffs. Since completing *Sunshine Cleaning* she has been based back in New Zealand but travels to the United States several times a year for development meetings and to direct commercials, being one of the stable of directors associated with the New York-based commercial production company Xenon.

There have also been suggestions that she direct television, including episodes of *True Blood* (created by Alan Ball, HBO, 2008–2014) and *Dexter* (created by James Manos Jr, Showtime, 2006–2013) but this would require a commitment to living outside of New Zealand for long periods of time. Jeffs knows some 'fascinating and intelligent and creative people in Hollywood but the work is quite isolating – in and out, busy while you are there', and prefers to be based in New Zealand, 'It is a privilege to be able to live here and to work overseas. Most people have to live where they work and I am very lucky not to have to do that' (Jeffs 2013).

Nevertheless, although making features is not necessary to earn a living as a director across the contemporary spectrum of multimedia and advertising outlets there are always new film projects that Jeffs is trying to bring to fruition, both in the United States and New Zealand: 'I want to make films because I like creating things in that way, not just for business, but because I love creating emotion through image-making' (Jeffs 2013). With the changes in the industry since the making of *Rain*, that has become so much more difficult for directors who want to work in national cinemas or the transnational independent sector:

> There is a great deal of emphasis on cost today in film-making. There are fewer films being made, fewer dramas, fewer independent films. The kind of film that is getting funded now is different, with a bias towards entertainment and spectacle. And today, still only a small percentage of directors are female. (Jeffs 2013)

In the reviews of *Rain* a decade ago, Christine's name was added to a list of female directors who were at that time enhancing local cinema: Jane Campion, Alison Maclean and Niki Caro. While there are numerous factors that pull directors into other territories, or other media, such as Campion's recent move into television (*Top of the Lake*, Sundance Channel, 2013) it is a loss to public culture that these and other directors now find it so difficult to get backing to make films within a New Zealand-cinema framework and need to search for funding overseas. In July 2013, Jeffs signed on to direct a forthcoming project, provisionally call *The Saltwater Solution*, which will be based on the founding of the Greenpeace organisation.

Ann Hardy

References

Appadurai, A (1996) *Modernity at Large: Disjuncture and Difference in the Global Cultural Economy*, Minneapolis: University of Minnesota Press.

Berardinelli, J (2009) 'Sunshine Cleaning' [Review], *Reelviews*, 17 March, http://www.reelviews.net/php_review_template.php?identifier=1534. Accessed 23 May 2013.

Campion, J and Lee, G (2013) *Top of the Lake*, See-Saw Films/Escapade Pictures/Screen Australia.

Campion, J (1993) *The Piano*, Australia/New Zealand/France: Australian Film Commission/CiBy 2000/Jan Chapman Productions.

Caro, N (2002) *Whale Rider*, New Zealand/Germany: South Pacific Pictures/ ApolloMedia DFistributors/Pandora Film Produktion.

Caro, N (1994) *Sure To Rise*, New Zealand: Frame up Films.

Ezra, E and Rowden, T (eds) (2006) *Transnational Cinema: The Film Reader*, Routledge, London and New York

Jackson, P (2012) *The Hobbit: An Unexpected Journey*, United States/New Zealand: New Line Cinema/MGM/Wingnut Films.

Jeffs, C (2013) interview, Auckland, New Zealand, 13 February.

Jeffs, C (2008) *Sunshine Cleaning*, United States: Overture Films/Big Beach Films/Back lot Pictures.

Jeffs, C (2005) *Sylvia*, Icon Films/BBC Films/Capitol/UK Film Council.

Jeffs, C (2000) *Rain*, New Zealand: Rose Road/Communicado/NZ Film Commission.

Jeffs, C (1994) *Stroke*, New Zealand: NZ Film Commission.

Kahi, TA (2013) *Mt Zion*, New Zealand: Small Axe Films.

Keller, L (n.d.) '*Sunshine Cleaning*' [Review], *Urban Cinefile*, http://www.urbancinefile. com.au/home/view.asp?a=15834&s=Reviews. Accessed 13 May 2013.

Maclean, A (1992) *Crush*, New Zealand: NZ Film Commission.

Maclean, A (1989) *Kitchen Sink*, New Zealand: NZ Film commission.

Matthews, P (2001) '*Rain*' [Review], *NZ Listener*, October, http://www.filmarchive.org.nz/ feature-project/pages/Rain.php. Accessed 13 May 2013.

Mita, M (1992) 'The Soul and The Image', in Jonathon Dennis and Jan Bieringa (eds), *Film in Aotearoa New Zealand*, Wellington: Victoria University Press.

Mulheron, D (2012) *Fresh Meat*, New Zealand: Gibson Group Fresh Meat/Gibson Group.

Neill, S and Rymer, J (1995) *Cinema of Unease: A Personal Journey*, New Zealand: BFI/ NZ Film Commission/NZ On Air.

Pivac, D, Stark, F and McDonald, L (eds) (2011) *New Zealand Film: An Illustrated History*, Wellington: Te Papa Press.

Reid, M (1988) *Send A Gorilla*, New Zealand: NZ Film Commission.

Travers, P (2009) '*Sunshine Cleaning*' [Review], *Rolling Stone*, 11 March, http://www. rollingstone.com/movies/reviews/sunshine-cleaning-20090311#ixzz2U5KQ1nc0. Accessed 13 May 2013.

Note

1. Acknowledgement needs to be given to the perseverance and achievements of both Gaylene Preston and Yvonne McKay within the New Zealand environment. The former has moved between feature dramas and feature-length documentaries to create the most extensive *oeuvre* of films by any New Zealand film-maker, while Yvonne McKay continues to be active in producing, especially in television.

EXPERIMENTAL & DOCUMENTARY FILM

THEATRICAL DOCUMENTARY IN NEW ZEALAND 2012: FUNDING, MARKETING AND DISTRIBUTION

At least nineteen documentary feature films were screened in cinemas throughout New Zealand in 2012, mainly in festivals:[1]

- Two Films at the World Cinema Showcase (Auckland, Wellington, Dunedin, Christchurch)
- Five films at the Documentary Edge Festival (Auckland and Wellington).
- Ten films at the New Zealand International Film Festival (NZIFF) (Auckland, Christchurch, Dunedin, Hamilton, Hawke's Bay, Masterton, Nelson, New Plymouth, Palmerston North, Tauranga, Wellington).
- Two major documentary features funded by the New Zealand Film Commission (NZFC) were released in cinemas nationwide.

The majority of these films were seen only by enthusiastic but relatively small festival crowds, but many of the documentary features that proved popular at film festivals (particularly the NZIFF) have gone on to have limited national or regional cinema releases due to popular demand, and several have enjoyed critical (if not commercial success) at prestigious international festivals.

Although the volume of feature-length documentaries released in 2012 may reflect the lower production barriers brought about by cheaper, more accessible production technologies, the most significant changes which are consistent with global trends relate to shifting dynamics between producers, audiences and intermediaries (distributors and exhibitors) as online and social media facilitate a more direct relationship between film-makers and the audience.

Focusing particularly on the impact of new technologies on New Zealand's documentary production ecology, this essay presents an overview of current trends in the funding, marketing, distribution and exhibition of New Zealand documentaries based on analysis of this group of nineteen films.

The films

One of the most important criteria that must be fulfilled in order to receive funding from either of the government organizations which provide the most support for New Zealand documentaries (the NZFC and NZ on Air), is that films or television programmes must focus on 'New Zealand stories'. This is a policy frequently bemoaned by film-makers wishing to tackle broader subjects, yet most of the films listed below do contain international elements, and films shot solely in New Zealand are in fact in the minority. Films such as *Brother Number One* (Annie Goldson, 2011), *The Last Dogs of Winter* (Costa Botes, 2011) and *Intersexion* (Grant Lahood, 2012), which all received significant public funding, are largely set outside New Zealand but present subjects framed from the perspective of a New Zealander as central protagonist and often are shaped by a New Zealand sensibility. While these are distinctly New Zealand films, they represent a perspective on the world that is far from insular.

To reflect this diversity of subject matter and style, films have been listed according to broad themes as follows:

Social/political/cultural

Films that cover a diverse range of social and political issues and cultural and historical subjects:

Brother Number One follows the journey of New Zealand athlete Rob Hamill to a war crimes tribunal in Cambodia where he confronts Comrade Duch, the man responsible for his brother's death under the Khmer Rouge regime.

Mental Notes (Jim Marbrook, 2012) exposes the historical failure of New Zealand's mental health institutions and celebrates the resilience of the five survivors of 'the Bins' who share their stories and revisit their traumatic pasts.

Nazi Hunter (Alex Behse, 2012) documents ex-policeman Wayne Stringer's secret investigation of 47 people suspected of being Nazi war criminals who sought refuge in New Zealand as 'displaced persons' after World War II.

Intersexion offers an insight into life as an intersex person through New Zealander Mani Bruce Mitchell's conversations with fellow intersex people around the world.

How Far is Heaven (Chris Loader and Shane Loader, 2011) is an intimate observational study of life in the rural village Jerusalem/Hiruhama, where the Catholic order the Sisters of Compassion have lived alongside the Maori community for 120 years.

Tatarakihi: The Children of Parihaka (Paora Joseph, 2012) is a 'journey of memory' undertaken by a group of Parihaka children following in the footsteps of their ancestors, who were transported to the South Island and jailed after the Taranaki land confiscations of the 1860s.

Maori Boy Genius (Pietra Brettkelly, 2012) is a portrait of a talented and politically ambitious Maori teenager Ngaa Rauuira Pumanawawhiti, who travels to Yale for intensive studies at the age of sixteen, carrying with him the weight of family expectations and sacrifice.

Yakel 3D (Rachael Wilson, 2012) is New Zealand's first 3D documentary, which aims to capture life in a remote village in Vanuatu where a 108-year-old chief is reaching the end of his life, presenting a challenge to the traditional way of life his people have preserved in isolation.

Tongan Ark (Paul Janman, 2012) pays homage to Futa Helu, the founder of the Atenisi Institute, an independent Tongan educational institution based on the teachings of ancient Greek philosophers and a love of classical Italian opera.

Environmental

While not solely environmental stories, three films focus on the natural world and environmental issues:

The Last Dogs of Winter takes us to the remote and harsh terrain of Churchill, Manitoba where a grizzly Canadian and his young Kiwi assistant rear Eskimo dogs alongside polar bears in a bid to preserve the endangered species of indigenous dogs.

Song of the Kauri (Mathurin Molgat, 2011) highlights issues of sustainability through the story of a master craftsman who uses Kauri timber to create guitars and violins.

The Last Ocean (Peter Young, 2012) is an activist film produced as part of a campaign to end commercial fishing in the Ross Sea (Antarctica).

Arts/music/performance

Beautiful Machine (Sam Peacocke, 2012) is a rockumentary about Shihad, one of New Zealand's most successful rock bands.

Te Hono ki Aotearoa (Jan Bieringa, 2012) follows the creation and handover of a *Māori waka taua* (Maori ceremonial canoe) commissioned for the Dutch Museum Volkenkunde in Leiden.

Disappear into Light (Leonie Reynolds, 2011) is an observational documentary that follows nine months in the life of acclaimed playwright Jo Randerson.

View from Olympus (Geoffrey Cawthorn, 2011) is a portrait of John Psathas, a composer born to Greek immigrants in New Zealand, which explores Psathas's life, cultural identity and music.

Persuading the Baby to Float (Keith Hill) captures the artistic collaboration between pianist Norman Meehan, poet Bill Manhire and singer Hannah Griffin.

Pictures of Susan (Dan Salmon, 2012) is the story of outsider artist Susan Te Kahurangi King, who does not speak but expresses herself through thousands of detailed and colourful drawings. The film follows Susan's artistic and personal rebirth as she resumes drawing after a silence of twenty years.

Village by the Sea (Michael Heath, 2012*)* is a follow-up to an earlier documentary about the artist Edith Collier, centred on an Irish fishing village where Collier lived and painted for two summers during 1914–15.

Funding

Funding for New Zealand documentary films comes from a variety of sources ranging from public investment, the support of community organizations, private philanthropic donations, to industry support in the form of free or discounted labour or goods. 2012 has seen the emergence of crowdfunding as a potentially significant new funding strategy, which two of the films in this group have used with some (modest) success.

The NZFC has gradually expanded its support for documentary features in recent years. Three films released in New Zealand in 2012 have received Feature Film Investment from the NZFC: *Brother Number One*, *Beautiful Machine* and *Last Dogs of Winter*. Funding for *Brother Number One* and *Beautiful Machine* was also augmented by NZ On Air, the government agency that supports free-to-air NZ broadcast content. Smaller NZFC Feature Film Finishing Grants (generally between NZ$10,000 to NZ$25,000) were awarded to a number of feature documentaries in this group for post-production costs necessary to enable theatrical distribution.

In addition to *Brother Number One* and *Beautiful Machine*, five films received funding from NZ On Air: *Intersexion*, *View from Olympus*, *Nazi Hunter*, *The Last Ocean* and *Maori Boy Genius*. As New Zealand's commercial television hour is a short 43 minutes, these films are usually significantly re-versioned for theatrical release.

Two films (*How Far is Heaven* and *Tongan Ark*) received their primary funding from combined NZFC/Creative New Zealand funds that have since been discontinued (the Independent Filmmakers Fund and the Screen Production Innovation Fund).

Funding for the documentaries on this list vary greatly. At one extreme, *Beautiful Machine* received NZ$813,900 from the NZFC and NZ$160,068 from NZ On Air, bringing its total public funding to NZ$973,968, a significant documentary budget even by international standards. NZ On Air funding for the films in this group ranged from NZ$80,000 to NZ$170,000. On the more modest end of the public funding scale, *Tongan Ark* received NZ$15,000 from the Screen Innovation Production Fund (NZFC/Creative NZ).

Philanthropic funding and crowdfunding

In addition to public funding, much of the support for documentary comes from goodwill in the form of labour, equipment and other resources donated or provided at significantly discounted rates. A number of films on the list above have been supported at least in part by various community and arts organizations with a special interest in the film's subject matter. *Tatarakihi*, for example, was partially funded by a grant from the TSB Community Trust; *How Far is Heaven* was partly funded by the Wanganui District Council; and *Mental Notes* received the support of the Frozen Funds Trust and a reTHiNK Grant from Mind and Body Consultants. As these films demonstrate, it is not uncommon for documentaries to receive some funding from philanthropic sources, but New Zealand lacks formalized systems to widely promote or reward such investment, as is the case in the United States and Australia, for example (Ministry for Culture and Heritage 2010). This seems set to change, due to a shift in cultural policy and in part due to the growing influence of crowdfunding.

Competition for public funding is intense, particularly in the midst of a sustained economic downturn, prompting the Minister for Arts, Culture and Heritage Hon.

Christopher Finlayson to establish a taskforce to explore ways to increase private investment in the arts (Ministry for Culture and Heritage 2010). The primary outcome of the work of the taskforce has been the launch in 2012 of a matched funding scheme administered by government organization Creative New Zealand called Creative Giving Matched Funding, which aims to aid arts organizations in attracting new sponsorship or donations. Almost concurrently, philanthropic organization the Arts Foundation has launched their own strategy for philanthropic funding, one that uses crowdfunding as the model for broadening and increasing private investment in the arts.

Crowdfunding 'involves an open call, mostly through the Internet, for the provision of financial resources either in form of donation or in exchange for the future product or some form of reward and/or voting rights' (Belleflamme, Lambert and Schwienbacher 2011: 5–6). Crowdfunding seemed to gain critical momentum and public awareness in New Zealand in 2012 when local film director Taika Waititi successfully raised US$110.796 on the US crowdfunding website Kickstarter to facilitate the American release of the film, *Boy* (Kickstarter 2012). New Zealand's first local crowdfunding platform, PledgeMe, had its official launch in January 2012 (following a soft-launch in 2011), raising a total of NZ$420, 000 in its first seven months (PledgeMe 2012). Australian crowdfunding platform Pozible and the US-based Indiegogo have also proved popular with New Zealand film-makers. The Arts Foundation's site, Boosted, will enable donors to receive tax rebates of 33 per cent on their donations to projects, rather than offering rewards as crowdfunding campaigns usually do (Arts Foundation 2012).

Crowdfunding offers film-makers an additional or alternative avenue for funding that offers film-makers the ability to reach a large pool of potential supporters. At the very least, it can be a more effective and less intrusive way to 'pass the hat' around a small crowd of friends and family, but a strong campaign supported by social media, grassroots outreach and publicity can garner a much wider crowd beyond the immediate social networks of the film-maker. Two of the films in this group, *Maori Boy Genius* and *Tatarakihi: The Children of Parihaka* have used crowdfunding campaigns with some success.

Maori Boy Genius was initially funded by NZ On Air and broadcast on Maori Television in the hour-long Pakipumeka Aotearoa New Zealand Documentary slot. The director, Pietra Brettkelly, wanted to re-cut and extend the television documentary as a theatrical work and was invited to screen the film in competition at the prestigious Berlin Film Festival in 2012. Brettkelly used Indiegogo to raise funds for a final edit, sound design and mix, music rights, film finishing costs and marketing. While Indiegogo is an international platform (unlike high-profile platform Kickstarter, which is limited to US and UK residents), the support of non-profit partner, From the Heart Productions, meant that donations were tax-deductible in the United States.

As is the norm for crowdfunding campaigns, incentives or rewards were offered in return for financial contributions, ranging from a signed DVD of the completed film for NZ$30 to an Associate Producer credit for $5,000. Funding came from 62 funders, most of whom either contributed $30 or $65, with seven people contributing $250 for a DVD set of films by Brettkelly.

The campaign raised only NZ$5,900 of its $10,000 goal but was able to keep this money as the campaign was run on a Flexible Funding basis (the project gets to keep all the funds raised but Indiegogo charges a higher commission for unsuccessful Flexible Funding campaigns) (Indiegogo n.d.).

Most other crowdfunding sites run campaigns on a fixed funding (all or nothing) basis, meaning that pledges are only processed when the funding goal is reached and campaigns that fail to reach their goal by the set deadline do not receive any of the money raised. The rationale for this mode of funding is that there is less risk for both creators and funders and that funders are more motivated to actively support a project when the stakes are higher (Kickstarter n.d.).

Tatarakihi: The Children of Parihaka ran two crowdfunding campaigns on Australian-based crowdfunding site Pozible on a fixed-funding basis, raising AU$8,494 in the first campaign (exceeding the AU$7,500 goal) and AU$1,750 in the second campaign (meeting the goal exactly). As with *Maori Boy Genius*, the *Tatarakihi* campaign was focused specifically on the request for funds needed to finish the film for a cinema release.

Tatarakihi offered a broader range of rewards; from AU$1 for the opportunity to be an 'outreach partner', $10 for a signed postcard, $20 for a CD of the film's soundtrack, and $100 for a limited edition DVD through to $500 for an overnight stay at Parihaka, $5,000 for a contributor credit and $10,000 for an associate producer credit. The highest value reward chosen was $500.

Neither crowdfunding campaign made a significant amount of money as a percentage of overall costs, but provided the film-makers with a small amount of much needed cash when it was most needed, and within a short space of time. Average pledges for both campaigns were slightly higher than average pledges for crowdfunding sites – AU$80 for Pozible (Pozible 2012), US$74 for Indiegogo (Baddour 2012) and NZ$70 for PledgeMe (PledgeMe 2012) – but the success of a crowdfunding campaign depends not on the size of individual donations, but on the size of the crowd. As the success of Taika Waititi's Kickstarter campaign for *Boy* demonstrates, traditional media 'gatekeepers' still influence the chances of crowdfunding success (Sørensen 2012). This article compares traditional and new ways of funding documentary film in the UK and asks what crowd financing, pay-if-you-want schemes and online distribution sites mean for documentary films and its industry today. How do online financing models impact on producers, traditional funding models and funders? And following the money, who really benefits? The first section of this article charts trends in British documentary budgets in the last decade and explores how changes in financing impact on the production of documentary films. The second focuses on new ways of funding and distributing documentary films online. Drawing on case studies of crowd investment schemes, crowdfunding and P2P distribution; interviews with documentary and multiplatform producers and commissioners, as well as on statistics and annual reports from broadcasters, lobbyists and regulators, I will argue that in real terms there has been a decline in and a polarization of documentary budgets in the UK. As a result, producers are increasingly looking to the internet to fund their documentaries. However, an online financing market suspended between ad hoc funding and long-term recuperation has consequences for the documentary industry, the kinds of documentaries made, the topics they explore and the ways in which they are produced as projects with a high-profile figure such as Waititi attached are able to generate publicity through traditional media channels, effectively reaching a much bigger 'crowd'.

Marketing, distribution and exhibition

For most film-makers, crowdfunding will supplement rather than replace traditional funding sources; but it serves an additional purpose as a valuable marketing and distribution tool, enabling film-makers to build an actively supportive audience base prior to a film's release. An online presence and use of some form of social media to promote and engage with audiences is now an essential aspect of film-making, as the film industry undergoes a process of disintermediation that increasingly requires the film-maker to play a more active role in distribution and marketing (Iordanova and Cunningham 2012).

Neither *Tatarakihi* nor *Maori Boy Genius* had a dedicated website at the time that their campaigns were running (though both had Facebook pages), so their campaign pages helped to increase their online presence, functioning as temporary promotional sites (featuring trailers, film descriptions and production information, and providing the film-makers with a mechanism for communicating with supporters via the site, social networks and e-mail). Social media sharing buttons on each project's campaign site enabled site visitors to easily share links to campaigns with their social networks. In the case of *Tatarakihi* for example, 735 people posted a link to the Pozible campaign as a Facebook status update.

Most of the nineteen films listed in this essay have some kind of stand-alone website that serves to promote the film, though some have a dedicated page as part of a production company website, and a few simply have Facebook pages.

Film websites typically feature a film trailer, reviews an EPK (Electronic Press Kit) for media, a list of screenings, a mailing list sign-up, links to Facebook and Twitter accounts, a blog, contact form and a shopping cart for DVD sales. For films that are connected with a broader social campaign or project such as *The Last Ocean* or *Tatarakihi*, a donate button is also a feature of the website. The website for *Brother Number One* offers a detailed study guide aimed at high school students; an occasional extra in New Zealand productions, but a standard feature for Australian documentaries where Screen Australia funds study guides as part of a programme, coordinated with ATOM (Australian Teachers of Media) and Screenrights, which assists film-makers in increasing revenue from the educational market.

Facebook pages serve as a useful interface between film-maker and audience, where regular updates and discussion can help fuel audience interest in a film over time. This is often a space where not just the film-maker, but the 'stars' or protagonists of films may directly engage with the audience, as is the case with, for example, *The Last Dogs of Winter* (www.facebook.com/Dogsofwinter) and *Brother Number One* (http://www.facebook.com/BrotherNumberOne.film).

Distribution and exhibition

The growing need for direct audience engagement via social media channels is one dimension of a shift in the role of the independent film-maker to encompass a range of activities that previously would have been undertaken by a number of individuals. Not only are film-makers increasingly performing a range of production tasks single-handedly, such as operating a camera and sound equipment while also producing, directing and editing, but they are increasingly involved in distribution.

At the time of writing, none of the films featured were offering Video on Demand (VOD) or other online viewing or download options, but many offer DVD sales (generally directly, rather than via a third party such as Amazon). While VOD sales would undoubtedly open up access to a global market for New Zealand documentary, the local market for VOD is limited as most international VOD services are not legally available in New Zealand and broadband data caps imposed by local ISPs are prohibitive.

Although at least two films (*Brother Number One* and *Beautiful Machine*) have agreements with local distributors such as Metropolis Film and Rialto Distribution, where films have gone on to screen in theatres post-festival, they are primarily self-distributed by the film-makers. With the shift from celluloid prints to digital formats, it is now more cost effective for multiple copies of a film to be in circulation and local documentaries tend to be circulated around a circuit of small independent cinemas or alternative community venues[2] such as Waiheke Cinemas on Auckland's Waiheke Island or the Village Theatre in Takaka, rather than the network of larger cinema chains such as Hoyts or Event Cinemas.

The market for locally produced theatrical documentaries is certainly modest (of the films included here, only three films, *Brother Number One*, *Beautiful Machine* and

How Far is Heaven even register in New Zealand box office statistics), but the volume of theatrical documentaries is impressive nonetheless. The 2009 documentary about the Topp Twins *Untouchable Girls* (Leanne Pooley) has been the most successful New Zealand-produced documentary to date, earning nearly NZ$2 million at the box office.

Festivals play a vital role in the circulation of these films, providing opportunities for limited exhibition across the breadth of New Zealand, from large cities to small towns, which otherwise would not be possible. With the exception of *Beautiful Machine*, all of these films have screened in New Zealand film festivals: two films screened at the World Cinema Showcase (*Te Hono ki Aotearoa* and *Mental Notes*), five films screened at the Documentary Edge Festival (*Disappear into Light*, *Intersexion*, *Yakel 3D*, *View From Olympus*, *Nazi Hunter*) and eleven films screened at the NZIFF (*The Last Dogs of Winter*, *How Far is Heaven*, *Song of the Kauri*, *Persuading the Baby to Float*, *The Last Ocean*, *Tatarakihi: The Children of Parihaka*, *Maori Boy Genius*, *Pictures of Susan*, *Tongan Ark*, *Village by the Sea* and *Brother Number One*.)[3]

International festivals are also responsible for the wider circulation of these films and several have had considerable critical success at high-profile international festivals including *Maori Boy Genius* (Berlin International Film Festival, Sheffield DocFest and Sydney International Film Festival), *Last Dogs of Winter* (Toronto International Film Festival 2011, International Documentary Film Festival Amsterdam [IDFA]), and *Brother Number One* (Melbourne International Film Festival, IDFA).

Television broadcast still plays an important role is supporting New Zealand documentary – as previously mentioned, seven of these films were originally commissioned for television – but the volume of documentaries produced and exhibited in theatres may be seen as a reflection, not only of a growing audience for theatrical documentaries, but of the decline of longer form television documentaries in favour of half-hour factual entertainment series.

Conclusion

The number of features screened in New Zealand cinemas in 2012, and the diversity and quality that this group of films represent, are positive signs of creative and cultural well-being in New Zealand's documentary production ecology; but it is yet to be seen whether this level of output is sustainable. However, local film-makers are increasingly adopting digital tools to support the funding, outreach, marketing and distribution of their work and will need to continue to be innovative and entrepreneurial to succeed in a complex, globalized and competitive media environment.

Anna Jackson

References

Baddour, Nic (2012) 'Indiegogo Insight: Nearly 40% of Active Campaigns Receive Money From Multiple Countries', *Indiegogo Blog*, http://www.indiegogo.com/blog/2012/05/indiegogo-insight-nearly-40-of-active-campaigns-receive-money-from-multiple-countries.html. Accessed 19 October 2012.

Indiegogo (n.d.) 'Fees & Pricing' [Support], http://support.indiegogo.com/entries/20492953-fees-pricing. Accessed 12 November 2012.

Iordanova, Dina and Cunningham, Stuart D. (2012) *Digital Disruption : Cinema Movies Online*, http://onlineshop.st-andrews.ac.uk/browse/extra_info.asp?compid=1&catid=87&modid=1&prodid=0&deptid=0&prodvarid=111. Accessed 9 November 2012.

Kickstarter (2012) 'BOY: The American release!', http://www.kickstarter.com/projects/18395296/boy-the-american-release. Accessed 12 November 2012.

Kickstarter (n.d.) 'Kickstarter Basics » Frequently Asked Questions (FAQ)', http://www.
kickstarter.com/help/faq/kickstarter%20basics. Accessed 12 November 2012.

Ministry for Culture and Heritage (2010) *Growing the pie: Increasing the level
of cultural philanthropy in Aotearoa New Zealand: Report of the Cultural
Philanthropy Taskforce to the Minister for Arts, Culture and Heritage, Hon.
Christopher Finlayson*, Ministry for Culture and Heritage, http://www.mch.govt.
nz/research-publications/our-research-reports/cultural-philanthropy. Accessed 14
April 2012.

Belleflamme, Paul, Lambert, T and Schwienbacher, A (2011) *Crowdfunding: Tapping
the right crowd*, CORE Discussion Paper, Belgium: CORE Center for Operations
Research and Econometrics, http://dial.academielouvain.be/vital/access/services/
Download/boreal:78971/PDF_01?view=true. Accessed 9 October 2012.

PledgeMe (2012) ;Infographic fun: Crowdfunding in New Zealand', *PledgeMe Blog*,
http://blog.pledgeme.co.nz/infographic-fun/. Accessed 19 October 2012.

Pozible (2012) '2 Million Reasons to Smile', http://www.pozible.com/index.php/help/
prpage_details/3. Accessed 19 October 2012.

Sørensen, IE (2012) 'Crowdsourcing and outsourcing: The impact of online funding
and distribution on the documentary film industry in the UK', *Media, Culture &
Society*, 34: 6, pp. 726–43.

Arts Foundation (2012) Boosted [Organization], http://www.boosted.org.nz/.
Aaccessed 12 November 2012.

Notes

1. The actual number of documentaries screened in limited venues may be higher,
   but this figure accounts for multiple screenings in at least two major centres.
2. See Geoff Lealand's website on independent and arthouse cinemas in New
   Zealand for more detail on the importance of such small local cinemas: http://
   cinemasofnz.info/.
3. *Brother Number One* premiered at the NZIFF in 2011, prior to its 2012 general
   theatrical release.

GENRES OF NEW ZEALAND EXPERIMENTAL FILM

Experimental film displays a continuous line of development in New Zealand since at least 1970, with several practitioners from the 1970s and 1980s still active today. Much of the New Zealand work can be grouped within six subgenres – landscape, psychodrama, identity politics, visual music, installed and expanded cinemas, and animation. Some of the artists move across genres and media being active also as composers, musicians, poets and visual artists.

Landscape

With a trend toward naturalism since the Italian Renaissance the depiction of nature and then landscape has become more important in western art.

Early forms of European landscape art in New Zealand were utilitarian cartographic charts, concerned with describing the land for geographic and settlement purposes. Over time this documentary approach developed an expressive edge, one that tended toward spiritual and subjective mappings of the self and environment. Whilst landscape came to play an important part in the history of New Zealand art and music it has not figured so prominently as an aesthetic concern for Kiwi industrial film-makers, except for the work of Vincent Ward. Only in the area of experimental film has the landscape really come to the fore.

Both Joanna Margaret Paul and Philip Dadson began addressing landscape in their experimental films in the early 1970s and it is today a genre that is on the ascendant and yet to reach its critical peak.

Kathryn Dudding's extended essay film *Asylum Pieces* (2010) is a landscape work that completes a photographic project left unfinished by her former partner after he committed suicide whilst being medicated for depression.

An accomplished and mature work *Asylum Pieces* proceeds through a series of contemplative shots which linger on the landscape setting and architecture of historic New Zealand mental asylums. These are contrasted with the transcendental Japanese concept of *Wabi Sabi*[1] and the eighteenth-century Italian artist Giovanni Battista Piranesi's etchings of imaginary prisons. The etchings appear as the prisons within the dark labyrinths of selfhood. Of a self that cannot reconcile itself with the demands of society, or a society which cannot quite meet the needs of its citizens. The film slowly, almost imperceptibly, leads the viewer toward the conclusion that evolving practices of mental health treatment in New Zealand are systemic only in their continuing dysfunction.

Tragically, Dudding died just weeks after *Asylum Pieces* premiered at the New Zealand International Film Festival in 2010. Circumscribed as it is by the death of its two unseen protagonists, *Asylum Pieces* survives Dudding as her tribute to love, commitment and hope.

Other film artists who address landscape in their work include Lissa Mitchell, PR Wareing, SJ Ramir and the author.

Psychodrama or trance films

The historic psychodramatic form of experimental film-making appeared in the work of David Blyth and George Rose in the late 1970s and was continued by artists such as Brent Hayward since the 1980s. Such forms of film-making tend to question the nature of reality and one's place within the world.

Working-class musician, painter, performance and outsider artist Brent Hayward got his screen education by working as a projectionist for the Auckland Film Society in the late 1980s.

The Everyman (1999) is Hayward's sermon for the marginalized, dispossessed and forgotten to images of butts, Buddhas and gun-toting strangers.

The film builds through repetitious sound and image sequences. A monk-like figure spins like a whirling dervish, a man with a megaphone, a tongue, a fire-eater, a purple reverend wearing a blonde wig and sunglasses. The mesmerizing audio rhythm intensifies, drawing the viewer in on images of flowers, tyres, the purple reverend dancing in a carwash, a strobe-lit woman brandishing a broadsword, a pyramidal mound, an ant crawling on a blue finger, a naked woman emerging from a tunnel, plumes of fire, megaphone man kick-boxing in an auto junkyard, a prayer to the God of Everyman.

Hayward's persistent repetition of images involves the viewer as an active participant in the work, predicting and questioning how, where and why actions and images reappear in relation to other visual elements.

Identity politics

Following the arrival of television in New Zealand more and more groups within society realized that they were subject to media neglect or misrepresentation.

In the early 1980s independent film-makers began addressing gay, women's and Maori issues. Their work extended the frame of reference towards social engagement and activism as well as an expanded sense of multiculturalism. These artists included Peter Wells, Shereen Maloney and Merata Mita.

Indigenous concerns have been continued in recent work by Maree Mills, Rose-Michelle Lee, Natalie Robertson and Rachel Rakena. They address issues of self and environment from a specific Maori perspective. Such concerns can be related to the evolution of the idea of New Zealand into Aotearoa, as a society that embraces Maori cultural and spiritual values as its foundation.

You Love My Fresh (2010) is a short three-channel installation work by Tano Gago addressing the complexity and diversity of the Samoan experience in the 'new villages' of South Auckland, New Zealand.

A Samoan, brought to New Zealand as a young child and brought up by an adoptive Palangi (European) mother and Tongan father Gago hankers after the 'authentic' Samoan experience and one in which a gay Samoan male can exist outside the *fafafingi* (transvestite) stereotype.

Set to a haunting, ambient soundtrack which hints at Polynesian hip hop *You Love My Fresh* opens on an image of the Otara Shopping Centre at night. Subsequent sequences show the almost Third World Otahuhu bus station and shopping centre, a church-based workshop to teach New Zealand-born Samoans how to prepare and cook a traditional Samoan *UMU* (earth oven), and high voltage pylons traversing the working-class Polynesian suburb of Otara. A succession of titles question Polynesians' status as anything more than token New Zealanders, valued as exotica but relegated to menial, minimum wage jobs, discount shopping centres, and thought of as the All Blacks of the ghetto. 'Your cultural experience shapes me, makes me cynical, violent and resentful […] I feel redundant as a citizen in your first world.'

The work ends on a choreographed Samoan dance set to an evocatively Polynesian rendering of the New Zealand national anthem. The loss or absence that Gago addresses is held equally by *i* Pakeha (European New Zealander) and Palangi (Samoan name for Europeans), though they may not yet know or recognize their loss or absence from the cross-cultural process.

Lisa Reihana's current work in progress, *In Pursuit of Venus* (aka *POV* – point of view) reconstructs a nineteenth-century French wallpaper, *Les Sauvages de la mer Pacifique* (Jean-Gabriel Charvet, 1806) , of idealized South Sea scenes as a contemporary moving-image work. Conceived of by Reihana as an installation work for several projectors, in *POV* the wallpaper becomes a setting for live-action Polynesian performers playing out various scenes against the Europeanized backdrop, refiguring the wallpaper in a sensual postcolonial discourse of Indigenous politics and reality.

Visual music

This is the tradition that in New Zealand has come down from Len Lye and, more recently, Michael Nicholson, Jed Town and Janine Randerson.

Notions of visual music can also be related to ideas of the spiritual in art as held by several late-nineteenth and early-twentieth-century artists. Kandinsky wanted to redirect humans away from what he considered to be the false values of materialism. His aim was to connect the visual aspect of art to one's inner life as a resonance of the musical and spiritual.

Although secular, and working at a far remove in space and time from his European predecessors, Michael Nicholson found inspiration in Kandinsky's ideas.

Seeing himself as a composer of images,[2] Nicholson conceived of his *Visual Music Project: Stage 3, Opus 1–4* (2008) as a piece of visual music akin to classical music. Drawing on precedents from film, music and art he fashioned self-referential video structures that exist parallel to external reality. The four movements begin tentatively, like a fragmented interplanetary transmission of optical vibrations. Vibrations that range from stark black and white through primary video shapes and colours, merging in and out of one another in a tenuous stability that evokes the very interior of a technological vision. (The colours are not naturalistic, they are electronic.) The energy, or forces, that Nicholson marshals, create patterns shaped in choreography of light, colour, shape and movement.

Straddling the divide between identity politics and visual music Lelani Kake's *Kiaora/Kiaorana* (2010) presented the viewer with text of New Zealand and Cook Island Maori (Rarotongan) greetings which transformed into flattened abstract black-and-white patterns, like a moving electronic tapa of swirling star patterns, doubled biomorphic images and evocations of flora – almost as the first organisms moving into and through life – accompanied by a rhythmic and at times almost ethereal ambient music track.

Video VJ's are today further re-posing notions of visual music within popular, at times spectacular and Bacchanalian, live music and dance events where music and images may be sampled and remixed. Increasingly, since the early 1990s, artists have been sampling and remixing the work of other artists and producers – appropriating and reworking objects that are already in circulation. Notions of authenticity and originality are given different currency, becoming devalued in a society in which extraction, production and consumption must now be equalled by recycling as we re-negotiate our pathways through economy, language and culture. Today the second-hand shop, surplus store and street market surpass the art gallery, concert hall and cinema.

This tendency was anticipated in the 1980s by Popular Productions when they began producing Bad Music Bad Sound and Bad Films in works such as *Dora's Lunch*, half of a double-screen work (1988–89), which parodies the concerns of Continental and other theories. Here High theorists find themselves in a very low setting, where notions of craft, artifice and preciousness hold little currency, almost as stained and chipped crockery in a second-hand emporium.

Installed and expanded cinemas

Driven by a desire to create immersive and experiential forms of cinema some media and performance artists create presentational environments which expand the notion of the film frame and the single projected image from one to many images which can play across screens, monitors or other objects placed throughout an exhibition environment.

For some artists expanded cinema projections provide a context for their musical performances, they appropriate an antique technology and found footage to create a setting for work that is conceived of more as experience rather than a finished product that cannot be altered.

Following on from Leon Narbey and Darcy Lange in the 1970s, contemporary artists such as Janine Randerson, The Parasitic Fantasy Band (Eve Gordon and Sam Hamilton), Alexandra Monteith and Rachel Rakena continue to enliven their installation and performance art with cinematic and digital imagery, at times presented as expanded cinema events.

Raewyn Turner worked with the band Split Enz from 1975 to 1983 touring extensively in Australasia, Europe and North America as an artist working with light and music. As an intermedia artist Turner explores the potential of new technologies to affect extra and sub-sensory awareness in work which includes video, aroma, coloured light and live performance with orchestras, jazz, contemporary music and dance.

In September 2010 Turner presented her installation piece *Re/Sense* at the Moving Image Centre in Auckland. This collaboration with the Canadian artist Diana Burgoyne presented electronic projections of atmospheric greens from mid-winter New Zealand and Western Canadian environments. Turner chose locations in North Taranaki including those contaminated by the chemical company Ivan Watkins Dow in the late 1960s. Here nature may seem imperilled by human activity.

In *Re/Sense* handmade perfumes were synaesthetically linked to specific colours engendered by specific environments. Perfume beads were placed on tiny upward-facing audio speakers mounted at the bottom of drinking glasses set on pedestals arranged in front of the projected colours. The colours triggered lonely, eerie sounds, like those of a space wind, causing vibrations which in turn activated the release of specific aromas.

Turner's installation evoked a sense of intimacy, fragility and domesticity both in the use of her materials and the way the spectator was drawn in to sniff the aromas, almost as quaffing on a wine glass (see image on p. 229).

Experimental animation

Much of New Zealand animation today employs a moving visual collage technique, not as in collage film-making, but in a cut-and-paste approach in which disparate images and filmic sequences are juxtaposed against one another in productions that are amongst the most sophisticated and visually inventive work by Kiwi film artists.

Hamilton animator Dan Inglis utilizes the wide-screen 16.9 aspect ratio as a technological representation of the human field of vision to play with the idea of framed vision and how our contemporary world-view may be framed by technology.

Inglis's *Mind Your Eyes: Observations from a Flatbed Scanner* (2007) opens with a mechanical sound, a white rectangle enters from screen right and fills the frame in a scanning motion, the titles appear. We see spinning pairs of cans, keys, a barcode, feline paws, fabric then a radio. A scan reveals the radio's interior circuitry. A banana appears on a plate then is flanked by a knife and fork, another banana is peeled by a scan before later disintegrating. A succession of model animals nonchalantly drift across the screen then are followed by a flying pig before twin cameras fade into view, their lenses fixing on the viewer and with a click the film finishes.

As with Inglis's *Mind Your Eyes*, Jill Kennedy's *At Home with the Ants* (2009) also begins with a scanning motion from a photocopy or scanning device. We see a package labelled 'live animals'; a rat emerges from paper wrapping then is picked up by a human hand. The background photographic imagery advances toward a human house. Kennedy creates dark associations with the idea of sub-urbanity and nuclear families. The ants which we have been led to expect from the title seem to have become rats and they live in a suburban house. From suburbia we are transported to a strangely lush desert location then follow a flying insect back to a house interior. Here we see the cross-sectional view of a 'pet' ant nest. As a child looks into the nest a train unexpectedly rushes through the scene. Another train criss-crosses the sky. The train stops, multiplies then sets off again in the opposite direction but this time through a landscape. The camera pulls back to reveal a little boy holding a model train in front of a mock-up of an ant nest that looks to be a school project. Is it scientific or just something that was all on TV in the comfortable home of a happy family with their chirping caged bird and decapitated dog?

In *Freeks Formuler* (c.2007) James Robinson layers words upon words and images upon images in the manner of a graffiti-scrawled cinematic report on the movements of his consciousness. Like a moving visual rant, *Freeks Formuler* works as an explicit and organic revelation of the thinking and creative processes through which the artist realizes his singular vision.

Robinson's initial conception of *X.O. Genesis* (2009) was as a way of continuing his childhood obsession with making model spaceships, vessels which he later came to see as vehicles of consciousness, dreams, escapism and alienation.

X.O. Genesis, Robinson's collaboration with Rowan Wernham, is an interplanetary creation and destruction myth which could have begun, 'A long time ago in a galaxy far away.' Its humanoid inhabitants are subjected to information overload, pollution – as alien eco abortion – over consumption and surveillance, in a petro-chemical night which leads ultimately to war.

Our film artists ask questions of the relationship between humans and nature, alternative realities and spiritual states, perception, abstraction, notions of social justice and equality, as well as the exercise of their imaginative, intellectual and perceptual faculties. Theirs is work that speaks of an engaged, at times contentious relationship with life.

Martin Rumsby

Note
1. *Wabi* and *sabi* refer to aesthetic ideals that are particularly associated with Zen Buddhism … *wabi* evokes rather poignant nuances of sparseness and quiet understatement, even poverty, while *sabi* has a connotation of age, patina and loneliness.
2. A visual artist since the 1940s, Nicholson completed and released the *Visual Music Project* in 2008 when he was 93 years of age.

'PRINCIPLED PATRIOTISM': NUCLEAR IMAGES AND THE CURATION OF NATIONAL MEMORY

Funny how history turns out, isn't it? How it twists and tangles. Who would have thought that the country that gave birth to 'the father of the atom' would take such a strong lead in the campaign against nuclear weapons, power and propulsion? Or that what started as a radical protest would become a foundation stone of national identity?

(Journalist Tim Watkin in his 2012 introduction to
the NZ On Screen 'Nuclear-free New Zealand' collection)

'Nuclear plumes of burnt orange against a crisp blue sky.
The Rainbow Warrior – the Greenpeace protest boat – submerged in an oceanic grave
    after sabotage by French operatives.
Streams of Wellington protestors bearing placards against French nuclear testing in the
    Pacific
A sign that reads, 'We don't pee in the Atlantic, so don't shit up our Pacific.'

These are some of the images that evoke New Zealand's traumatic nuclear legacy. While there has been no nuclear testing in New Zealand itself, the country's national identity has become very much tied to a nuclear-free ethos. NZ On Screen, the online digital resource that promotes New Zealand's visual culture, affirmed this nuclear-free heritage through the launch of the 'Nuclear free New Zealand' collection in 2012. This commemorated the 25th anniversary of the New Zealand Nuclear Free Zone, Disarmament, and Arms Control Act 1987, which established New Zealand as a nuclear-free zone.

Film, television, news reports and music videos across four decades depict a strong stance and contribute to the body of New Zealand anti-nuclear visual culture. What emerges is a coherent anti-nuclear voice, generated across the multiple media platforms displayed in the collection. This essay reflects particularly on the role of film in this collection, as it most aptly demonstrates the diversity of screen productions which promote anti-nuclear sentiment.

The focus is on science fiction films *The Quiet Earth* (Geoff Murphy, 1986), and *Nutcase* (Roger Donaldson, 1980), and the 1988 documentary *Niuklia Fri Pasifik/A Nuclear Free Pacific*, directed by Lesley Stevens, and the sound performance group From Scratch's rhythmic 1993 experimental short *Pacific 3-2-1-Zero* (directed by Gregor Nicholas). These films, read individually and as part of the NZ On Screen collection, emphasize the ways in which the archive creates a popular 'ethical community by bring[ing] testifiers and testimonial witnesses together at the audiovisual interface' (Sarkar and Walker 2010: 1). The films use moving images to protest and testify against the use of nuclear weapons and nuclear power in the South Pacific and bear witness to the consequences. While the films span a number of different genres encompassing adult and children's science fiction, documentary, and experimental forms, together they demonstrate a prominent distrust of foreign political powers.

Nuclear-free is engrained in New Zealand's national consciousness, and the move towards anti-nuclear legislation played a significant role in developing strong national identity. This identity was solidified through a number of historical altercations with world superpowers. In 1985 New Zealand refused port entry to a potentially nuclear-abled US military ship, thus leading to the disintegration of the formal Australia, New Zealand and the United States military alliance ANZUS, founded in 1951 (for further discussion of the political implications, see Brown 1999). This culminated in 1987 legislation, which established New Zealand as nuclear-free. The impact of nuclear testing in our oceanic 'backyard' was also felt through the sustained history of nuclear testing in the Pacific. Both the United States and Britain had conducted extensive tests in the region post-World War II, but this ceased in 1963. However, the French shortly began intensive testing in the region after a move from Algeria, with fallout from atmospheric nuclear bombs impacting a number of Pacific locations, including Mangareva. French testing finally ceased and a Comprehensive Test Ban Treaty (CTBT) was signed in September 1996 (see Claudia Pond Eyley's 1997 insider's point of view). One of New Zealand's most traumatic events was the sinking of the Greenpeace protest boat, the Rainbow Warrior, in Auckland in July of 1985. The boat was destroyed by French secret operatives, with the intention of destroying it so it could not be used for further protests against French nuclear testing in Mururoa in French Polynesia. Such incidents and accompanying citizen and state protest within the country are indicative of a move in New Zealand toward a more localized, Pacific-centric ethos. This 'principled patriotism', to cite journalist Tim Watkin (2012), also manifests in audio-visual activist material that shows a mainstreaming of anti-nuclear sentiment. This mistrust of foreign political influence, particularly from France and the United States, serves as a strong ideological theme in a number of films in the NZ On Screen 'Nuclear-free New Zealand' collection.

NZ On Screen (www.nzonscreen.com) was launched in 2008 by NZ On Air as part of its digital media strategy, which seeks to disseminate content through a number of diverse channels. The site offers extensive curated material of New Zealand's cultural heritage in the form of archival film, television, music videos and practitioner profiles. As a result the site ensures media that may have limited screening are invested with an afterlife – especially important for stories controversial or peripheral in nature. According to NZ On Air's Digital Strategy, digital media creates 'extension and expansion […] allowing [our] stories to evolve, expand and develop in new directions' (2012). Artefacts of national memory are dematerialized due to the nature of NZ On Screen's digitality, thus demonstrating the convergence of historical collections with new media platforms.

However, the 'Nuclear-free New Zealand' collection also represents a successful transmediated approach to telling the nation's stories. The collection includes science fiction film (*The Quiet Earth*; *Nutcase*) co-existing with experimental film (*Pacific 3-2-1-Zero*) and documentary (including *A Nuclear Free Pacific*). However, these films are contextualized, expanded, (arguably) legitimized and situated historically and culturally through the collection's inclusion of links to televised key speeches and debates by political leaders, such as with former New Zealand Prime Minister David Lange's forceful Oxford Union debate against Reverend Jerry Falwell in March 1985, in which he insisted, 'nuclear weapons are morally indefensible' (Lange, 1985). This transmediated approach means that fiction and experimental film are shown to be critically vital in the nuclear-free debate. Indeed, the camp children's film *Nutcase*, with its French dominatrix-esque villain who threatens to explode a nuclear bomb in Auckland's volcanoes, seems all the more important as a nuclear-free ideology when read against Lange's speech.

Given that the 'internet [can be interpreted] as a vehicle of memory', as Ekaterina Haskins proposes, the collection ultimately reads as an official historiography and memorializing of and in the popular sphere (2007: 401). NZ On Screen legitimizes the anti-nuclear movement through the transmediated memory of digital space, although interestingly the site maintains an apolitical stance. While Haskins proposes the 'function of hyperlinking facilitates interconnectedness among different sources, producing a cacophonous heteroglossia of public expression' (2007: 405). Arguably in the NZ On Screen nuclear-free resources such hyperlinking is demonstrable of a unified expression of protest across not only media forms (for example, a 1995 reggae music video from the band Herbs; and unaired public service announcements by Spike Milligan from 1976) and media practices, but also through communities, both national and within the Pacific region (such as Peter Turei's 1988 television documentary *Hotu Painu*, which directly relates the bombing of the Rainbow Warrior with the suffering of Pacific peoples at the hands of the French). This may be the unexpected benefit of the 'nuclear-free' collection – while the repository seeks to promote New Zealand history and culture, the archive selection also results in a strong Pacific identity, which is characteristic of New Zealand's cultural identity.

In *Documentary Testimonies: Global Archives of Suffering*, Bhaskar Sarkar and Janet Walker argue the 'vocation of the archive is ethical' (2010: 5). While *Documentary Testimonies* focuses on grassroots testimonies of witnessing and suffering, their call to recognize the ethical dimension of media collection, dissemination and curation is useful in the context of NZ On Screen's 'Nuclear-free' collection. Sarkar and Walker's multidimensional investigation not only considers the role of citizen-led audio-visual testimony, but it also values the role state-funded agencies play in curating national and public memory. Sarkar and Walker suggest

> These archives [...] are benefiting from the emergence of new media technologies for the capture, assembly, storage, and circulation of the gathered materials. In our latter twentieth and twenty-first century 'era of witness,' media testimonial initiatives – be they official, grassroots, guerrilla, transitory, insistent, or any combination thereof – participate in the creation of ethical communities by bringing testifiers and testimonial witnesses together at the audiovisual interface. (2010: 1)

This ethical – and arguably moral – impetus to use media testimony as a critique of nuclear colonization is present in both the moving images themselves and the wider collection. The NZ On Screen collection includes selections where media makers act as political watchdogs and witnesses on *behalf* of other nations. For example, Gregor Nicholas's experimental short film *Pacific 3-2-1-Zero*, with the sound performance group From Scratch, offers a critical defence of a number of Pacific countries, which have been exposed to nuclear testing. The musical short, which shows rhythmic drumbeats and repetitive shouting of inhabitants of islands in the Pacific, including Mururoa (also known as Moruroa) and Fangataufa, depicts the ritualistic nature of protest. The title itself gives a sense of urgency, calling up a countdown to a bomb blast but also simultaneously is reminiscent of the vitality of protest call and response chants. Of note, From Scratch's activism extended to a live performance of *Pacific 3-2-1-Zero* in France when invited to perform there. Feeling like the performative protest was limited to a sympathetic art audience, the group re-performed the piece outside, amongst French citizens, in order to fully realize the activist dimension of the work (for a lively recounting of this event, see Nina Seja's 1999 documentary *Let the Earth Hum: Articulating Philip Dadson*).

Like *Pacific 3-2-1-Zero*, the documentary *Nuclear Free Pacific* also contributes to an explicit critique of the impact of testing in Pacific locales. The film offers a long history of the effects of nuclear testing in the Pacific. One of the strengths of the documentary is to localize and indigenize the experiences on the ground during tests. One subject on Tanna Island in Vanuatu, John Louhman, argues,

> The volcano is like the bomb that the French are testing at Mururoa. Mururoa is in the Pacific. If they continue testing, all our ground will be poisoned in the end. All our water will be poisoned, all our fish will be poisoned, eventually ruining life in the Pacific.

By including the film in the collection, the broader narration of New Zealand's nuclear-free identity moves further away from the historic political western alliance of ANZUS and locates New Zealand's nuclear-free identity as part of a local Pacific one.

However, while activism through documentary clearly sets out promotion of a nuclear-free Pacific, it is likewise important to see the activist contours of fiction film-making, which are also included in the NZ On Screen collection. Geoff Murphy's *The Quiet Earth*, and children's film *Nutcase* by Roger Donaldson, offer further claims for an anti-nuclear ideology. *The Quiet Earth* imagines the New Zealand after-effects of a disaster (which can be read as a metaphor for nuclear fallout) due to American-led scientific research gone wrong. The only apparent people to survive include Zac Hobson, who worked on the experiment, Joanne, and Api, a Maori man. The film offers extensive opportunities for analysis, including the growing triangulated hostility and sexual tension, which clearly highlights racial politics as Zac demands to be leader of the trio while Api challenges this white privilege (see, for example, Jonathan Rayner's discussion of the 'male landscape' in Geoff Murphy's work [2007: 152–68]). However, in the context of this focus on New Zealand's anti-nuclear stance in a global milieu, the role of the United States as a proponent of nuclear technology is historically significant.

The film alludes to the legacy of US nuclear testing in the Pacific – as co-writer and producer Sam Pillsbury states, 'It was about then me and some of my friends had what was called the peace squadron and would go out and blockade American nuclear boats that tried to get into Auckland Harbour' (Heinemann 2010). In the film, Zac believed that Project Flashlight, the experiment on which he was working, was not ready, so much so that his guilt led him to commit suicide at the time of the disaster (which was reversed during 'The Effect'). While Joanne argues that the experiment is gendered – 'an exclusive all-male club playing God with the universe' – Zac tries to displace blame by proposing, 'Besides, we might not have been responsible. God may have just blinked.' However, Zac also defends himself because of US dishonesty – 'The Americans withheld information […] we trusted them, they were on our side.'

A key theme in *The Quiet Earth* is the ethics of scientific development (and implicitly nuclear research) and the transparency surrounding such experiments. Mistrust is an undercurrent of the film, as the characters dance around intimacy and withdrawal, deciding in what ways to depend on the others. For example, referring to Zac, Api states, 'He tells lies.' However, while the trio learn to negotiate their ambivalence toward each other, a core message of the film is that external powers cannot be trusted. Zac states the experiment 'was an American idea'. While he could remove himself from all responsibility, he eventually takes full culpability by driving the truck loaded with dynamite in order to halt 'The Effect'. However, as the film demonstrates, it was the US that refused to stop the research, regardless of Zac's warnings. A sense of betrayal permeates the film, as the emptied streets and vanished victims are the outcomes of New Zealand being used for an 'American idea'. The film ultimately offers a meditation on the psychological cost of trusting a foreign power, which claims to be an ally.

The children's film *Nutcase*, directed by Roger Donaldson, reads as a campier rendition of *The Quiet Earth* – the failures of bureaucracy and authority mean nuclear obliteration looms. *Nutcase* – which should by all means attain cult status due to its indigenized *Rocky Horror Picture Show*-esque features – is an unlikely addition to the theme of political activism. What it does indicate, however, is that the anti-nuclear ethos is multigenerational. In the film, three children – backyard creators of an anti-gravity machine – save Auckland from nuclear obliteration. The female villain Evil Eva, a French faux-dominatrix in cat eyes make-up, tight black vinyl clothing and gold shoulder pads – threatens to drop a nuclear device into Auckland's volcanoes unless police pay her 5 million dollars. Through technological wizardry and sharp thinking, the children are the ones left to foil her plan, given the incompetence of the adults. The children's father, Chief Inspector Cobblestone, and his police team are incapacitated, stoned and left dancing like chickens on tables due to being secretly drugged with 'Happy Chappy Powder' by Evil Eva's goons.

In amongst the conga lines, stubbies-wearing, warbling rubbish collectors and the disco lights of the musical numbers, there exists a serious call that youth are the ones responsible for anti-nuclear activism. It is children who are the most plan-oriented, making forward movement to prevent certain death by bomb. While adult authority is incapable of realizing the severity of the situation, the group of children know that non-conventional means are the best way to circumvent disaster. In the climax of the film, grassroots action to stop the bomb takes the form of a swarm of children surrounding the villains, giving a clear interpretation of mass civic protest by the most vulnerable.

In an eerie precursor to the bombing of the Rainbow Warrior, Evil Eva is also French (or at least coded to be). One of Evil Eva's songs emphasizes this: 'As the world is turning and you're drifting in your sleep / my master plan is tick tick ticking and will go up with a bang / just like a mushroom in a cloudy sky. / You'll be okay if you obey.'

A key message from the film is the importance of being vigilant, particularly against those who appear foreign. The risk of not doing so is certain obliteration at the hands of outsiders who slip into the country unnoticed. Likewise, the foreigners' antipathy is not only toward institutions of power such as the police, but it also extends to children, who in fact pose more of a threat to the villains and who recognize the severity of the evil plan. While playful, the film is also ideological, emerging from a time in which the nuclear movement was gaining momentum. It is important to acknowledge that children's films can be politically credible. As Marc G Doucet argues, 'Children's popular films […] help to craft and restore certain perspectives for each new generation of young minds during the crucial years' (2005: 291). *Nutcase* orients the child viewer to broader global power structures, where New Zealand is at the mercy of (nuclear) violence from the French. 'Films are pedagogically powerful […] because they can help us teach International Relations,' Doucet suggests (2005: 290). Thus it is important to read *Nutcase* not only as a shimmying science fiction adventure, but one in which the juvenile learns to mistrust outsiders who seek to disrupt and destroy New Zealand's nuclear-free peace.

After the sabotage of the Rainbow Warrior, those considered allies – specifically Great Britain and the United States – feigned indifference. As David Lange states in another 'Nuclear-free' collection television documentary *Revolution* (John Carlaw, 1996), 'We never had a peep out of those people we were allegedly in a western alliance with.' This betrayal is present in the NZ On Screen collection, particularly *The Quiet Earth*. However, the anti-nuclear movement became a defining moment for New Zealand's cultural identity and self-determination. This, too, resonates in the archive – the wide-ranging films show we scrap, we plot and we fight against nuclear colonization. But they also demonstrate allegiance – disintegrating with former allies and rebuilding new ones in the great South Pacific.

Nina Seja

References

Brown, Bruce (ed.) (1999) *New Zealand in World Affairs III 1972–1990*, Wellington: Victoria University Press.

Doucet, Marc G (2005) 'Child's Play: The Political Imaginary of International Relations and Contemporary Popular Children's Films', *Global Society*, 19: 3, pp. 289–306.

Haskins, Ekaterina (2007) 'Between Archive and Participation: Public Memory in a Digital Age', *Rhetoric Society Quarterly*, 37, pp. 401–22.

Heinemann, Andreas (2010) '"The Quiet Earth" Interview,' *The Flicks Interviews*, http://www.flicks.co.nz/blog/amazing-interviews/the-quiet-earth-interview/. Accessed 20 January 2013.

Lange, David (1985). www.publicaddress.net/great-new -zealand-argument/nuclear-weapons-are-morally-indefensible/. Accessed 2 October 2013.

NZ On Air (2012) *NZ on Air Digital Strategy 2012–2015*, Wellington: NZ On Air.

Pond Eyley, Claudia (1997) Protest at Moruroa: First-hand Accounts from the New Zealand-based Flotilla, North Shore City: Tandem Press.

Rayner, Jonathan (2007) 'Embodying the Commercial: Genre and Cultural Affect in the Films of Geoff Murphy', in I Conrich and S Murray (eds), *New Zealand Filmmakers*, Detroit: Wayne State University Press, pp. 152–68.

Sarkar, Bhaskar and Walker, Janet (2010) 'Introduction: Moving Testimonies', in B Sarkar and J Walker (eds), *Documentary Testimonies: Global Archives of Suffering*, Routledge: New York and London, pp. 1–34

Watkin, Tim (2012) 'Background: How We Learned to Start Worrying and Loathe the Bomb', Nuclear-free New Zealand, NZ On Screen, http://www.nzonscreen.com/collection/nuclear-free-new-zealand/background. Accessed 20 January 2013.

Acknowledgements

Special thanks to Irene Gardiner at NZ On Screen for answering questions about the 'Nuclear-free New Zealand' collection.

EMERGING ASIAN NEW ZEALAND FILM-MAKERS IN NEW ZEALAND CINEMA

Since the arrival of Chinese immigrants with the nineteenth-century Gold Rush and Indian immigrants soon after them, New Zealand has become the home of many Asians from various parts of that vast continent. The Statistics New Zealand Census conducted in 2006 shows that Asians are one of the major ethnic groups in New Zealand consisting mainly of ethnic Chinese, Indian and Korean. There are also many immigrants from other parts of the world and Pacific Islanders who enhance the multicultural nuances of the New Zealand nation, despite New Zealand's officially bicultural policy implementation which privileges the relationship between Maori and Pakeha (European New Zealanders) in definitions of the nation's identity.

This 'multicultural' New Zealand has embedded several diasporas in its demographic composition.[1] One of the key elements in the formation of a diaspora or a diasporic community and its appearance in the demographic structure of a host country is through the immigrants' social, cultural, economic, educational and political practices. One of the main implications of this diasporic formation is the ability of migrants and their succeeding generations to be visible as a part of the creative and cultural production of the new homeland which enhances their involvement in social and political domains of the host society. In fact, some of the most creative sites for contemporary cultural production belongs to diasporic people where they 'are obliged to live together, struggle for space and speak across cultural languages' (Hall 2010: ix). The presence of the creative potential of diaspora is what Homi Bhabha (1994: 326) calls bringing 'newness […] into the world'. The cultural production of diaspora is, therefore, manifested in 'hybrid, syncretic and creolized cultural forms' as the result of intermingling and blending of cultural traditions (Hall 1989). Diasporic cultural products are more than mere recreations of traditions or a reproduction of social forms in a new place, because they are the creative product of experiences of living in a new place and conditions (Hall 1989).

The demographic shift in New Zealand's population and its increasingly multicultural composition especially in the largest city, Auckland, have also been reflected in the New Zealand film industry in the last decade. It is only recently that the members of the Asian diaspora in New Zealand have found a space in New Zealand cultural production and attracted public attention, such as Stephen Kang, the Korean New Zealand film-maker who received an award during Critics' Week at the Cannes Film Festival 2011 for his short film *Blue* (2011) and *My Wedding and Other Secrets* (2011), a romantic comedy feature directed by Roseanne Liang (a New Zealand-born Chinese) which reached number three in the New Zealand box office. Liang's and Kang's successes illustrate the public emergence of a new category in New Zealand cinema in which film-makers originating from the various Asian immigrant communities relate their own versions of life, experience and reality. This unrecognized but exciting body of work that I would call 'Asian New Zealand cinema', can be defined as an emerging body of films including both works by New Zealanders of Asian descent and New Zealand films producing images of Asian diasporic people.[2] These works include features, short films, documentaries and television series produced in New Zealand in the last few decades. The New Zealand Film Commission Act (1978) defines 'a New Zealand film' as the one with 'a New Zealand story'. Asian New Zealand films are the film-makers' 'New Zealand stories' that reflect upon the Asian diaspora and migratory and diasporic experiences of living in New Zealand by expressing various dimensions of contact and relationships with the host society and culture as well as the deterritorialized conditions and lives of diasporic individuals and communities.

Being able to speak of an 'Asian New Zealand' arena is a relatively recent possibility. In the 1990s, there were only a few migrant New Zealand film-makers. Among them there were two women film-makers of Asian descent: Helene Wong and Mandrika Rupa. Helene Wong has been described as the first New Zealand woman who brought a Chinese perspective to the New Zealand screen. She worked as a Development Consultant with the New Zealand Film Commission, also on a variety of television dramas and short and feature-length films, including *Illustrious Energy* (1998), Leon Narbey's acclaimed feature about Chinese gold miners in Otago, and a documentary for television, 'Footprints of the Dragon' (Helene Wong, 1994), for the series *An Immigrant Nation* (1994–1996) screened on TV One. Wong's personal reflection on her film-making journey in New Zealand, best describes the forces behind the emergence of Asian New Zealand film-makers today:

> Obviously, the majority culture dominates when it comes to types of films to be made or types of stories to be told. [The] New Zealand film industry started in the late 70s and probably it took 30 odd years for Roseanne's film [director of *My Wedding and Other Secrets*] to be made. So for two decades the focus was really on 'white New Zealand stories', and then bringing in Maori stories and then Pacific stories and Chinese (Asian) stories. If you were like me [a Chinese] born in New Zealand, you wouldn't make films but you would be watching anything other than your own faces on the screen […] not only you would accept what you would be seeing, you never even considered along with a lot of generations, *being* a filmmaker. (Helene Wong, personal communication, 21 February 2012)

In the first *Directory of World Cinema: Australia and New Zealand* (2010), Harriet Margolis reminds us that 'One would not know about [New Zealand] multiculturalism, though, from New Zealand films made prior to this century' (290). *Illustrious Energy* (1988) directed by Leon Narbey and *Broken English* (1997) directed by Gregor Nicolas were the only two features which incorporate New Zealand immigrant stories and 'provided pre-millennial images that suggested New Zealand's national stories might include people other than Maori, Islanders and Pakeha' (Margolis 2010: 290). The shift in the demographic population of New Zealand towards becoming more culturally diverse, and its manifestation in New Zealand film in the last decade is a new trend which has been created through the emergence of Asian New Zealand talents. The Asian talents in New Zealand have dared to dream of being film-makers – a cultural space in which they are able to create their own images and tell their own New Zealand stories. This can also be conceived as a new development that contributes in making the multicultural dimensions of contemporary New Zealand society more widely sensed, acknowledged and recognized. The paucity of film-making practices and resources by Asians in New Zealand in the past can be traced in the factors that caused Asian migration to New Zealand, chiefly for trade, economic and educational reasons. These also explain Wong's description of and positioning as a film-maker in the early stages of her career and that film (cultural) production by members of a diaspora is influenced by a relationship between socio-political forces and trajectories of diasporic consciousness. Asian parents in New Zealand may not have considered film-making as an occupation for the future of their children and instead wanted them to be doctors, lawyers, accountants and engineers integrated into the host society (Helene Wong, personal communication, 21 February 2012), and their children would not, therefore, consider other ways to form and maintain cultural identities inherited from their ethnic ancestors. This latter progress refers to a developmental stage when members of a diaspora start interacting with the question of identity and visibility after overcoming their preliminary financial and social struggles for survival in the new environment. The outcome is a cultural product, 'a film' in this case, or what Naficy, the theorist of accented cinema,[3] calls the film-maker's 'performativity of identity' (2001).

The second figure in the 1990s of Asian New Zealand film-making, Mandrika Rupa, introduces herself as an independent film-maker and social worker who utilizes the medium of film for personal and social expressions. Rupa was born in Gujarat, India and emigrated as a child with her family from an Indian village to Newton Gully, Auckland in 1960 (Mandrika Rupa, 20 February 2012, personal communication). In most of her short films, notably *Naya Zamana* (*Modern Times*, 1996), *Poonam* (1994) and her recent documentary *Hidden Apartheid: A Report on Caste Discrimination* (2011), Rupa gives priority to the class and caste system, arranged marriage, hybrid identities and gender issues (particularly women) and focuses on the social dimensions of diasporic communities and the effects that a new home has on their lives. Women in Rupa's films present themselves in a struggle to be free from the claustrophobic confinements of their inner and ethnic community and its prescriptions for their behaviour and identity.

Unlike Rupa who turns her lens on the problems faced by Indian immigrants living in the West, and creates representations which bear explicit nuances of identity politics, feminism, critical nationalism and global humanitarianism, Shuchi Kothari's films allude to the simple difficulties of daily life for common people who happen to be living in their new adopted land. Kothari is metaphoric and poetic in representing diasporic consciousness and the social circumstances of migrant life in New Zealand. Shuchi Kothari, originally from Ahmedabad, India, is an example of a film-maker who has both 'settled' in New Zealand and has managed to make her presence felt in New Zealand public culture. Kothari moved first to the United States and then to New Zealand in 1997, where she works as a lecturer in the Department of Film, Television and Media Studies, at the University of Auckland. Kothari and Sarina Pearson established a production company Nomadz Unlimited in 1999 that aimed to foster projects that reflect their nomadic experience. Pearson also migrated to New Zealand a long time ago and since then been involved with several projects mainly in collaboration with Kothari. Kothari's output may be divided into three categories: one category consists of short film, documentary, feature and TV series or episodes that incorporate representations of diasporic experiences and feature the Indian diaspora in New Zealand. She has previously been associated with the short films *Fleeting Beauty* (2005) directed by Virginia Pitts and which Kothari scripted and co-produced, *Clean Linen* (2007) written by Kothari and directed by Zia Mandviwalla (also a New Zealand film-maker of Indian origin), and her most acclaimed feature *Apron Strings* (2008) co-written with Dianne Taylor and directed by Sima Urale, the renowned Samoan New Zealand film-maker. In her documentary *A Taste of the Place: Stories of Food and Longing* (2001) co-directed by Susan Pointon and produced by Sarina Pearson, Kothari interviewed women from various diasporas in New Zealand. This is the nature of the second category of her output which includes the projects relating to more than one diaspora where Kothari plays various roles cooperating with creative artists and outputs of other diasporic communities in New Zealand; for instance her role as the executive producer of short film *Take 3* (2005), directed by Roseanne Liang (a New Zealand-born Chinese), which focuses on tokenism experienced by three actresses of Chinese origin going for a New Zealand audition. The third category includes film projects which seem not to have diasporic subjects but show Kothari's professional and personal connection to her homeland India while settled in New Zealand, such as the feature *Firaaq* (2008) which she co-scripted. *Firaaq* is an Indian film about the victimization of ordinary people after the 2002 violence in Gujarat, India.

Being involved with more than one diaspora is one the fascinating characteristics of diasporic film-making in New Zealand. Zia Mandviwalla, a New Zealander of Zoroastrian-Indian origin made her short film *Eating Sausage* (2008) about a Korean family and their challenges of settlement and displacement in New Zealand. Her short film *Night Shift*, which brought her recognition in 2012 at the Cannes Film Festival, tells a story of a Samoan woman and her mundane life and struggles as an airport cleaner. Similarly, *Coffee and Allah* (2007), which is about an Ethiopian Muslim woman in New Zealand, was written by Kothari, an Indian New Zealand scriptwriter and directed by Sima Urale, a Samoan New Zealand director. Urale also directed *Apron Strings* which features the Indian diaspora in New Zealand. The series *A Thousand Apologies*, which was aired on the national television channel TV3 in 2005, is a good example of a group of minority artists working together, among whom were Shuchi Kothari, Roseanne Liang, Angelin Loo (also the co-scriptwriter of *My Wedding and Other Secrets*) and Zia Mandviwalla. It is a satirical comedy of the diversity of the Asian experience in the New Zealand context. This admirably collaborative film process and cultural capital investing exercise in diasporic film-making in New Zealand is a significant observation of the above occurrence. It seems that the cast and crew, scriptwriter, producer, director; every link in the film production chain who belongs to or identifies with a minority group in New Zealand, feels internally and emotionally related to a film that showcases a diasporic subject.

The film-maker most successful in reaching mainstream audiences in this emerging category is Roseanne Liang already known to New Zealand audiences and film industry through her first documentary *Banana in a Nutshell* (2005), aired on national television, and the short film *Take 3* which had its premiere at the 2008 New Zealand International Film Festival (NZIFF). Liang gained fame in New Zealand cinema in 2011 as the director and co-writer of *My Wedding and Other Secrets*, co-written by the Chinese New Zealand script-writer Angeline Loo, and produced by Paul Davis and John Barnett from South Pacific Pictures New Zealand.

My Wedding and Other Secrets was developed as a romantic comedy and extended version of Liang's documentary and has been selected for several festivals. It is a story of a Chinese New Zealand girl, Emily Chu (played by a New Zealand actress of Chinese extraction, Michelle Ang), when she has to decide between love for her Chinese parents and her love for a Kiwi boy, James Harrison (played by popular New Zealand actor Matt Whelan). The film portrays the first and second generations of the Chinese diaspora in New Zealand and the conflicts that may arise in maintaining and negotiating the traditions and customs of their original culture with that of the new country. Though targeted at mainstream New Zealand audiences, there are several moments in the film, which can largely be felt and internalized on an emotional level by diasporic people identifying themselves with such dilemmas, issues and identities. *My Wedding and Other Secrets* is positively involved with the question of cultural identity and construction of Chinese (Asian) New Zealand identities. It draws attention to a Chinese-looking girl who speaks with a Kiwi accent and behaves like a Kiwi girl; however, her diasporic consciousness provides an awareness of difference. This sense of difference may appear from a very early age as can emblematically be observed in the film's opening when Emily as a child declines to eat Weet-Bix – typical Kiwi fare – for breakfast. At the end of the film, Emily is shown having her Chinese breakfast while

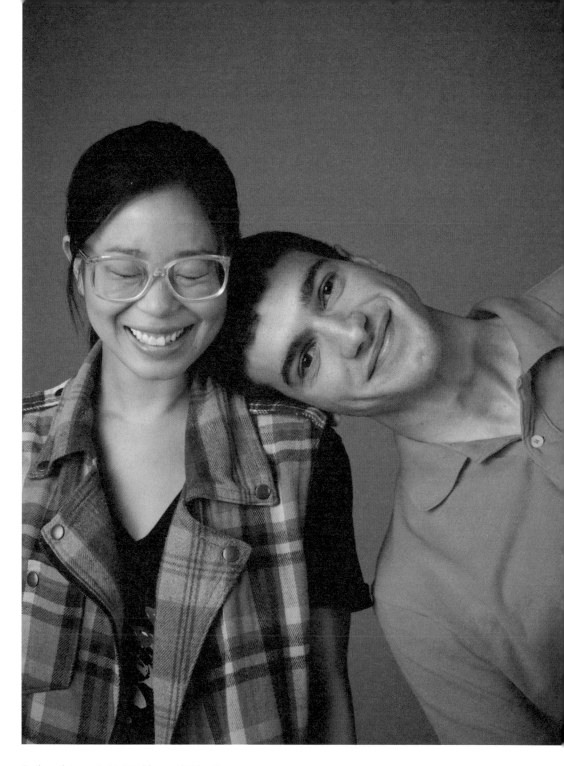

Emily and James in *My Wedding and Other Secrets*
(Roseanne Liang, 2011). Image courtesy of the director.

her Kiwi husband is enjoying his Weet-Bix at their home in Auckland. The sense of difference may also arise due to the language her family speaks at home, and the traditions they abide by. Emily's internal conflicts to decide to get married to her Kiwi boyfriend without her parents' knowledge, is an act or decision that Chinese culture (within the context of this film) would not approve such a girl to do. The film does not contemplate on how to reconcile the sense of difference and the ways it can be transformed to a harmonious whole, to feel belonging to two cultures. Nevertheless, it attempts to offer a unifying strategy through its narrative cliché of cross-cultural marriage and comedy genre. Embracing a charming romance summed up by the 'girl meets boy' structure, this film satisfies the audience through a happy ending (Zalipour 2011) – which initially made it compatible for a commercial and industrial mode of production.

Liang reminisces about her early experience of film-making in New Zealand and her thrill when she was approached by South Pacific Pictures to make *My Wedding and Other Secrets*:

> I really wanted to make something so I decided to turn the camera on myself and what that meant to me and I made the documentary *Banana in a Nutshell* […] I'd been talking about the project to a friend of mine, Alistair Kwun, and he said 'You really need to submit it to the New Zealand International Film Festival and then if you get in I will publicize it for you.' Amazingly, the film at the very early stages got accepted. In the screening of the documentary, lots of people wanted to share their own experiences that film had spoken to them about and John Barnett saw that. John Barnett of South Pacific Pictures strolls up to me, shakes my hand and says, 'Do you want to make a feature film of this movie?' […] In production of *My Wedding and Other Secrets*, I was very well taken care of. It was a tremendously charmed process for me. (Roseanne Liang, personal communication, 2 March 2012)

Liang's success with *Banana in a Nutshell*, the universality of its story, and more importantly its market potential were the reasons for John Barnett, a significant figure in the New Zealand film industry, to approach the young Chinese New Zealand director. Furthermore, as per Liang's account, the film's cultural value attracted Barnett who has been involved with many successful New Zealand films which feature different cultural voices, such as *Whale Rider* (Niki Caro, 2002) and *Sione's Wedding* (Simon Bennett, 2012).

Not all the emerging moments in the history of New Zealand cinema which have been created by Asian New Zealand film-makers are as charmed as that of Liang. Some of the film-makers in this category are independent film-makers and their film-making is driven by the film-maker's search for financial support. The 'smallness, imperfection, amateurishness, and lack of cinematic gloss' (Naficy 2001: 45) in diasporic film-making are the forces that shape and influence some of the existing films within the category of Asian New Zealand cinema. In other words, these isolated film-makers live on the periphery of the New Zealand film industry and in the face of cultural, logistical or funding challenges, are nevertheless managing to make their presence felt in mainstream New Zealand film culture.[4]

One example of the employment of an unorthodox mode of film production by Asian New Zealand film-makers due to insufficient funding and budget is in the 2007 feature film {Dream} Preserved by Stephen Kang, a Korean New Zealand film-maker. Kang spoke of the process he adopted in making this film as a 'one-man-production' (Stephen Kang, personal communication, 18 April 2012). {Dream} Preserved was screened in 2007 as part of the Desktop Cinema: 8 Recent New Zealand Digital

Features season. This film narrates the story of Mark and his fridge, which seems to be the only space he can claim – a place where he feels safe and has a sense of belonging. Mark's sense of loss, his ambivalent and unsettled life conditions, doing odd jobs such as standing in long queues at the New Zealand immigration office for other people, are portrayed in the story with an acrimonious tone that can be grasped from Mark's paranoid dreams and the open ending of the film – where he finds himself in a typical New Zealand field we saw at the start of the film. Kang's films deploy motifs of the struggles of immigrants to overcome their predicaments and obstacles of settlement in New Zealand through deterritorialization of identity, language, self and culture.

Kang, who is trying to find his voice in New Zealand cinema, has recently attracted local and international recognition with his short film *Blue* (2011). This occurred at the same time as the long awaited screening of his digital feature *Desert*, in the cinemas of Auckland. *Desert* was one of the low-budget moving-image projects which was supported by the final round of the 2009/2010 Independent Filmmakers Fund because it matched the IFF's 'emphasis on innovation, uniqueness and emerging talent' (NZFC 2010: 12).[5] While *Desert* did not manage to reach New Zealand audiences due to lack of distribution and screenings, it was nevertheless premiered at the Pusan International Film Festival in October 2010 and also selected as one of the three New Zealand films to screen in the Panorama section of the 14th Shanghai International Film Festival in June 2011.

Similar to Kang's previous feature, *Desert* is the story of unsettled conditions of life when the road taken does not promise a settled future, peace and security. Jenny, a young Korean girl living in New Zealand is baffled when she is left to fend for herself after being abandoned by her Kiwi boyfriend. The film cannot be called 'another' cross-cultural marriage but rather a journey to Jenny's mind and life when she has no one to count on in a foreign land; her Asian community also rejects her for the shame of getting pregnant to a westerner out of wedlock. *Desert* depicts the emptiness that one's soul can reach when the external sources are absent in a place where one cannot see many familiar faces.

Kang's New Zealand Film Commission (NZFC)-financed short film, *Blue*, produced by Tara Riddell, co-produced by Matt Noonan and Leanne Saunders, production of AKA Film and Curious Film, was the winner at the 50th Semaine De La Critique Grand Prix Canal and Du Meilleur Court Metrage Best Short Film at the Cannes Film Festival 2011. The short centres on a disillusioned character, Blue, a waiter in an Asian restaurant in New Zealand where he has to work hard to keep his job. He is depicted as being occasionally recognized from his popularity in a children's television show before migrating to the West; however, he is mostly ignored and forgotten now. Being reduced to a waiter, Blue symbolically can stand for many Asian artists who migrate to the West for better opportunities and are, indeed, left disillusioned about not being able to do what they have come for – art. Though *Blue* was shot in central Auckland, the film does not specify any particular country or nation for its protagonist, Blue, except that he is Asian (possibly Korean) and he is in a western country (possibly New Zealand). Kang describes Blue as representing anyone:

> A large number of immigrants here in New Zealand, make a living out of something that they have not done before. They start doing business in laundry, cleaning and restaurant in which they never had experienced before. This is because either they do not qualify in New Zealand to continue their original profession or simply due to the language barrier. (New Zealand Film Commission 2011)

The financial and logistic limitations and cultural and social constraints faced by young Asian New Zealand film-makers have led them to respond creatively to their deterritorialized conditions. Asian New Zealand film should not be located in authorship per se, nor film production or audiences but in the interstices of the New Zealand film industry and the society. My aim was to foreground an emerging group of Asian New Zealand films and film-makers that have delineated important aesthetic, cultural, social, gendered and political complexities over the last decade. It is an attempt to speak of the untapped terrain of New Zealand film history and national memory. Asian diasporic New Zealanders' cultural representations and production of themselves and by themselves create a platform for a negotiation of relationships that exist or emerge and the identities that are constructed in a multicultural or cross-cultural context, the relationships that may have been taken for granted or overlooked not because they were not significant, but because they never claimed any public space.

Arezou Zalipour

References

Bhabha, Homi (1994) *The Location of Culture*, London and New York: Routledge.

Hall, Stuart (1989) 'Ethnicity: Identity and difference', *Radical America*, 23: 4, pp. 9–20.

Hall, Stuart (2010) 'Foreward', in YR Isar and HK Anheier, *Cultures and Globalization Creativity and Art*, London: Sage, pp. ix–xii.

Margolis, Harriet (2010) 'Directors, Shuchi Kothari and multiculturalist New Zealand films', in B Goldsmith and G Lealand, *Directory of World Cinema: Australia and New Zealand*, Bristol: Intellect, pp. 290–93.

Naficy, Hamid (2001) *Accented Cinema: Exilic and Diasporic Filmmaking*, New Jersey: Princeton University Press.

NZFC (New Zealand Film Commission) (2010) *Annual Report*, http://www.nzfilm.co.nz/sites/nzfc/files/NZFC%20Annual%20Report%202009-10.pdf. Accessed 15 June 2012.

New Zealand Film Commission (NZFC) (2011) *Blue Press Kit*, http://www.nzfilm.co.nz/sites/nzfc/files/Blue%20Presskit%20-%202012.pdf. Accessed 3 December 2012.

Parliamentary Council Office (2011) *Immigration Act 1987*, http://www.legislation.govt.nz/act/public/1987/0074/latest/DLM108018.html. Accessed 23 August 2011.

Parliamentary Council Office (2005) *New Zealand Film Commission Act 1978*, http://www.legislation.govt.nz/act/public/1978/0061/latest/DLM22640.html. Accessed 23 August 2011.

Statistics New Zealand (2006) *2006 Census Data: Ethnic Groups in New Zealand*, http://www.stats.govt.nz/Census/2006CensusHomePage/QuickStats/quickstats-about-asubject/culture-and-identity/ethnic-groups-in-new-zealand.aspx. Accessed 25 June 2011.

Zalipour, Arezou (2011) '*My Wedding and Other Secrets*: A true story of women of the Asian diaspora in New Zealand' [Review], *Women's Studies Journal*, 25: 2, pp. 117–18.

Notes

1. The contemporary notion of diaspora refers to a population who voluntarily or involuntarily have left their countries and resided in a new land. Currently, the Asian diaspora in New Zealand consists of three main communities: the Chinese, Indian and Korean.

2. This definition is based on the findings of my current research project on 'The Asian Diaspora in New Zealand Film: Conceptualizing Asian New Zealand Cinema' commenced in May 2011 at the University of Waikato.

3. Diasporic film-making has been comprehensively discussed in Naficy's book: *Accented Cinema: Exilic and Diasporic Filmmaking* (2001). Theoretically, I would rather use 'diasporic cinema' or 'diasporic film' here as a generic term that includes Naficy's three types of accented films (for further information on this, see Arezou Zalipour's forthcoming publications on diasporic film and audiences).

4. Another example of this in New Zealand film is Rupa's recent documentary *Hidden Apartheid: A Report on Caste Discrimination* (2011) which was made mainly based on her own budget and financial help from her friends who love films as a medium of social and cultural articulation (Mandrika Rupa, personal communication, 20 February 2012).

5. The IFF, formerly Screen Innovation Production Fund, is a partnership between the NZFC and Creative New Zealand which was founded to support independent film-makers in New Zealand.

RECOMMENDED READING

Aveyard, Karina (2011) 'Australian Films at the Cinema: Rethinking the Role of Distribution and Exhibition', *Media International Australia*, 38, pp. 36–45.

Babington, Bruce (2007) *A History of the New Zealand Fiction Feature Film*, Manchester: Manchester University Press.

Barclay, Barry (1992) 'Amongst Landscapes', in Jonathan Dennis and Jan Bieringa (eds), *Film in Aotearoa New Zealand*, Wellington: Victoria University Press, pp. 116–29.

Barclay, Barry (2003) 'Celebrating Fourth Cinema', *Illusions*, 35, pp. 7–11.

Bartlett, Myke (2010) 'Sex, Violence and Cultural Anxiety: *Tomorrow when the War Began*', *Screen Education*, 60, pp. 113–18.

Becchio, Penny (2006) 'Interview with Brian Trenchard-Smith', *Metro*, 149, pp. 174–77.

Bennet, James and Rebecca Beirne (2011) *Making Film and Television Histories: Australia and New Zealand*, London: Tauris.

Bertrand, Ina (1978) *Film Censorship in Australia*, St Lucia: University of Queensland Press.

Bertrand, Ina (ed.) (1989) *Cinema in Australia: A Documentary History*, Kensington, NSW: University of New South Wales Press.

Bertrand, Ina (1999) 'The Anzac and *The Sentimental Bloke*: Australian Culture and Screen Representations of World War One' in Michael Paris (ed.) *The First World War and Popular Cinema: 1914 to the Present*, Edinburgh: Edinburgh University Press, pp. 74–95.

Bertrand, Ina (2004) '"Good Taste at Hanging Rock"? Historical Nostalgia in the Films of the Australian Revival', *Metro*, 140, pp. 42–7.

NDED

Blackwood, Gemma (2007) 'Wolf Creek: An UnAustralian Story?', Continuum: Journal of Media & Cultural Studies, 21:4, pp. 489–97.

Blythe, Martin (1994), Naming the Other: Images of the Maori in New Zealand Film and Television, Metuchen, NJ: Scarecrow Press.

Bradbury, Keith (2001) 'Australian and New Zealand Animation', in Lent, J. (ed.), Animation in Asia and the Pacific, Bloomington and Indianapolis: Indiana University Press.

Brodie, Ian (2006) A Journey Through New Zealand Film, Auckland: HarperCollins.

Brophy, Philip (2008) The Adventures of Priscilla, Queen of the Desert, Australian Screen Classics series, Sydney: Currency Press.

Buckley, Anthony (2009) Beyond a Velvet Light Trap: A Filmmaker's Journey from Cinesound to Cannes, Prahan, Vic: Hardie Grant.

Bullock, Emily (2011) 'Rumblings from Australia's Deep South: Tasmanian Gothic On-screen', Studies in Australasian Cinema, 5: 1, pp. 71–80.

Burnside, Sarah (2011) 'Red Dog Whitewashes The Pilbara', New Matilda, 16 August, http://newmatilda.com. Accessed 12 November 2012.

Burton, Geoff and Raffaele Caputo (eds) (1999) Second Take: Australian Film-Makers Talk, St Leonards, NSW: Allen & Unwin.

Burton, Geoff and Raffaele Caputo (eds) (2002) Third Take: Australian Film-Makers Talk, St Leonards, NSW: Allen & Unwin.

Butterss, Philip (2000) 'Australian Masculinity on the Road', Media International Australia, 95, pp. 227–36.

Cairns, Barbara and Helen Martin (1994) Shadows on the Wall: A Study of Seven New Zealand Feature Films, Auckland: Longman Paul.

Cameron, Allan (2010) 'The Locals and the Global: Transnational Currents in Contemporary New Zealand Horror', Studies in Australasian Cinema, 4: 1, pp. 55–72.

Cao, Benito (2012) 'Beyond Empire: Australian Cinematic Identity in the Twenty-First Century', *Studies in Australasian Cinema*, 6: 3, pp. 239–50.

Caputo, Raffaele (1995) 'The Animated Features of Yoram Gross', in Scott Murray (ed.), *Australian Film 1978–1994*, Melbourne: Oxford University Press, pp. 398–400.

Chan, Queenie Monica (2008) 'Reconstructing Images of History: Christopher Doyle, *Rabbit-Proof Fence* and Postcolonial Collage', *Studies in Australasian Cinema*, 2: 2, pp. 121–40.

Chauvel, Charles (1938) *Screen tests for Errol Flynn and Mary Maguire and the grooming for stardom of Betty Pike and Patricia Firth*, Sydney: Expeditionary Films, http://www.nfsa.gov.au/site_media/uploads/file/2011/12/05/NFSA_Charles_Chauvel_amended.pdf. Accessed 3 January 2013.

Churchman, Geoffrey B (ed.) (1997) *Celluloid Dreams: A Century of Film in New Zealand*, Wellington: IPL Books.

Collins, Felicity (2008) 'Historical Fiction and the Allegorical Truth of Colonial Violence in *The Proposition*', *Cultural Studies Review*, 14: 1, pp. 55–71.

Collins, Felicity and Therese Davis (2004) *Australian Cinema After Mabo*, Cambridge, UK: Cambridge University Press.

Conor, Brigid (2011) 'Problems in "Welliwood": Rethinking the Politics of Transnational Cultural', *LabourFlow TV*, 13 (7), 27 January, http://flowtv.org/2011/01/problems-in-wellywood/. Accessed 23 February 2012.

Conor, Liz (2010) 'A Nation So Ill-Begotten: Racialized Childhood and Conceptions of National Belonging in Xavier Herbert's *Poor Fellow My Country* and Baz Luhrmann's *Australia*', *Studies in Australasian Cinema*, 4: 2, pp. 97–113.

Conrich, Ian and Stuart Murray (eds) (2007) *New Zealand Filmmakers*, Detroit: Wayne State University Press.

Conrich, Ian and Stuart Murray (2008) *Contemporary New Zealand Cinema: From New Wave to Blockbuster*, London: I. B. Taurus.

Coyle, Rebecca (ed.) (2005) *Reel Tracks: Australian Feature Film Music and Cultural Identities*, Eastleigh: John Libbey.

Craven, Allison (2011) 'Dual Occupancy: Melbourne and the Feminist Drama of Dwelling in *Monkey Grip*', *Studies in Australasian Cinema*, 5: 3, pp. 333–342.

Craven, Allison (2013) 'Heritage Enigmatic: The Silence of the Dubbed in *Jedda* and *The Irishman*', *Studies in Australasian Cinema*, 7: 1, pp. 23–34.

Craven, Ian (ed.) (2001) *Australian Cinema in the 1990s*, London: Frank Cass.

Crimmings, Emma and Rhys Graham (2004) *Short Site: Recent Australian Short Film*, Melbourne: Australian Centre for the Moving Image.

Cunningham, Stuart (1991) *Featuring Australia: The Cinema of Charles Chauvel*, Sydney: Allen & Unwin.

Dalziell, Tanya (2009) 'Gunpowder and Gardens: Reading Women in *The Proposition*,' *Studies in Australasian Cinema* 3:1, pp. 121–31.

Delamoir, Jeanette (2004) 'The First "Gum-Leaf Mafia": Australians in Hollywood, 1915–25', *Screening the Past*, 16, http://tlweb.latrobe.edu.au/humanities/screeningthepast/firstrelease/fr_16/jdfr16.html. Accessed 10 May 2013.

Dennis, Jonathan and Jan Bieringa (eds) (1996) *Film in Aotearoa New Zealand*, Wellington: Victoria University Press.

Dermody, Susan (1980) 'Action and Adventure', in Scott Murray (ed.), *The New Australian Cinema*, West Melbourne: Thomas Nelson Australia, pp. 79–95.

Dermody, Susan and Elizabeth Jacka (1987) *The Screening of Australia: Anatomy of a Film Industry*, Paddington: Currency Press.

Dermody, Susan and Elizabeth Jacka (1988a) *The Screening of Australia: Anatomy of a National Cinema*, Paddington: Currency Press.

Dermody, Susan and Elizabeth Jacka (1988b) *The Imaginary Industry: Australian Film in the Late 1980s*, North Ryde, NSW: Australian Film, Television and Radio School.

Dixon, Robert (2009) 'Peter Carey's and Ray Lawrence's *Bliss* (1985): Fiction, Film and Power', *Studies in Australasian Cinema*, 3: 3, pp. 279–94.

Dunleavy, Trisha and Hester Joyce (2011) *New Zealand Film and Television: Institution, Industry and Cultural Change*, Bristol: Intellect.

Edwards, Sam and Helen Martin (1997) *New Zealand Film 1912–1996*, Auckland: Oxford University Press.

Eisenberg, Daniel (2011) 'Shooting Cinematic Outlaws: Ned Kelly and Jesse James as Viewed Through Film', *Studies in Australasian Cinema*, 5: 2, pp. 145–54.

Ellis, Katie (2006) 'Rehabilitating 1990s Australian National Cinema', *Senses of Cinema*, 39, http://sensesofcinema.com/2006/39/rehab_australian_cinema_1990s/. Accessed 5 November 2012.

Formica, Serena (2011) 'When It All Started: Politics and Policies of the Australian Film Industry from the Revival to the International Breakthrough', *Studies in Australasian Cinema*, 5: 1, pp. 43–57.

Fox, Alistair (2011) *Jane Campion: Authorship and Personal Cinema*, Bloomington and Indianapolis: Indiana University Press.

Fox, Alistair, Radner, Hilary and Barry Keith Grant (eds) (2011) *New Zealand Cinema: Interpreting the Past*, Bristol: Intellect.

French, Lisa (ed.) (2003) *Womenvision, Women and the Moving Image In Australia*, Melbourne: Damned Publishing.

French, Lisa (2009) 'Poetry In Motion: The Short Film Form In Australia', in Amit Sarwal and Reema Sarwal, (eds.) *Creative Nation: Australian Cinema and Cultural Studies Reader*, SSS Publications: New Delhi, pp. 83–98.

French, Lisa and Mark Poole (2009) *Shining a Light: 50 Years of the Australian Film Institute*, The Moving Image no. 9, St Kilda: Australian Teachers of Media.

Fresno-Calleja, Paloma (2011) 'Reel New Zealanders: Contesting Tokenism and Ethnic Stereotyping in Roseanne Liang's *Take 3*', *Studies in Australasian Cinema*, 5: 1, pp. 19–29.

Gallasch, Keith (2007) *Dreaming in Motion: Celebrating Australia's Indigenous Filmmakers*, Sydney: Australian Film Commission.

Gaunson, Stephen (2010) 'International Outlaws: Tony Richardson, Mick Jagger and Ned Kelly', *Studies in Australasian Cinema*, 4: 3, pp. 255–65.

Gaunson, Stephen (2012) 'Australian (Inter)national Cinema: The Royal Commission on the Moving Picture Industry in Australia, 1926–1928, Australasian Films Ltd. and the American Monopoly' *Studies in Australasian Cinema*, 6: 3, pp. 291–300.

Gibson, Ross (1992) *South of the West: Postcolonialism and the Narrative Construction of Australia*, Bloomington and Indianapolis: Indiana University Press.

Gillard, Garry (2007) *Ten Types of Australian Film*, Perth: Murdoch University.

Gillett, Sue (2004) *Views from Beyond the Mirror: The Films of Jane Campion*, St Kilda: Australian Teachers of Media.

Goldsmith, Ben (1997) 'Government, Film and the National Image: Reappraising the Australian Film Development Corporation', *Australian Studies* 12: 1, pp.98–114.

Goldsmith, Ben (2009) 'Settings, Subjects and Stories: Creating Australian Cinema', in Amit Sarwal and Reema Sarwal (eds) *Creative Nation: Australian Cinema and Cultural Studies*, New Delhi: SSS Publications, pp. 13–26.

Goldsmith, Ben (2010a) 'Introduction: Australian Cinema', in Ben Goldsmith and Geoff Lealand (eds), *Directory of World Cinema: Australia and New Zealand*, Bristol: Intellect, pp. 9–21.

Goldsmith, Ben (2010b) 'Outward-looking Australian Cinema', *Studies in Australasian Cinema*, 4: 3, pp. 199–214.

Goldsmith, Ben and Geoff Lealand (eds) (2010) *Directory of World Cinema: Australia and New Zealand*, Bristol: Intellect.

Goldsmith, Ben and Tom O'Regan (2005) *The Film Studio: Film Production in the Global Economy*, Lanham: Rowman and Littlefield.

Goldsmith, Ben, Ward, Susan and Tom O'Regan (2010) *Local Hollywood: Global Film Production and the Gold Coast*, Brisbane: University of Queensland Press.

Gottschall, Kristina (2011) '"Trashing the Suburban Streets": Learning about "Bad" Youth With/in *Idiot Box* and *Suburban Mayhem*', *Studies in Australasian Cinema*, 5: 3, pp. 293–306.

Hall, Ken G (1977) *Directed by Ken G. Hall: Autobiography of an Australian film-maker*, Melbourne: Lansdowne Press.

Hall, Sandra (1985) *Critical Business: The New Australian Cinema in Review*, Adelaide: Rigby.

Hamilton, Peter and Sue Mathews (1986) *American Dreams, Australian Movies*, Sydney: Currency Press.

Handel, Jonathan with Pip Bulbeck (2013) *The New Zealand Hobbit Crisis: How Warner Bros. Bent a Government to Its Will and Crushed an Attempt to Unionize 'The Hobbit'*, Los Angeles: Hollywood Analytics.

Harding, Bruce (2011) '"The Donations of History": *Mauri* and the Transfigured "Māori Gaze": Towards a Bi-national Cinema in Aotearoa', in Alistair Fox, Hilary Radner and Barry Keith Grant (eds), *New Zealand Cinema:Interpreting the Past*, Bristol: Intellect, pp. 218–37.

Hardy, Ann (2012) 'Hidden Gods – Religion, Spirituality and Recent New Zealand Cinema', *Studies in Australasian Cinema*, 6: 1, pp. 11–27.

Harris, Hilary (2006) 'Desert Training for Whites: Australian Road Movies', *Journal of Australian Studies*, 29: 86, pp. 99–110.

Helms, Michael (1998) '*Dark City*' [interview with Andrew Mason and Alex Proyas], *Cinema Papers*, 124, pp. 18–21.

Hocking, Scott (ed.) (2006) *100 Greatest Films of Australian Cinema*, Richmond, Vic: Scribal Publishing.

Hoeveler, Diane Long (1998) 'Silence, Sex, and Feminism: An Examination of *The Piano*'s Unacknowledged Sources', *Literature/Film Quarterly*, 26: 2, pp. 109–16.

Hoskins, Dave (2011) 'Familiar Territory: *Red Hill* Rides into Town', *Metro*, 167, pp. 12–15.

Isaacs, Bruce (2009) 'The Birth of a Nation: Living on the Land in *Lucky Country*', *Metro*, 161, pp. 36–40.

Jayamanne, Laleen (2010) 'The Drover's Wives and Camp Couture: Baz Luhrmann's Preposterous National Epic', *Studies in Australasian Cinema*, 4: 2, pp. 131–43.

Jennings, Karen (1993) *Sites of Difference: Cinematic Representations of Aboriginality and Gender*, Melbourne, Vic.: Australian Film Institute, Research and Information Centre.

Johinke, Rebecca (2009) 'Not Quite Mad Max: Brian Trenchard-Smith's Dead End Drive-In', *Studies in Australasian Cinema*, 3: 3, pp. 309–18.

Kevin, Catherine (2010) 'Solving the Problem of the Motherless Indigenous Child in *Jedda* and *Australia*: White Maternal Desire in the Australian epic Before and After *Bringing Them Home*', *Studies in Australasian Cinema*, 4: 2, pp. 145–57.

Kevin, Tony (2010) 'Australian Invasion Anxiety in Adolescent Fantasy', *Eureka Street*, 20: 17, pp. 8–9.

Khoo, Olivia (2010) 'Tokyo Drifting: Toei Corporation's *The Drifting Avenger* and the Internationalization of the Australian Western', *Studies in Australasian Cinema*, 4: 3, pp. 231–41.

Khorana, Sukhmani (2012) 'Film Festivals and Beyond: Activist Discourses in the Reception of *Samson and Delilah* and *The Tall Man*', *Studies in Australasian Cinema*, 6: 2, pp. 217–227.

Kunze, Peter C (2013) 'Out in the Outback: Queering Nationalism in Australian Film Comedy', *Studies in Australasian Cinema*, 7: 1, pp. 49–59.

Lagerberg, Robert and Andrew McGregor (2012) 'Inside the Outside: Aspirations of Authenticity in the Representation of Lebanese-Australian Youth in Serhat Caradee's *Cedar Boys*', *Studies in Australasian Cinema*, 6: 3, pp. 251–61.

Landman, Jane (2006) *The Tread of a White Man's Foot: Australian Pacific Colonialism and the Cinema, 1925–1962*, Canberra: Pandanus Books.

Langton, Marcia (1993) *Well, I Heard It On the Radio and I Saw It On the Television…: An Essay for the Australian Film Commission on the Politics and Aesthetics of Filmmaking By and About Aboriginal People and Things*, Woolloomooloo: Australian Film Commission.

Lent, John A (ed.) (2001) *Animation in Asia and the Pacific*, Bloomington and Indianapolis: Indiana University Press.

Leotta, Alfio (2009) 'Framing the Beach: A Tourist Reading of *The Piano*', *Studies in Australasian Cinema*, 3: 3, pp. 229–38.

Leotta, Alfio (2011) *Touring the Screen: Tourism and New Zealand Film Geographies*, Bristol: Intellect.

Levy, Wayne (1995) *The Book of the Film, and the Film of the Book: A Bibliography of Australian Cinema and TV 1895–1995*, Melbourne: Academia Press.

Limbrick, Peter (2007) 'The Australian Western, or A Settler Colonial Cinema Par Excellence', *Cinema Journal*, 46, pp. 68–95.

Lucas, Rose (1998) 'Dragging it Out: Tales of Masculinity in Australian Cinema, from *Crocodile Dundee* to *The Adventures of Priscilla, Queen of the Desert*', *Journal of Australian Studies*, 22: 56, pp. 138–46.

Malone, Peter (ed.) (2001) *Myth & Meaning: Australian Film Directors In Their Own Words*, Strawberry Hills: Currency Press.

Malone, Peter (2012) 'Thinking about *Far East*', *Studies in Australasian Cinema*, 6: 1, pp. 87–96.

Margolis, Harriet (2010) 'Directors, Shuchi Kothari and Multiculturalist New Zealand Films', in Ben Goldsmith and Geoff Lealand (eds), *Directory of World Cinema: Australia and New Zealand*, Bristol: Intellect, pp. 290–93.

Marsh, Pauline (2012) 'The Primitive, the Sacred and the Stoned in Richard J Frankland's *Stone Bros.*', *Studies in Australasian Cinema*, 6: 1, pp. 29–43.

Martin, Adrian (2003) *The Mad Max Movies*, Sydney: Currency Press.

Martin, Adrian (2010) 'Ozploitation Compared to What? A Challenge to Contemporary Australian Film Studies', *Studies in Australasian Cinema*, 4: 1, pp. 9–21.

Martin, Helen and Sam Edwards (1997) *New Zealand Film, 1912–1996*, Oxford, Melbourne and Auckland: Oxford University Press.

Mayer, Geoff (1983) 'Turkey Shoot', *Cinema Papers*, 42, pp. 69–71.

Mayer, Geoff and Keith Beattie (2007) *The Cinema of Australia and New Zealand*, London: Wallflower.

McCredden, Lyn (2012) '*Ten Canoes*: Engaging Difference', *Studies in Australasian Cinema*, 6: 1, pp. 45–56.

McDonald, Neil (2002) 'Getting It Right – Damien Parer, Osmar White and Chester Wilmot on The Kokoda Track', *The Sydney Papers*, 14: 2, pp. 96–1109.

McDouall, Hamish (2009) *100 Essential New Zealand Films*, Wellington: Awa Press.

McFarlane, Brian (1980) 'Horror and Suspense', in Scott Murray (ed.), *The New Australian Cinema*, West Melbourne: Nelson.

McFarlane, Brian (1987) *Australian Cinema 1970–85*, Melbourne: William Heinemann Australia.

McFarlane, Brian (2009) 'Genres and Generalities' *Meanjin*, 68: 1, pp. 79–84.

McFarlane, Brian and Geoff Mayer (1992) *New Australian Cinema: Sources and Parallels in American and British Film*, Cambridge: Cambridge University Press.

McFarlane, Brian, Mayer, Geoff and Ina Bertrand (eds) (1999) *The Oxford Companion to Australian Film*, Melbourne and New York: Oxford University Press.

McGregor, Andrew (2010) *Film Criticism as Cultural Fantasy: The Perpetual French Discovery of Australian Cinema*, Bern: Peter Lang.

McHugh, Kathleen (2007) *Jane Campion*, Urbana and Chicago: University of Illinois Press.

McKinnon, Scott (2011) 'The Emerald City of Oz: The City of Sydney as a Gay Space in Australian Feature Films', *Studies in Australasian Cinema*, 5: 3, pp. 307–19.

McMullen, Sean (2010) 'Science fiction and Fantasy', in Ben Goldsmith and Geoff Lealand (eds), *Directory of World Cinema: Australian and New Zealand*, Bristol: Intellect, pp. 224–35.

Mills, Jane (2012) *Australian Screen Classics: Jedda*, Strawberry Hills, NSW: Currency Press.

Milner, Johnny (2013) 'Australian Gothic Soundscapes: *The Proposition*', *Media International Australia*, 148, pp. 94–106.

Mita, Merata (1996) 'The Soul and the Image', in Jonathan Dennis and Jan Bieringa (eds) *Film in Aotearoa New Zealand*, Wellington: Victoria University Press, pp. 36–54.

Mitchell, Robert (2010) 'My Interview with Brian Trenchard-Smith', http://soldierofcinema.blogspot.com.au/2010/12/my-interview-with-brian-trenchard-smith.html. Accessed 17 October 2012.

Mitchell, Tony (1985) 'A Dangerous Independent: An Interview with Merata Mita', *Filmviews Quarterly*, 124, pp. 6–7.

Molloy, Bruce (1990) *Before the Interval: Australian Mythology and Feature Films, 1930–1960*, St Lucia: University of Queensland Press.

Moore, Tony (2005) *The Barry McKenzie Films*, Sydney: Currency Press.

Moran, Albert (1991) *Projecting Australia: Government Film Since 1945*, Sydney: Currency Press.

Moran, Albert (ed.) (1993) *Film Policy: An Australian Reader*, Brisbane: Institute for Cultural Policy Studies.

Moran, Albert and Tom O'Regan (eds) (1985) *An Australian Film Reader*, Sydney: Currency Press.

Moran, Albert and Tom O'Regan (eds) (1989) *The Australian Screen*, Ringwood, Vic: Penguin.

Moran, Albert and Errol Vieth (2005) *Historical Dictionary of Australian and New Zealand Cinema*, Lanham, MD: Scarecrow.

Moran, Albert and Errol Vieth (2006) *Film in Australia: An introduction*, Cambridge, UK: Cambridge University Press.

Morgan, Stephen (2011) 'Woolloomooloo or Wapping? Critical Responses to *The Sentimental Bloke* in 1920s London and the Normalization of the Inner-City Working Class', *Studies in Australasian Cinema*, 5: 3, pp. 321–32.

Morton, John (2010) 'Redeeming the Bastard Child: Exploring Legitimacy and Contradiction in *Australia*', *Studies in Australasian Cinema*, 4: 2, pp. 159–72.

Murray, Scott (ed.) (1980) *The New Australian Cinema*, West Melbourne: Thomas Nelson.

Murray, Scott (ed.) (1994) *Australian Cinema*, North Sydney: Allen and Unwin, in association with the Australian Film Commission.

Murray, Scott (ed.) (1995) *Australian Film 1978–1994: A Survey of Theatrical Features*, Melbourne: Oxford University Press in association with the Australian Film Commission.

Murray, Stuart (2007a) 'Activism, community and governance: Barry Barclay's *The Kaipara Affair* (2005)', *Studies in Australasian Cinema*, 1: 2, pp. 147–59.

Murray, Stuart (2007b) 'Images of Dignity: The Films of Barry Barclay', in Ian Condrich and Stuart Murray (eds), *New Zealand Filmmakers*, Detroit: Wayne State University Press, pp. 88–102.

Nowra, Louis (2003) *Walkabout*, Australian Screen Classics series, Sydney: Currency Press.

O'Regan, Tom (1996) *Australian National Cinema*, London and New York: Routledge.

O'Regan, Tom and Rama Venkataswamy (1999) 'A Tale of Two Cities: *Dark City* and *Babe: Pig in the City*', in Deb Verhoeven (ed.), *Twin Peeks: Australian and New Zealand Feature Films*, Melbourne: Damned Publishing, pp. 187–203.

Peters, Geraldene (2007) 'Lives of Their Own: Films by Merata Mita', in Ian Conrich and Stuart Murray (eds), *New Zealand Filmmakers*, Detroit: Wayne State University Press, 2007, pp. 103–20.

Petrie, Duncan (2007) *Shot in New Zealand: The Art and Craft of the New Zealand Cinematographer*, Auckland: Random House.

Pihama, Leonie (2000) 'Ebony and Ivory: Constructions of Maori in *The Piano*', in Harriet Margolis (ed.), *Jane Campion's 'The Piano'*, Cambridge: Cambridge University Press, pp. 114–34.

Pike, Andrew and Ross Cooper (1998 [1980]) *Australian Film, 1900–1977: A Guide to Feature Film Production*, Melbourne: Oxford University Press.

Pivac, Diane, Stark, Frank and Lawrence McDonald (eds) (2011) *New Zealand Film: An Illustrated History*, Wellington: Te Papa Press.

Polan, Dana (2001) *Jane Campion*, London: BFI.

Porter, Eric and Ray Edmondson (1976) 'Eric Porter interviewed by Ray Edmondson' [sound recording], Australia: National Library Australia, http://nla.gov.au/nla.oh-vn4610506. Accessed 1 October 2013.

Probyn, Fiona (2005) 'An Ethics of Following and the No Road Film: Trackers, Followers and Fanatics', *Australian Humanities Review*, http://www.australianhumanitiesreview.org/archive/Issue-December-2005/Probyn.html. Accessed 1 October 2013.

Radner, Hilary, Fox, Alistair and Irène Bessière (eds) (2009) *Jane Campion: Cinema, Nation, Identity*, Detroit: Wayne State University Press.

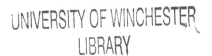

Rattigan, Neil (1991) *Images of Australia: 100 Films of the New Australian Cinema*, Dallas: Southern Methodist University Press.

Rayner, Jonathan (2000) *Contemporary Australian Cinema: An Introduction*, Manchester and New York: Manchester University Press.

Rayner, Jonathan (2007) 'Embodying the Commercial: Genre and Cultural Affect in the Films of Geoff Murphy', in Ian Conrich and Stuart Murray (eds), *New Zealand Filmmakers*, Detroit: Wayne State University Press, pp. 152–68.

Rayner, Jonathan (2009) 'Adapting Australian Film: Ray Lawrence from *Bliss* to *Jindabyne*', *Studies in Australasian Cinema*, 3: 3, pp. 295–308.

Reade, Eric (1971) *History and Heartburn: The Saga of Australian Film 1896–1978*, Sydney: Harper and Row.

Reis, Brian (1997) *Australian Film: A Bibliography*, London: Mansell.

Reynaud, Daniel (1999) 'Convention and Contradiction: Representations of Women in Australian War Films 1914–1918', *Australian Historical Studies*, 29: 113, pp. 215–30.

Reynaud, Daniel (2005) *The Hero of the Dardanelles and Other World War I Silent Dramas*, Canberra: Research and Academic Outreach National Film and Sound Archive Monographs.

Reynaud, Daniel (2007) *Celluloid ANZACs: The Great War Through Australian Cinema*, Melbourne: Australian Scholarly Publishing.

Reynaud, Daniel (2010) 'War', in Ben Goldsmith and Geoff Lealand (eds), *Directory of World Cinema: Australia and New Zealand*, Bristol: Intellect, pp. 102–13.

Robertson, Pamela (1997) 'Home and Away: Friends of Dorothy on the Road in Oz', in Steven Cohan and Ina Rae Hark (eds), *The Road Movie Book*, London and New York: Routledge, pp. 271–86.

Robson, Jocelyn and Beverley Zalcock (1997) *Girls' Own Stories: Australian and New Zealand Women's Films*, London: Scarlet Press.

Routt, William D (1989) 'The Fairest Child of the Motherland: Colonialism and Family in Australian Films of the 1920s and 1930s', in Albert Moran and Tom O'Regan (eds), *The Australian Screen*, Ringwood: Penguin, pp. 28–52.

Routt, WD (2003) 'Bush Westerns? The Lost Genre' [lecture delivered at the Australian Centre for the Moving Image], Melbourne, 3 February, http://www.routt.net/Bill/BushWesterns.htm. Accessed 12 September 2012.

Rutherford, Leonie (2003) 'Australian Animation Aesthetics', *The Lion and the Unicorn*, 27: 2, pp. 251–51.

Ryan, Mark David (2008) *A Dark New World: Anatomy Of Australian Horror Films*, PhD dissertation, Queensland University of Technology, Brisbane. http://eprints.qut.edu.au/18351/1/Thesis.pdf. Accessed 1 October 2013.

Ryan, Mark David (2008) 'Writing Aussie horror: An interview with Shayne Armstrong and Shane Krause', *Metro*, 159, pp. 46–48.

Ryan, Mark David (2009) 'Whither Culture? Australian Horror Films And The Limitations Of Cultural Policy', *Media International Australia, Incorporating Culture and Policy*, 133, pp. 43–55.

Ryan, Mark David (2010a) 'Australian Cinema's Dark Sun: The Boom In Australian Horror Film Production', *Studies in Australasian Cinema*, 4: 1, pp. 23–41.

Ryan, Mark David (2010b) 'Towards An Understanding Of Australian Genre Cinema And Entertainment: Beyond The Limitations Of "Ozploitation" Discourse', *Continuum: Journal of Media & Cultural Studies*, 24: 6, pp. 843–54.

Ryan, Mark David (2012) 'A Silver Bullet For Australian Cinema? Genre Movies And The Audience Debate', *Studies in Australasian Cinema*, 6: 2, pp. 141–57.

Sabine, James (ed.) (1995) *A Century of Australian Cinema*, Port Melbourne, Victoria: William Heinemann.

Screen Australia (2011) *Convergence 2011: Australian Content State of Play: Informing Debate*, Sydney: Screen Australia.

Screen Australia (2012) 'Number of Australian and overseas films released in Australian cinemas 1984–2011', http://www.screenaustralia.gov.au/research/statistics/ wcfilmxcountry.asp. Accessed 13 October 2012.

Shelton, Lindsay (2005) *The Selling of New Zealand Movies*, Wellington: Awa Press.

Shirley, Graham and Brian Adams (1989) *Australian Cinema: The First Eighty Years*, Sydney: Currency Press.

Sibley, Brian (2006), *Peter Jackson: A Film-Makers Journey*, London: HarperCollins.

Sigley, Simon (2013) *Transnational Film Culture in New Zealand*, Bristol: Intellect.

Simmons, Rochelle (2013) 'Suburban Metropolis: The City in Peter Wells' Cinema', *Studies in Australasian Cinema*, 7: 1, pp. 77–86.

Simpson, Catherine (2010) 'Australian Eco-Horror and Gaia's Revenge: Animals, Eco-Nationalism and the New Nature', *Studies in Australasian Cinema*, 4: 1, pp. 43–54.

Simpson, Catherine, Murawska, Renata and Anthony Lambert (eds) (2009) *Diasporas of Australian Cinema*, Bristol and Chicago: Intellect.

Smaill, Belinda (2013) 'Asianness and Aboriginality in Australian Cinema', *Quarterly Review of Film and Video,* 30: 1, pp. 89–102.

Sowry, Clive (1984), *Film Making in New Zealand: A Brief Historical Survey*, Wellington: New Zealand Film Archive.

Speed, Lesley (2008) 'The Comedian Comedies: George Wallace's 1930s Comedies, Australian Cinema and Hollywood', *Metro*, 158, pp. 76–82.

Stadler, Jane and Peta Mitchell (2010) 'Never-Never Land: Affective Landscapes, the Touristic Gaze and Heterotopic Space in *Australia*', *Studies in Australasian Cinema*, 4: 2, pp. 173–87.

Starosielski, Nicole (2011) '"Movements that are Drawn": A History of Environmental Animation from *The Lorax* to *FernGully* to *Avatar*', *International Communication Gazette*, 73: 1–2, pp. 145–63.

Stockwell, Stephen (2011) 'Crime Capital of Australia: The Gold Coast on Screen', *Studies in Australasian Cinema*, 5: 3, pp. 281–92.

Stratton, David (1980) *The Last New Wave: The Australian Film Revival*, London, Sydney: Angus and Robertson.

Stratton, David (1990) *The Avocado Plantation: Boom and Bust in the Australian Film Industry*, Chippendale, NSW: Pan Macmillan.

Sunderland, Sophie (2012) 'Grieving Secularism: Jane Campion's Secular Daughters in Spiritual Spaces', *Studies in Australasian Cinema*, 6: 1, pp. 73–85.

Thomas, Deborah (2009) 'Tarantino's Two-Thumbs up: Ozploitation and the Reframing of the Aussie Genre Film', *Metro*, 161, pp. 90–95.

Thoms, Albie (1985) 'Ken Hall', in Albert Moran and Tom O'Regan (eds), *An Australian Film Reader*, Sydney: Currency Press, pp. 48–54.

Thornley, Davinia (2012) 'Maori Identity By Way of New Zealand Film or Why "I Don't Have to be a Particular Skin Colour to Feel Beige"', *Studies in Australasian Cinema*, 6: 2, pp. 203–15.

Torre, Dan and Lienors Torre (2009) 'Recording Australian Animation History', *Animation Studies–Animated Dialogues 2007*, pp. 115–24.

Treacey, Mia (2000) 'Bitumen, Dirt Tracks and Lost Highways – Australian Road Movies – A Select Bibliography and Filmography,' *Metro*, 124/25, pp. 144–51.

Tulloch, John (1981) *Legends on the Screen: The Narrative Film in Australia 1919–1929*, Sydney: Currency Press, Australian Film Institute.

Tulloch, John (1982) *Australian Cinema: Industry, Narrative and Meaning*, Sydney: George Allen & Unwin.

Turcotte, Gerry (1998) 'Australian Gothic', in Mulvey Roberts (ed.), *The Handbook to Gothic Literature*, Basingstoke: Macmillan.

Turner, Graeme (1986) *National Fictions: Literature, Film, and the Construction of Australian Narrative*, Sydney: Allen & Unwin.

Turner, Graeme (1997) 'Australian Film and National Identity in the 1990s', in Geoffrey Stokes (ed.) *The Politics of Identity in Australia*, Melbourne: Cambridge University Press, pp. 185–92.

Venkatasawmy, Rama, Simpson, Catherine and Tanja Visosevic (2001), 'From Sand to Bitumen, From Bushrangers to Bogans: Mapping the Australian Road Movie, *Journal of Australian Studies*, 25: 70, pp. 75–84.

Verevis, Constantine (2010) 'Dead on Arrival: The Fate of Australian Film Noir', *Studies in Australasian Cinema*, 4: 3, pp. 243–53.

Verhoeven, Deb (ed.) (1999) *Twin Peeks: Australian and New Zealand Feature Films*, Melbourne: Damned Publishing.

Verhoeven, Deb (2006) *Sheep and the Australian Cinema*, Carlton: Melbourne University Press.

Verhoeven, Deb (2009) *Jane Campion*, London: Routledge.

Verhoeven, Deb (2010) 'It Was An Experience That Totally Blew Up In My Face: Steve Railsback and *Turkey Shoot*', *Studies in Australasian Cinema*, 4: 1, pp. 73–79.

Wexman, Virgina Wright (ed.) (1999) *Jane Campion: Interviews*, Jackson: University Press of Mississippi.

White, David (1984) *Australian Movies to the World: The International Success of Australian Films Since 1970*, Sydney and Melbourne: Fontana Australia and Cinema Papers.

Wiles, Mary M (2010) '"A Gentle Voice in a Noisy Room": An Interview with New Zealand Filmmaker Gaylene Preston', *Senses of Cinema*, 58, http://www.sensesofcinema. com/2010/feature-articles/%E2%80%9Ca-gentle-voice-in-a-noisy-room%E2%80%9D-an-interview-with-new-zealand-filmmaker-gaylene-preston/. Accessed 2 October 2013.

Williams, Deane (2007) '*The Overlanders*: Between Nations', *Studies in Australasian Cinema*, 1: 1, pp. 79–89.

Williams, Marise (2009) 'The White Woman's Burden: Whiteness and the Neo-Colonialist Historical Imagination in *The Proposition*', *Studies in Australasian Cinema*, 3: 3, pp. 265–78.

Zimmermann, S (2012) 'I suppose it has to come to this ... How a Western Shaped Australia's Identity', in T Klein, I Ritzer and PW Schulze (eds), *Crossing Frontiers: Intercultural Perspectives on the Western*, Marburg: Schüren Verlag.

AUSTRALIA &
NEW ZEALAND
CINEMA
ONLINE

AUSTRALIAN CINEMA ONLINE

Asian Australian Cinema
http://asianaustraliancinema.org
   This website was set up to accompany a research project on the history of Asian Australian
   cinema conducted by Audrey Yue (University of Melbourne), Belinda Smaill (Monash
   University) and Olivia Khoo (Monash University). The website contains information on over 500
   films, 499 directors and 620 production companies. The project has also produced a book,
   Transnational Australian Cinema by Audrey Yue, Belinda Smaill and Olivia Khoo, published by
   Lexington Books in 2013.

Australian Centre for the Moving Image
http://www.acmi.net.au/default.aspx
   ACMI evolved from the Victorian State Film Centre to become a major cultural venue in
   Melbourne dedicated to the moving image – cinema, television and digital culture. The
   Centre hosts exhibitions, film festivals, live events, educational programs and creative
   workshops. ACMI is also a major archive, with substantial holdings of film prints and related
   materials.

Australian Cinematographers' Society
http://www.cinematographer.org.au/home
   The ACS is the professional association for Australian cinematographers. The website
   contains information about the society, technological developments and discussion of the
   past and present of Australian cinema from a cinematographer's perspective. See also
   The Shadowcatchers, a website to accompany the ACS-sponsored book on the history of
   cinematography in Australia – http://www.shadowcatchers.com.au.

Australian Directors' Guild
http://www.adg.org.au
   The ADG (formerly the Australian Screen Directors' Association) is the professional association
   for film, television and digital media directors, documentary makers, animators, assistant
   directors and independent producers. The website contains information about events of
   interest to members including the guild's annual conference, news and resources for directors.

Australian Film Critics Association
http://www.afca.org.au
> AFCA is a professional association for film critics, film reviewers and film journalists. The Association hosts annual Film Writing Awards, and annual Film Awards, as well as hosting events in support of the Australian film industry and international screen culture. The site includes reports on film festivals around the world.

Australian Film Institute/Australian Academy of Cinema and Television Arts
http://www.aacta.org
> Founded in 1958, the AFI/AACTA is Australia's foremost screen culture organization. The website contains information about the annual AFI/AACTA Awards, Australian films currently screening in cinemas and a collection of short films available for viewing by members. AACTA also hosts a blog – http://blogafi.org.

Australian Film Institute Research Collection
http://www.afiresearch.rmit.edu.au/
> The Australian Film Institute Research Collection is a non-lending, specialist film and television industry archive. The Collection is open to the public and housed at RMIT University in Melbourne. The website contains information about the collection, and a searchable catalogue.

Australian Film, Television and Radio School
http://www.aftrs.edu.au
> The AFTRS is the national centre for professional education and advanced training in film, broadcasting and interactive media for Australian citizens and permanent residents. The school's main campus is at Moore Park in Sydney, adjacent to the Fox Studios Australia site. The school also has offices in each Australian state. The website contains information about current courses, research and events, news about the achievements of alumni, video and audio content, and the searchable catalogue of the Jerzy Toeplitz library which contains a large collection of scripts, books, magazines and journals on Australian and international cinema.

Australian Film Trailers
http://www.youtube.com/playlist?list=PL931D34363575F35D
> YouTube channel maintained by Screen Australia containing trailers of Australian films currently or recently in cinema release.

Australian Screen
http://aso.gov.au/
> Australian Screen is an outreach program of the National Film and Sound Archive. The site provides access to information and educational resources about Australian film and television, including excerpts from a broad range of feature films, documentaries, television programs, newsreels, short films, animations and home movies. Many of the entries are accompanied by teachers' notes to enable their use in secondary and tertiary programs.

The Cinema and Theatre Historical Society
http://www.caths.org.au/
> CATHS is a non-profit organization dedicated to the history of cinemas and theatres in Australia. The website contains a database of current and former cinemas and theatres, and information on meetings and events.

Culture and Communication Reading Room
http://wwwmcc.murdoch.edu.au/ReadingRoom/
> This website, developed by students at Murdoch University, is no longer updated, but is still a valuable archive of writing, reviews and analyses of Australian film, radio and television, cultural policy and cultural studies.

Currency Press: Australian Screen Classics
http://www.currency.com.au/australian-screen-classics.aspx
> Website for the book series 'Australian Screen Classics', in which leading critics and scholars critically analyse selected Australian feature films. Each book focuses on a single film, with titles including *The Adventures of Priscilla Queen of the Desert*, the Mad Max movies, *Walkabout* and *The Piano*. The website contains information and brief extracts from each title in the series.

Directory of World Cinema
http://worldcinemadirectory.org/
> The website for the Directory of World Cinema series featuring film reviews and biographies of directors. It is an ideal starting point for students of world cinema.

Encore Magazine
http://encore.com.au
> Founded in 1983, *Encore* Magazine is one of Australia's leading media and marketing publications. It has recently become available in free Android and iPad editions.

Film Ink
http://www.filmink.com.au
> *Film Ink* is a monthly Australian film magazine. The website contains news, features and reviews, as well as a blog and a 'Videos' section that includes trailers and short documentaries on current films.

Inside Film
http://www.if.com.au
> *Inside Film* is a monthly magazine that covers the production, distribution and exhibition of Australian films, as well as technological developments. The website contains news stories, employment information, video content and information about Australian films currently in production.

Metro
www.metromagazine.com.au
> A site for the glossy magazines *Metro* and *Screen Education*, published by the Australian Teachers of Media (ATOM). Both magazines regularly feature in-depth analysis of Australian and New Zealand films and television. Over the last few years, each issue of *Metro* has featured a long article on one of the films in the National Film and Sound Archive Kodak/Atlab collection of 50 Australian feature films that have been restored to a quality superior to their original release prints. The full list of films is at http://www.nfsa.gov.au/collection/film/film-partnerships/kodakatlab/.

National Film and Sound Archive
http://www.nfsa.gov.au/
> The NFSA is Australia's principal audio-visual archive, based in Canberra. The website contains information about the Archive's national screening and access programs, information about preservation activities, educational and online learning resources, and a searchable catalogue of the Archive's collection of over 1.3 million items.

Popcorn Taxi
http://www.popcorntaxi.com.au
  Popcorn Taxi regularly hosts events, screenings and Q&As, mostly in Sydney, with leading local and international film personalities. The website includes information on forthcoming events, transcripts of past events, and a blog containing feature articles and reviews on Australian and international cinema.

Roadshow Entertainment
http://www.roadshow.com.au
  The website for leading Australian screen entertainment company Village Roadshow contains news and videos relating to content the company has produced or is distributing, as well as links to corporate information.

Rouge
http://www.rouge.com.au
  Online journal edited by Helen Bandis, Adrian Martin and Grant McDonald. Irregular volumes (the last in 2009) containing fascinating articles on world cinema.

Screen Australia
http://www.screenaustralia.gov.au/
  Screen Australia is the principal federal government agency assisting the production, promotion, development and distribution of Australian films, documentaries and television programs. The agency was formed in 2008 following the merger of the former agencies the Australian Film Commission, the Film Finance Corporation, and Film Australia. The agency also conducts research and collects statistics on aspects of Australian film, television and animation, with much of this work published online via the annual *National Production Survey*, and the regularly updated statistical service *Get the Picture*.

Screen Hub
http://www.screenhub.com.au
  Screen Hub is a subscription-based service for industry professionals and researchers. The site provides news about the industry in Australia and overseas, and regular jobs and events bulletins.

Screening the Past
http://www.latrobe.edu.au/screeningthepast/
  Screening the Past is an international refereed online journal of screen history. The journal publishes articles on all aspects of world cinema history, with a particular interest in Australian cinema and screen culture.

Screen Producers Association of Australia
http://www.spaa.org.au/
  SPAA is the principal association for screen producers in Australia. It plays an active role in advocacy and policy, negotiates industrial agreements and commercial arrangements, and holds an annual conference in November each year. Website contains information on current activities, copies of submissions to government and details of industrial agreements, terms of trade, tax arrangements, and more.

Senses of Cinema
http://www.sensesofcinema.com
  Senses of Cinema is an Australian-based online journal of cinema. The journal includes articles on all aspects of world cinema, though it has a particular interest in Australian cinema past and present. The journal also focuses on particular films or bodies of work

(through articles and regular sections 'Cteq Annotations' and 'Great Directors'), as well as on film theory and philosophy, and reports on film festivals.

The Society of Australian Film Pioneers
http://cinemapioneers.com.au/
    The SAFP is a non-profit association dedicated to the recognition of people who have worked in the Australian film industry.

Studies in Australasian Cinema
http://www.tandfonline.com/loi/rsau20#.VH--18mjj78
    Studies in Australasian Cinema is an academic journal published by Taylor and Francis. The publication provides an important forum for the critical discussion of all aspects of cinema from Australia, New Zealand and the Pacific region. The journal focuses upon postcolonial and political contexts as well as issues around production, distribution/ exhibition and reception.

Urban Cinefile
http://www.urbancinefile.com.au
    Website covering world cinema, from an Australian perspective. The site is edited by Australian critic and film writer Andrew Urban, and contains news and reviews of films and DVDs released in Australia (including over 400 reviews of Australian films), interviews with film-makers and competitions.

Women in Film and Television
http://www.wift.org/index.html
    WIFT was founded in 1982 to support women working in the screen industries in Australia. The website contains information about membership, the annual WOW Festival, a calendar of events and information about the Mentor Scheme, a program established to provide opportunities for women entering the screen industries to gain professional mentoring, with the aim of redressing the gender imbalance in Australian film and television.

NEW ZEALAND CINEMA ONLINE

Cinemas of New Zealand
http://cinemasofnz.info
    Geoff Lealand's site about the many arthouse/independent cinemas in New Zealand. Includes full information on cinemas, as well as discussions of film distribution and film audiences.

Film New Zealand
http://www.filmnz.com/default.aspx
    Film New Zealand is New Zealand's international film business agency. Oriented principally towards international film-makers wanting to work in New Zealand, the site contains information on current New Zealand film policies and incentives, general information about New Zealand, a guide to New Zealand's screen production industry, industry contacts and a gallery of film locations.

Illusions
http://www.illusions.org.nz
> A fairly rudimentary online version of the New Zealand print journal, which is dedicated to scholarly criticism of New Zealand moving image and performing arts sectors.

The Lumiere Reader
http://www.lumiere.net.nz/
> *The Lumiere Reader* is New Zealand's leading online journal of film and arts criticism. Website includes commentary and editorials, features, interviews, reviews and essays on cinema in New Zealand and abroad.

Maori Television Service
http://www.maoritelevision.com
> Dual language (Maori and English) site promoting the two state-funded, free-to-air channels which were established in 2003 to promote and sustain Maori language and culture. The channels often feature New Zealand and foreign films and television, from non-traditional sources, and are generally regarded as essential parts of the New Zealand mediascape.

The New Zealand Film Archive
http://www.filmarchive.org.nz/
> The Film Archive is the home of New Zealand's moving image history with over 150,000 titles spanning feature films, documentaries, short films, home movies, newsreels, TV programmes and advertisements.

New Zealand Film Commission
http://www.nzfilm.co.nz/
> NZ Film is the principal New Zealand film financing and development agency. The website contains news of locally-made film, box office statistics, teaching resources, information on funding opportunities, past funding decisions, career development resources, distribution advice, information for international film-makers wanting to work in New Zealand, a monthly industry bulletin, and trailers and synopses for many new and recent New Zealand films.

New Zealand: Home of Middle Earth
http://www.nzhomeofmiddleearth.com/
> All you ever wanted to know and more about the production of the Hobbit films, the contributions made by people across New Zealand, and the impact of the films and their production on the country.

New Zealand Journal of Media Studies
www.nzmediastudies.org.nz
> A scholarly online journal which sometimes includes film analysis.

New Zealand On Air
http://www.nzonair.govt.nz
> Government-funded agency which finances local television programming, public service radio and New Zealand-made music. Often invests in local film-making, in the expectation that such films will get television screenings.

NZ On Screen
http://www.nzonscreen.com/
> *NZ On Screen* is the online showcase of New Zealand film, television and music video. The website offers access to the back catalogue of the best of New Zealand-produced film and television, for both local and overseas users. Content is arranged under themes, and contains full-length short films, television programs and music videos, excerpts and trailers from New Zealand feature films, video interviews with leading New Zealand film-makers, a user-generated locations map, all accompanied by detailed notes and commentaries. The new companion site *Audio Culture* – www.audioculture.co.nz – describes itself as 'The noisy library of New Zealand music'.

Onfilm
http://www.onfilm.co.nz
> Website for the long-established, monthly print magazine for the New Zealand screen industry, with features, profiles and full in-production details. The site features supplementary material to the magazine. The *Onfilm* site appears to have been archived from 2013.

Screen Directors Guild of New Zealand
http://www.sdgnz.co.nz/
> Website for the New Zealand directors' guild.

Screen Production and Development Association
http://www.spada.co.nz/home/home.html
> SPADA is an advocate for independent New Zealand screen practitioners, provides training opportunities and hosts events. The website contains links and resources, with more information and resources available for members.

The Sorta Unofficial New Zealand Film Awards
http://www.nzfilmawards.co.nz/
> New Zealand Film Awards – the Moas – resurrected by passionate film folk after the demise of the Aotearoa Film and Television Awards. Site contains information on winners, and full-length video of previous awards ceremonies.

1. Name the two Australian directors who won the Camera d'Or at the Cannes Film Festival in 2009 and 2010.

2. What breed was *Red Dog*, and what was the name of the dog that played him?

3. Which renowned Australian cinematographer is the subject of Cathy Henkel's documentary *Show Me the Magic* (2013)?

4. Who played the starring roles in *Charlie & Boots*, and where does their road trip take them?

5. What is the term coined by Stuart Cunningham in his biography of Charles Chauvel to describe on-location production designed to showcase the Australian landscape?

6. Where was Errol Flynn born?

7. What was the name of the short film for which Jane Campion won the Palme d'Or in 1986?

8. What number(s) was the last issue of *Cantrills Filmnotes*?

9. Was Ken G Hall (a) Director and Producer; (b) Writer and Director; (c) Writer and Editor; or (d) Producer and Editor of *Kokoda Front Line*, the first Australian film to win an Academy Award?

10. What did Brian Trenchard-Smith describe as 'the universal currency of the movie market'?

11. Which two films, released on the same day in 1983, featured Nicole Kidman in her first big screen roles?

12. What was the first film made under the official Australia-China co-production agreement?

13. Which valuable commodity did 'Sharkeye' Kelly discover in the highlands of New Guinea at the start of *Walk into Paradise*?

14. What is the title and who was the director of Australia's first animated feature film?

15. Which character has the last line of dialogue spoken in *Babe*, and what is it?

16. Which late 1980s television series, which also ran for six years as a breakfast radio show, is the common link between comedian comedies *The Castle*, *Bad Eggs* and *Kath and Kimderella*?

17. What is the name of the dating show in *The Craic*, and where do Fergus and Margo travel to for their date?

18. What is the name of the company for which the eponymous *Kenny* works?

19. At which film festival did *Animal Kingdom* win the Jury Prize in 2010?

20. Who is the screenwriter and main actor of David Field's *The Combination*?

21. How does Jimmy lose $10,000 in *Two Hands*?

22. Who are the Hobyahs in Ann Turner's *Celia*?

23. Which short film directed by Roman Polanski was one of the inspirations for Jane Campion's *The Piano*?

24. Who or what did director Greg McLean say was the 'fifth main character' in *Wolf Creek*?

25. Kimble Rendall, director of *Bait*, was a guitarist in which iconic Australian rock band?

26. What, according to Stephan Elliot, writer/director of *The Adventures of Priscilla: Queen of the Desert*, is the 'key to all road trips'?

27. What is the name of Alex Proyas's 1981 student film that foreshadowed the themes and style of *Dark City*?

28. Where have Nazis been hiding for over seventy years in *Iron Sky*?

29. Name the eight types of Australian suspense thriller identified by Albert Moran and Errol Vieth?

30. What is the subject of the title character's quest in David Nettheim's *The Hunter*?

31. What was the name of the Sydney anti-development campaigner and newspaper publisher whose disappearance in 1975 is referenced in both Donald Crombie's *The Killing of Angel Street* and Phillip Noyce's *Heatwave*?

32. Which film about World War II marked Russell Crowe's feature film debut?

33. Which World War I battle is the focus of Simon Wincer's *The Lighthorsemen*, and when did the battle take place?

34. What causes the injury to the father, Nat, which presages tragedy in Kriv Stenders's Australian western *Lucky Country*?

35. Name the two characters played by Kirk Douglas in George Miller's *The Man from Snowy River*?

36. What role does NZ On Air play in New Zealand film production?

37. Who directed *River Queen*?

38. Jane Campion's most recent *Top of the Lake* series for television was filmed where?

39. *The Orator* is the first feature film made in what language?

40. What 1997 mockumentary featured an early collaboration between Peter Jackson and Costa Botes?

41. Roseanne Liang's *My Wedding and Other Secrets* explored what aspects of contemporary New Zealand life?

42. Name one of New Zealand film-maker Annie Goldson's political documentaries?

43. What is the primary funding source for documentary production in New Zealand?

44. Who directed the New Zealand documentary *The Feathers of Peace*?

45. Name the director of *Boy*, one of New Zealand's most successful films.

46. Where did New Zealand documentary film-maker Cecil Holmes go on to for a later career?

47. Who and what is the subject of Gaylene Preston's *Home By Christmas*?

48. Name New Zealand director Christine Jeff's first American film?

49. Who directed the New Zealand feature film *The Strength of Water*?

50. What is the central premise of Geoff Murphy's New Zealand feature *The Quiet Earth*?

answers on next page

Answers

1. Warwick Thornton (*Samson and Delilah*), Michael Rowe (*Leap Year*).
2. Kelpie; Koko.
3. Don McAlpine.
4. Paul Hogan ('Charlie'), Shane Jacobson ('Boots'); they drive from Victoria up the eastern coast of Australia to Cape York.
5. Locationism.
6. Hobart, Tasmania.
7. *Peel*.
8. 93–100.
9. (d) Producer and Editor.
10. Action.
11. *BMX Bandits* and *Bush Christmas*.
12. Mario Andreacchio's *The Dragon Pearl*.
13. Oil.
14. *Marco Polo Jnr Versus the Red Dragon*; Eric Porter.
15. Farmer Hoggett, 'That'll do, Pig. That'll do.'
16. *The D-Generation*.
17. 'The Meet Market'; the Gold Coast.
18. Splashdown.
19. Sundance.
20. George Basha.
21. The money is stolen while Jimmy goes for a swim at Bondi Beach.
22. The Hobyahs are monsters in a fairy tale.
23. *Two Men and a Wardrobe*.
24. The Australian landscape.
25. The Hoodoo Gurus.
26. 'Don't stay on the main roads.'
27. *Strange Residues*.
28. The dark side of the moon.
29. Erotic thriller; 'thriller of acquired identity'; 'psychotraumatic thriller'; 'thriller of moral confrontation'; 'innocent-on-the-run'; 'thriller of time'; 'thriller of place'; political thriller.
30. The thylacine, or Tasmanian tiger.
31. Juanita Nielsen.
32. Stephen Wallace's *Blood Oath* (aka *Prisoners of the Sun*).
33. The Battle of Beersheba; 31 October 1917.
34. Nat falls on a rusty nail.
35. Spur; Harrison.
36. Contributes funding to documentaries and some features, on condition of free-to-air television screenings.
37. Vincent Ward
38. In the Queenstown region of New Zealand.
39. Samoan.
40. *Forgotten Silver*.
41. Second-generation Chinese-New Zealanders and cross-cultural relationships.
42. *CounterTerror: Framing the Panthers*; *Georgie Girl*; *Seeing Red*; *An Island Calling*; *Punitive Damage*; *Brother Number One*.
43. New Zealand Film Commission.
44. Barry Barclay.
45. Taika Waititi.
46. Australia.
47. The war experiences of her father.
48. *Sunshine Cleaning*.
49. Armagan Ballantyne.
50. A post-apocalyptic world where the main character (Bruno Lawrence) appears to be the sole survivor.

NOTES ON CONTRIBUTORS

Batoul Amhaz recently completed her Honours thesis and practical project in Film Studies at the School of the Arts and Media, University of New South Wales. The project was a two-channel video installation exploring Arab-Australian identity representation in screen culture. Her interests include film, representations of identity, and the politics of 'otherness'.

Karina Aveyard is a Lecturer in the School of Film, Television and Media Studies at the University of East Anglia. She is co-editor of *Watching Films: New Perspectives on Movie-Going, Exhibition and Reception* (Intellect, 2013). Karina's research interests include film exhibition and distribution, rural and community cinemas, and Australian films.

Anna Blagrove is a PhD researcher at the University of East Anglia. Her MA Film Studies dissertation was entitled 'Dreamtime to Screen-Time: An Exploration of the Representation of Aborigines in Contemporary Australian Road Movies' and her PhD thesis is an audience study of youth engagement with non-mainstream cinema in the United Kingdom. She is also employed as Film Education Officer at Cinema City in Norfolk.

Marco Bohr is a photographer, academic and researcher in visual culture. After completing a Visiting Fellowship at the Australian National University, Marco was appointed Lecturer in Visual Communication at Loughborough University. His blog can be found at www.visualcultureblog.com.

Matthew Campora is Screen Studies Lecturer at the Australian Film, Television and Radio School and Honorary Research Fellow at the Centre for Critical and Cultural Studies at the University of Queensland. His area of expertise is complex narrative cinema and he is the author of *Subjective Realist Cinema*.

Chris Carter is a Lecturer in Animation for the Creative Industries Faculty, Queensland University of Technology. He is a digital media expert with over fourteen years experience in animation, games and visual effects production. He is currently completing his PhD research on 3D character animation theory and practice.

Ilana Cohn is a PhD candidate in Theatre and Performance Studies at the University of New South Wales. Her current research focuses on contemporary performance art practices and the institutionalization of live art.

Adrian Danks is Director of Contextual Studies (including Cinema Studies) in the School of Media and Communication, RMIT University. He is co-curator of the Melbourne Cinémathèque, co-editor of *Senses of Cinema*, and is currently writing a monograph devoted to the history and practice of home movie-making in Australia, a book examining 'international' feature film production in Australia during the period 1945–75 (*Australian International Pictures*, with Con Verevis), and an edited companion to the work of Robert Altman (Wiley/Blackwell).

Greg Dolgopolov teaches and researches at UNSW in video production, film and television theory. Greg's research interests include post-Soviet cinema and the crime genre. Greg has written extensively on historical television detective serials, reality game shows, contemporary cinema, Australian vampire films, documentary films, international horror, and mafia representations. He is the curator and associate director of the Russian Resurrection Film Festival.

Daniel Eisenberg is Assistant Curator of Film at the Australian War Memorial and is currently completing his PhD at the Australian National University. His thesis is an explorative study navigating and negotiating the idea of the 'Australian western'. Other areas of academic interest include graphic novels on-screen, American cinema, and documentary. He is also a trained film archivist and projectionist, sporadic film reviewer and insatiable fan of all things cinema.

Elizabeth Ellison is a researcher and sessional academic at Queensland University of Technology. She recently completed her doctoral thesis, exploring film and fiction of the Australian beach and how the beach is a complex space of the mythic and the ordinary. Other research interests include gender studies, Indigenous stories, and international beach narratives.

Marian Evans's autoethnographic PhD in Creative Writing explored gender inequity within New Zealand state-funded feature film development. Her almost-complete postdoctoral *Development Project* explores global issues around screen storytelling by and about women. She tweets as @devt and @7R4SM.

Ben Goldsmith is Senior Research Fellow at Queensland University of Technology. He is the author of many articles on Australian cinema, and co-edited the first volume of the Intellect *Directory of World Cinema: Australia and New Zealand* (2010).

Ann Hardy is a Senior Lecturer in the Screen and Media Studies Programme at the University of Waikato, New Zealand. She is the author of numerous articles on New Zealand film and media, with particular interests in women's film-making, audience research and in the role that Maori spirituality plays in the popular imagination in New Zealand. She first met Christine Jeffs when the two of them worked on a documentary project for Television New Zealand in the late 1980s.

Lauren Carroll Harris is a PhD candidate at the University of New South Wales and an arts and film writer. Her research centres on film distribution, exhibition, screen business and Australian national cinema.

Zachary Ingle is a PhD student in Film and Media Studies at the University of Kansas. He has written for several volumes of Intellect's Directory of World Cinema, as well as for the World Film Locations and Fan Phenomena series. He is the editor of three books: *Robert Rodriguez: Interviews*; *Identity and Myth in Sports Documentaries*; and *Gender and Genre in Sports Documentaries*.

Anna Jackson is currently undertaking a joint PhD at the University of Auckland and the University of Melbourne, researching innovation and change in New Zealand's documentary production ecology. She is also the co-director of Transmedia NZ, an organization that seeks to promote the development of transmedia production in New Zealand.

Sylvia Lawson writes cultural history, critical journalism and fiction. Her most recent books are *Demanding the Impossible: Seven essays on resistance* (Melbourne University Press, 2012) and *The Back of Beyond*, on John Heyer's 1954 documentary, for the Australian Screen Classics series (Currency Press with the National Film and Sound Archive, 2013). She is currently film critic for the online and print journal *Inside Story*.

Geoff Lealand is Associate Professor in Screen and Media Studies at the University of Waikato, New Zealand. He contributed the chapter 'The Jackson Effect: The late 1990s to 2005' in *New Zealand Film: An Illustrated History* (2011) and is currently working on a research project about Shirley Temple 'double' competitions in New Zealand in 1935–36.

Alfio Leotta teaches Film Studies at Victoria University of Wellington. His primary research interests focus on the relation between film and tourism, the history of New Zealand cinema, and New Italian Cinema. His book *Touring the Screen: Tourism and New Zealand Film Geographies* examines the representation of landscape in a number of film productions shot in New Zealand which have subsequently been used as marketing tools to attract tourists to the country.

Harriet Margolis is the author of *The Cinema Ideal* (1988; reprinted by Routledge, 2013), editor of *Jane Campion's "The Piano"* (2000) and co-editor of *Studying the Event Film: "The Lord of the Rings"* (2006; paperback edition forthcoming). A collection of interviews with women cinematographers around the world, co-edited with Alexis Krasilovsky, is currently with publishers.

Helen Martin has written extensively on New Zealand film since the 1980s, most recently for *Onfilm* Magazine, Te Ara – the online Encyclopedia of New Zealand, and the book *Black: The history of black in fashion, society and culture in New Zealand*.

Tony Mitchell is a Senior Lecturer at the University of Technology, Sydney. He was born in New Zealand and has published widely on New Zealand music and cinema. He co-edited *Home, Land and Sea: Situating Music in Aotearoa New Zealand* in 2011.

Tom O'Regan is a Professor in Cultural and Media Studies at the University of Queensland and co-founder of *Continuum: Journal of Media & Cultural Studies*. His research interests include international film production and 'Global Hollywood'.

Jonathan Rayner is Reader in Film Studies at the University of Sheffield, United Kingdom. He researches in the areas of Australasian cinema, genre films and auteur studies. His publications include *The Films of Peter Weir* (Continuum, 2003 [1998]), *Contemporary Australian Cinema* (Manchester University Press, 2000) and *Cinema and Landscape* (ed. with Graeme Harper, Intellect, 2010).

Daniel Reynaud is Associate Professor in the Faculty of Arts and Theology at Avondale College of Higher Education. His research includes publications on Australian war cinema, and he has worked with the National Film and Sound Archive on recovering and partially reconstructing several silent war films.

Martin Rumsby is a self taught curator, film-maker and writer. Excerpts of films by and about Martin Rumsby can be viewed on YouTube.

Mark David Ryan is a Senior Lecturer in film and television studies for the Creative Industries Faculty, Queensland University of Technology. He is a national expert on Australian horror films and genre cinema, and a media commentator on anything horror, cult film or cinema related. He has written extensively on popular genre cinema, industry dynamics of cultural production, and cultural policy.

Peter Schembri is a Lecturer in film and television studies in the Creative Industries Faculty, Queensland University of Technology. He is completing a PhD on historical miniseries and has taught extensively in screen and genre studies.

Nina Seja is a doctoral candidate at the Department of Cinema Studies at New York University, and lectures in the fields of new media at Unitec (Auckland). Her research focuses on human rights atrocity and social movements. Her writing on subjects such as documentary photography after Chernobyl, cellphone witnessing during political revolution, and the political possibilities of humour has been featured in journals including *Afterimage* and *Continuum*.

Jane Stadler is Associate Professor of Film and Media Studies in the School of English, Media Studies and Art History at the University of Queensland. She is Chief Investigator of a collaborative Australian Research Council project on landscape and location in Australian narratives (2010–13), author of *Pulling Focus* (2008), co-author of *Screen Media* (2009) and *Media and Society* (2012) and co-editor of an anthology on adaptation, *Pockets of Change* (2011).

Deborah J Thomas has a PhD in Screen, Media and Cultural Studies. She has previously published on American and Australian cinema, and is currently working as a researcher on the Australian Research Council-funded Discovery Project 'Worldwide: The History of the Commercial Arm of the British Broadcasting Corporation' at the University of Queensland.

Mandy Treagus is Senior Lecturer and Head of English and Creative Writing at the University of Adelaide, Australia. She researches Victorian, Australian and Pacific literatures and film, and cultural history. Her current project explores the display of Pacific peoples in colonial exhibitions, and is especially concerned with the agency of the performers.

Sharn Treloar is a teacher in secondary education and cinephile who has also worked on film and theatre productions in a variety of roles from crew to performance. He holds a Bachelor of Contemporary Arts in Performing Arts and Media Studies, Post-Grad Diploma of Education, and is currently completing a Master of Arts degree.

Tess Van Hemert is completing a PhD on film festivals and female film-makers at the Queensland University of Technology. She has taught extensively in screen studies and has published articles on film pedagogy and film festivals.

Deb Verhoeven is Chair and Professor of Media and Communication at Deakin University. She was inaugural Deputy Chair of the National Film and Sound Archive of Australia, CEO of the Australian Film Institute and President of the online film journal *Senses of Cinema*. She is the author of *Jane Campion* (Routledge, 2009).

Susan Ward is a researcher in film and television for the University of Queensland. She has written extensively on film and television production cultures in Australia, including the socio-spatial dynamics of the screen industries in Australia; and more recently in relation to environmentalism. She is co-author of the book *Local Hollywood: Global Film Production and the Gold Coast* with Ben Goldsmith and Tom O'Regan (2010).

Dr Mary M Wiles is Senior Lecturer in Cinema Studies at the University of Canterbury. She recently published her first book, *Jacques Rivette* (2012), in the University of Illinois Press's Contemporary Directors Series. Since her arrival in Christchurch in 2003, she has developed a secondary area of research specialization in New Zealand film, and is currently working on a study of film-maker Christine Jeffs's *Rain* (2001), which will become part of the New Zealand Film Classics series.

Scott Wilson is a Senior Lecturer at Unitec Institute of Technology in the Department of Performing and Screen Arts. He has most recently served as the Visiting Fulbright Scholar in the Centre of Australian, New Zealand and Pacific Studies, Georgetown University, Washington DC.

Arezou Zalipour (PhD Literary Studies) is based in the Faculty of Arts and Social Sciences at the University of Waikato, New Zealand. Her research focuses primarily on relations between diaspora and cultural production, with a secondary research in poetics. The former encompasses current work on the Asian diaspora and its impact on the film industry in New Zealand. The latter represents a long-standing interest in the phenomenology of imagination.

Ruth Zanker teaches and researches at the New Zealand Broadcasting School, Christchurch Polytechnic Institute of Technology. Her recent research focuses on young people's media use, in particular the opportunities and challenges presented by digital media.

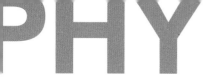

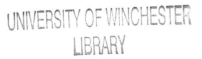

EXPLORING THE CITY ONSCREEN

A film book series from Intellect / **www.intellectbooks.com**

The World Film Locations series explores and reveals the relationship between the city and cinema by using a predominantly visual approach perfectly suited to the medium of film. The city continues to play a central role in a multitude of films, helping us to frame our understanding of place and of the world around us. Whether as elaborate directorial love letters or as time specific cultural settings, the city acts as a vital character in helping to tell a story.

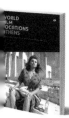

World Film Locations: Athens
Edited by Anna Poupou, Afroditi Nikolaidou and Eirini Sifaki
ISBN 9781783203598
Paperback 128 pages
Price £15.50
Published September 2014

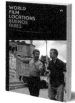

World Film Locations: Buenos Aires
Edited by Michael Pigott and Santiago Oyarzabal
ISBN 9781783203581
Paperback 128 pages
Price £15.50
Published October 2014

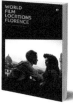

World Film Locations: Florence
Edited by Alberto Zambenedetti
ISBN 9781783203604
Paperback 128 pages
Price £15.50
Published September 2014

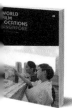

World Film Locations: Singapore
Edited by Lorenzo Codelli
ISBN 9781783203611
Paperback 128 pages
Price £15.50
Published September 2014

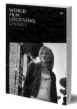

World Film Locations: Sydney
Edited by Neil Mitchell
ISBN 9781783203628
Paperback 128 pages
Price £15.50
Published October 2014

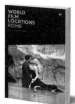

World Film Locations: Rome
Edited by Gabriel Solomons
ISBN 9781783202003
Paperback 128 pages
Price £15.50
Published Autumn 2014

LIKE WORLD FILM LOCATIONS ON FACEBOOK

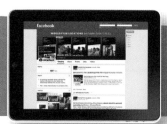

NEW BOX SET

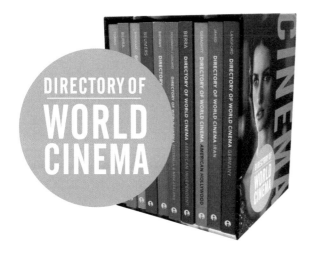

This unique box set brings together 10 volumes of the Directory of World Cinema series in a colorful, collectable box and is the perfect gift for any cinema buff or bibliophile. The series moves intelligent, scholarly criticism beyond the academy by building a forum for the study of film that relies on a disciplined theoretical base. Each volume of the Directory takes the form of a collection of reviews, longer essays and research resources, accompanied by film stills highlighting significant films and players.

GERMANY ITALY SPAIN IRAN JAPAN AMERICAN INDEPENDENT RUSSIA AUSTRALIA & NEW ZEALAND EAST EUROPE AMERICAN HOLLYWOOD

Intellect is an independent academic publisher of books and journals, to view our catalogue or order our titles visit www.intellectbooks.com or E-mail: orders@intellectbooks.com. Intellect, The Mill, Parnall Road, Fishponds, Bristol, UK, BS16 3JG. Telephone: +44 (0) 117 9589910.